ABOUT THE AUTHOR

Like so many homœopaths, Grahame Martin prescribed remedies long before attending a college and when he did get there he was taught by practitioners who were never taught in a college themselves. This underlines his belief that homœopathy is a means to health that belongs to all and, therefore, in the principle that the protection of lay homœopathy is also the protection of the nature of a free human being.

Having studied various levels of spiritualism it was to be the visualisation of miasmatic energy that became the glue that pulled his beliefs together. This philosophy was then expanded upon through the influence of Martin Miles and Robert Davidson, it being a river - the source of which can be traced back to the extraordinary teachings of Thomas Maughan and long before him.

Grahame is a member of the Guild of Homeopaths and continues to prove the new Guild remedies. Under the training of Janice Micallef, he has learnt how to apply his psychic perception to healing. He teaches both the philosophy of using chakras within homœopathy and the new remedies of the Guild using esoteric knowledge and psychic reception. He also holds meditative circles that encompass chakra healing.

Grahame has his practice in South London.

CHAKRA PRESCRIBING AND HOMŒOPATHY

by
Grahame Martin

Winter Press
16 Stambourne Way
West Wickham
Kent BR4 9NF
e-mail: cpah@winterpress.net

First published by Winter Press in 2007
Reprinted 2009, 2016

Copyright © Grahame Martin 2007

ISBN 9781 874581772

Cover design by the author, Sue Smith and Colin Winter
Illustrations by the author and Kerri Pritchard

Printed by Grosvenor Group, UK

All rights reserved. No part of this publication may be reproduced, stored in a retrieval system, or transmitted, in any form or by any means, electronic, mechanical, photocopying, recording or otherwise, without the prior permission of the publishers.

This book is presented as a collection of natural remedies and as an aid in understanding their use. It is intended for use by professional homœopaths and not as a replacement for professional consultation or treatment.

CONTENTS

Acknowledgments. 7
Foreword 8
Introduction 12
    How to use this book. 17
Miasms. 21
1 The Base Chakra. 27
    Incarnation. 31
    Kundalini 39
    Aspiration 44
    Saturn. 46
2 The Sacral Centre .57
    DNA and Growth. 63
    Sex 66
    Gender and Generation 73
    The Kidneys 79
    The Adrenals. 84
    The Sacral Centre, Transmutation and
        the Throat Centre 86
    Jupiter 88
3 The Solar Plexus. .93
    The Spleen: Gateway to the Vital Body 101
    Blood and the Ego. 104
    The Stomach, Feelings and the War of Digestion. . . 114
    The Liver, the GallBladder and the Astral World . . . 115
    The Pancreas and the Cosmos 124
    Mars. 126
4 The Heart Chakra 131
    Light. 142
    The Thymus Gland, the Blueprint of Karma 152
    The Heart, Syphilis and Self. 161
    The Love School 173
    The Sun and its Radiance as Number One 179
5 The Throat Chakra 183
    Art 197
    Prophecy 199
    The Thyroid 211
    The Parathyroid 218
    Sound, Breath and Akasha 220

6 The Brow Chakra 235
  Wisdom. 236
  The Kama Manas and the Manas 239
  Intuition. 244
  The Monads 246
  Elementals and Entities 254
  Evolution 256
  The Disease Process 260
  The Third Eye 263
  The Pituitary and the Hypothalamas Glands 284
  Mercury was a Thief 292
7 The Crown Chakra 301
  Healing the Spirit Within 348
  The Pineal Gland 349
  The Moon and Purple 353

FIGURES

1. The Star of David 33
2. Forming the Star of David 34
3. The Second Crucifixion 40
4. The Tree of Life 41
5. The Ascending Triangle 111
6. The Solar Cross 137
7. The Rosicrucian Fellowship 145
8. The Egyptian God Aten 174
9. The Four Chambered
   Human Heart. 176
10. The Pentagram 188
11. The Descending Triangle. 201
12. The Circumscribed Pentagram . 203
13. Transcendent circle of spirit
    risen above cross of matter. . . 225
14. Ankh 230
15. Earth's Life Chain. 248
16. The Globe Stage 249
17. The Planetary Manvantara. 249
18. Spirit overlapping matter 250
19. The Crosier 267
20. The Caduceus. 270
21. The Tau Cross 271
22 The Cross Bottony 272
23. Thousand-petalled lotus 311
24. The Star of Bethlehem 314
25. Circumscribed Square 315
26. Diamond formed by two
    Equilateral Triangles. 316
27. The Exchange of the Ascending
    and Descending Triangles . . . 317
28. The Superellipse 318
29. The Amalgamation of Spirit
    into Matter 325
30. Spirit Amalgamates with Matter 326
31. The Triad of the Pyramids 327
32. The Earthed Lightning Bolt
    on the Tree of Life 330
33. The Horseshoe 358
34. Sun, Earth and Moon
    during a Full Moon 362

ACKNOWLEDGMENTS

Many thanks to all those who have supported me both as a homœopathic practitioner and in writing this book. Especially to Jennifer Maughan for her guidance, Peter Firebrace for his patient teaching and Martin Miles for years of homœopathic insights. A big thank you and much gratitude to Janice Micallef, for not only enabling me to understand, but to equip me with the tools to turn around and make use of what I thought was a hindrance. I would also like to thank Susan Curtis, for without being prepared to undertake the journey of the seven chakras with me, there would be no book. And to all the members of the Guild of Homeopaths. I would further like to thank Natalie Greiff for her love and hard work during endless hours of constructing this book and all the friends that gave up their time to read first drafts and participate in feedback. Finally, to the artist Bernard Cohen for helping to establish my path – for being Saturn.

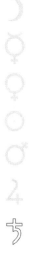

Dedicated to the memory of
Patricia Mary Hood

Michael Miles
who, during late night talks,
contributed so much

Martin Miles
for the love he gave,
the knowledge he shared
and the encouragement
he offered to so many people.

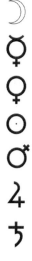

FOREWORD

Grahame, through long, hard and dedicated work on himself, his own life experiences and many years of meditative discipline on his own chakras has written this wonderful account on the chakra system. It holds a wealth of deep understanding, inner knowledge and experience on all levels that will help us all.

This book, as well as giving us a wider picture and deeper understanding of the chakra system, is bound to inspire us into looking within ourselves and enabling us to work with our own energy centres more deeply and with awakening consciousness.

Knowledge and understanding of the chakra system is an amazing gift and as we search and experience our own energy centres it is incredible how our lives are enriched, unfold and change for the better. This process will help us to understand that the more we 'know' and experience, the more in the wider context we 'know' nothing. The journey will keep us in humility; allow our hearts and minds to open to the truth; show us that we should never judge each other; allow us to have unconditional love; and how to live in the moment and surrender to God at all times; and to realise that the universe is ultimately benevolent.

Life is an interesting journey, moving us through many different states of consciousness. Throughout this journey we all grow and evolve according to the karma that we have developed: God presents the lessons to us that we require to fulfil our karmic responsibilities in each lifetime.

The blueprint of our karma is grafted into our energy centres or chakras that lie in the subtle body of man. The chakras therefore act as a bridge between physical and subtle matter.

Chakra is a Sanskrit word, meaning vortex or wheel. Chakras, therefore, are wheels or vortices of energy, spinning and vibrating at all times in the etheric body. The etheric body is invisible (to all but the psychic eye) and is the vehicle through which energy flows to keep the physical, mental and emotional bodies alive. The chakras are points of connection allowing vital energy to flow from one vehicle or body to another.

Chakras are active at all times, whether or not we are aware of it, and vital energy constantly moves through the chakras to produce different states of being. These wheels of fate and destiny are as individual and unique as we are. They evolve and open naturally over a long period of time according to our understanding and our life experiences: we are these energies and we evolve according to our experiences and the energy changes within our chakras.

Each chakra is related to a nerve plexus, an endocrine gland, a colour, a sound, a sense organ, a planet, a plane of consciousness and of course a bodily organ or organs. There is also a moral quality held in each chakra and as that quality develops and evolves, the centre becomes more refined.

Modern science will explain this process as chemical changes produced by the endocrine system, or ductless glands, that produce secretions directly from the gland into the bloodstream. This is certainly part of the process, but its cause originates from the energy of the vital force vibrating through the chakras; stimulating the nerve plexus and the endocrine secretions to alter the individual consciousness.

It is, remember, the balance of these secretions within the body that determines who we are as individuals and that enables us to fulfil our karma.

Whilst we are incarnate, man is ultimately a soul occupying many bodies: physical, mental, emotional and spiritual. The physical body is the part of the soul that manifests and completes its karma through the lower world in each incarnation. Indeed, man chases in each lifetime the vehicle of expression that enables him to journey through his chosen lessons and responsibilities.

Each chakra corresponds to a different layer of the auric field. The seven main chakras therefore link with the seven main layers within the auric field. Hence, if there is a disturbance in a chakra, there will also be a disturbance in the corresponding level of the aura; blocking the flow of life force energy and therefore dis-ease on some level will inevitably

Foreword

occur. This can be 'healed' by working with the chakra energy positively and as the energy begins to spin correctly the block and disease in the chakra and the aura will clear and health and vitality will return.

Ultimately we are all masters of our own destiny. The blueprint of this destiny lies hidden within our individual chakra system. By becoming aware of this enables us to be who we are and to follow our own destiny. This information lies within these secret wheels of fate and the energy field flowing through the life force within our chakra system.

We can awaken to evolve our chakras by individual or group meditation practice, through the lessons that life presents us, through genetic predisposition and conscious awareness of our path, and through complete trust and faith in life's unfolding patterns of change. It is important to remember that we are individuals so none of our experiences will be completely identical.

Through a deeper experiential understanding of the chakras we can help ourselves, each other and the planet and also positively effect the universal consciousness.

As we move through a deeper understanding of ourselves, we radiate light and positive vibrations into our chakras and our auric field, which is a wonderful experience. We become more conscious, healing occurs and we are given God's wisdom and power to use with integrity. On this journey we can only move and work with complete humility, with an open heart and mind to all humanity. We experience new horizons and belief systems and welcome change. We recognise that every soul has a special place within universal consciousness and that we are all an integral part of that whole.

We must at all times work without personal ego and for the greater good of all mankind. To journey into these spheres with wrong intention is never a good idea.

Chakra unfoldment is not an easy journey: it makes us face ourselves; and it makes us responsible for ourselves and for our health on all levels. However, it broadens our horizons, makes us much less judgemental of our fellows and we become more humble and heart-centred.

Grahame has experienced an inordinate amount of change on his adventure through these mystical wheels of fate. We must thank him for his journey that has allowed this book to unfold and come into our lives. Grahame has worked individually and in groups, experientially and intuitively, 'listening' to his guides and teachers on the higher levels. We thank him sincerely for his dedication, integrity, humility and especially for the healing and inspiration that this work contains and will bring to many lives.

This is an amazing book, let it inspire you to journey into your inner realms and the realms of universal consciousness and let your experiences unfold according to God's Will.

May God bless you all

Janice Micallef, Bexley, 2007

INTRODUCTION

A chakra is nothing more than an area of consciousness. There are many different schools of thought that differ in the position and number of both the major and minor chakras. This book concerns itself with the seven major chakras that are central to the spiritual practices that have been native to the people that have visited, participated in and inhabited the island of Britain for a long, long time. They are however, to be found in practices all over the world. These seven chakras pertain to seven differing regions of the body and all that is contained within those regions. They act on the physical body or matter, and on the etheric body, the astral body and the spiritualised bodies via the endocrine glands and the nervous system. So they are in effect master to all that is possible and not simply agents of the particular sphere to which they belong. Their interaction is the making of the whole human being, for in truth they cannot be separated.

The seven major chakras line up along the spine in order that spirit can dip in and out of them. Being manifested conscious energy, they are associated with each of the seven levels of awareness that make up the human constitution whilst here on Earth. Together and when in balance, they are the factory for producing purpose which manifests both in the physical world and the spiritual one. When balanced they enable Self to be in a state of 'now', not complete but at one and in focus with the task in hand, which may be to heal: this is to produce what is known as divine intervention or the spiritual purpose. Being centres of consciousness means that we add and subtract from them constantly and therefore they have the means to heal all locked away inside their mystery. Other than these seven chakras and the subdivisions of these chakras located elsewhere around the body, there is nothing more to being human. This may be why homœopaths have become so fascinated in their study, for their philosophy provides a structure for the prescribing of a homœopathic remedy.

The notion of a chakra can be traced back to many various sciences, spiritual beliefs, philosophies and religions. The wisdom as to their relationship to the energies of the body is as old as language itself. Like religions, languages have common factors for they originate from primal sources. Within them will be the crystallisation of wisdom of which the mystical knowledge of the seven energy centres – the chakras – is a major attribute in deciphering what lies behind human existence.

The purpose of this book is to be both a source of information and also primarily within the energy it evokes, a journey book for the development of the reader. Each chapter has been written both to instil knowledge and the essence of each chakra in an energetic way, which is not only homœopathic, but is also the very nature of working on each chakra. Therefore, contained in each chapter is the means for the reader to work on their own equivalent chakra and this will happen during the progression of this book.

When anything new is formed, be it in any medium, (just so happens to be a book here) it will evoke a response, as it contains its own energy so there is nothing new in my intention here. What has been intended though, is to try and evoke the pure energy of each chakra in order that the homeopath or any other practitioner or simply the spiritually curious who wishes to further their path, may receive a sense of its presence. Through this the feel of a chakra can be recognised. Its language and communication, not to mention its resonance and its aura, can reveal qualities that if out of balance can be understood and worked on. One is able to perceive disharmony within and it is hoped that in healing, these imbalances can be seen in one's patients, not just intellectually but intuitively. This imbalance may be observed within individual chakras or as a collective. In doing so, one is instantly projected to a point from which to prescribe or simply to send healing energy or light. Balance is the refining of both strengths and weaknesses, so both will require exploring but it will be the weaknesses that will require the most attention.

If there is information within this book that is unclear or difficult to understand, then this is an opportunity to meditate on it and thus allow understanding to filter through on some level, for the chakra will

Introduction

still continue to be worked on whether you are fully conscious of the process or not. This is the same for patients as they often present what is confusing to us, so one can just stop and meditate on it in order to receive an answer. However, simply allowing each chapter to wash over the reader will enable a communication to be energetically established and this will reveal itself when it is ready or necessary. This often happens during prescribing and this book will help the practitioner to think in the way of chakras or enable the intuition to open up to the chakras, the prescription, or hopefully both. When meditating on anything, one opens oneself up as a channel. It is thus very important to visualise and maintain in your mind's eye a circle of white light rotating anticlockwise around yourself or around the whole group if meditating together. This will provide protection whilst being in such an open state. This light should be dispersed when closing down from the meditation and the person should concentrate on being back in their body and back down on Earth, re-establishing their natural protective aura, completely sealed around them. This is a necessity and should be achieved before once again opening the eyes, as it is not safe to be in this kind of open state in what is essentially an uncontrollable world.

Each chakra contained in this book is a reflection of my discovery, research, what I've been taught, and that which I have channelled. To achieve this, I myself also had to work extensively through each of the seven main chakras, such is the nature of how this energy is obtained and thus how universally important it is in the healing process. The seven main chakras and their contents are central to all health, vision and wisdom through the expansion of consciousness that is the course of planetary development. Thus their inclusion makes inroads into all forms of healing and homœopathy is no exception. To understand the human constitution, an understanding of the seven chakras, along with each of their glands that make up the endocrine system, is imperative. This becomes clearer when studied next to the body's functions. Both are fundamental to existence and without the endocrine system being balanced, it is impossible to truly know who you are. Therefore, it stands to reason that the wisdom unlocked by an understanding of the chakras will become a necessity for all healers. Like the miasmatic philosophy of homœopathy, their essence is all encompassing and of course understanding the nature of the seven chakras inevitably widens miasmatic knowledge and thus aids in the perception of them, both in our minds and also as a tool for prescribing.

This book is intended to be a support for those who wish to ally their prescribing to using the seven chakras in order to heal. There is no particular method as it is the very engagement in energy work that is the key and what is required comes through the practitioner. The practitioner is not the healer but somœone who is able to allow healing energy to come through, which in homœopathy reveals itself in the remedy selection. The purpose of understanding the seven chakras, which can only come from working through them, is the means by which one's personal development unfolds and thus the experience is used to help others: it is this that makes homœopathic prescribing easier. This book is designed to offer the information and the means to develop in order that the chakra structures may become clearer, stronger and deeper as they are aligned with the human development of consciousness. This will then help open up the portals to enlighten perception.

    The book is not intended to be an intellectual pursuit, even though the intellect will benefit from it. Consciousness only occurs when the pursuer is ready. This is part of the development that will come clear when working on the ideas within the book. This book, therefore, is not only for health practitioners and homœopaths but also for all those who wish to work through their seven chakras and these people will come to it when they are ready. As already stated, it is a journey book to which homœopathic philosophy has been applied. Take the homœopathy away and it contains that which will enable everyone's development, so there are two ways of reading it. If you pass it on, do so with love.

Introduction

Lastly, the order of colours for each chakra are as follows: starting at the base chakra – yellow, the sacral centre – blue, the solar plexus – red, the heart chakra – green, the throat chakra – dark blue, the brow chakra – orange and finally the crown chakra – purple. This system is different from that of the rainbow, which is a system of colours that are said to make a direct bridge to the emancipation of Earthly existence. The colour system used here is ancient and the reason why they pertain to a particular chakra will become clear as each chapter is read but the key to their understanding is to be found in the concept of service. Coupled with the energetic resonance and information within each chakra, they are, about releasing and transforming the difficulties and stubborn patterns of human karma that inhibit us all. This ability to release human karma means that the seven chakras and their purpose are found in the centre of the majority of faiths and religions. The chakras are imperative in both esoteric and occult philosophy. This book helps the reader to understand some of the connections and harks back to the origins of such philosophies that have often been lost. Locked inside the true meaning will be the energy that has the power to induce the flow that we all need, offering a different way of perceiving the world.

If you have any questions during your journey through this book, please contact me by email via www.grahamemartin.com

HOW TO USE THIS BOOK

The Short Version
1. Read the book from beginning to end, rather than dipping in and out.
2. Start a new chakra chapter on a new day.
3. Observe the thoughts and events that occur when you are reading/working on a particular chakra.
4. Be careful to 'close down' after each reading.

The Longer Version
Just as the chakras overlap energetically, so a similar structure has been necessary in the creation of this book. There will be information or terms mentioned in a chapter, which may not be explained fully until in a later chapter. Though not easy on the reader, this is unavoidable, so as to avoid distraction away from the pure energy of the chakra: the detail will surface as the book progresses.

When evoking the energy of each chakra it is of the upmost importance to focus as specifically as possible on the quality of that chakra and pick up what it contains even on its periphery. However, it can be a thin line between what is starting to spread into another chakra and maintaining its own integrity. This can, of course, be the very nature of the chakra. For instance, the sacral centre, being ruled by Jupiter, is very expansive so one may get confused in knowing where the boundaries lie. The reader may benefit from writing down a term that is not explained when they come across it and either exploring a definition online or waiting to see how I have used the term later on in the book. Alternatively, one can allow the essence to simply wash over oneself whilst reading.

This book is designed to take the reader through each of the seven chakras and thus enable them to work on each chakra sequentially. This has been carefully constructed in order that the flow of this process is maintained. For the flow to be achieved, this book has had to steer away from being merely an intellectual exercise: it is rather a 'journey book' that uses the knowledge of ancient energies to evoke deep healing in the reader. If this is denied, and if it is judged solely intellectually, then its purpose, which is to induce the chakras energetically, will be missed. The book works and has to be accessed and thus assessed by other means. The intellect will, however, be required to assimilate the process as it unfolds, although this will become superseded by 'direct knowing': the intellect should never be used to hold back this process.

It will often be the subtleties, and even the areas that seem initially to make no sense within this book, that create the energy of the journey, for they prompt the unconscious. This is the point to the book – it reminds us of what we have forgotten but that is held in the unconscious and by making conscious – by remembering, we grow. There is no doubt that the reader has to work at it, but regular meditation will greatly help with the clarity required.

Like all journeys, this book has to build and this is how the chakras interrelate, so the next chapter will explain more about the previous one. As with all chakra work, one needs to be patient and this book has been written to develop patience. It also enables the reader to pace oneself, for with this work one needs time to absorb and adjust. It is a process and one simply cannot handle everything at once. The end result should be of a collective, in which all the parts of the book, where possible, have been fully covered. This ties together the seven chakras in a holistic way. It is this unification that completes the journey. One recognises this completion when the seven chakras are perceived as one.

It is imperative to 'switch off' the chakra and close it and yourself down not only after you have finished reading for a time, but also at the end of each chakra section to give yourself a break. This is the most important point within the 'How to Use this Book' section. The opening up of one's chakras will be a natural occurrence that happens during the process of reading each chapter. I suggest this is done in a comfortable place in which one has control of ones environment. The emphasis here must be in the closing down, as it is not wise to keep a chakra open all the time. The chakra, however, will remain active as one works through the consequences of it having been called on.

It is advisable to close down regularly, by first closing one's eyes and imagining that each chakra is a coloured light or candle. This should be visualised as this light belonging to the part of the body where the chakra lies. For example, the throat chakra would maintain the light at the throat, so it is from this position that it should be closed down. The colour should pertain to the colour of the chakra and in your mind's eye it should be switched off or blown out. Depending on the chakra and your relationship to it, this can prove difficult at times, but you should persist until confident that it has closed down completely. Once this is achieved, your aura should be re-sealed using the mind's eye, making sure there are no holes. Finally, you should feel completely back in your body with the feet firmly on the ground. It can be useful to remove your shoes and really feel the earth under the feet. Again, it is good practice to do this each time you finish reading and most importantly at the end of each chapter. It is also good to have a rest.

If you are confused and unable to understand a particular chakra, then this may be because you are working very deeply with the energy of that chakra. By closing down and leaving the chakra for a while, you can then re-read the chapter without the initial intensity and this should help. This refers particularly to the brow chakra, as the pituitary gland may not be able to both adjust to the process and absorb the information into the brain at the same time: it's as if the mind goes blank. Rest will cure this occurrence.

When this book is read initially, it should be in the sequence in which it is written - chronologically in the same way the chakras run up the spine, from base to crown. Only after this process is completed should an individual chakra be delved into at random. During this initial read and subsequently, if a chakra is dipped into and out of as pleased, it is necessary to make sure the light of the chakras prior to the one presently being read are also switched off when closing down. This should be achieved by starting with the most recent - the present chakra and working one's way back down to the base. This is because where one is on the evolution of chakra work is also an amalgamation of the work done on all the stations before, so the previous chakras will automatically light up to support the current position. For example, if one finishes at the end of or during the heart chakra, that should be switched off using the exercise above, and then switch off the solar plexus, followed by the sacral centre, and finishing with the base. A simple way to remember this is that whenever you close down, finish with the base chakra.

How to use this book

So, to summarise, by the simple act of reading this book one becomes open to its energy. The reader does this naturally because this energy is not in reality new but is the making of them. The process is constructed to be taken in a chapter at a time, and then once having absorbed the energy of the chapter, one waits.

> Pausing provides the time and the space to allow the consequences of the absorbed energy to develop. This cannot be rushed.

The information contained in Chapter One will explain this, as this is, in part, how one forms a good base chakra. As each chapter is read, its consequence will provide the tools to enable the reader to progress to the next chapter. For example, a good base is required to explore each chapter.

We live in fast adrenal driven times but in order to get the most out of the latter chapters, the discipline gained in the first few chapters should be adhered to. Once again, this is not achieved intellectually but by appointing the time and the space for the energy of each chapter to be integrated, achieving stability. This is like painting a picture, as each brush stroke is the making of the final image. How one starts anything will determine the finish. Each brush stroke needs to fit with its adjacent, each colour should add to the whole. But the surface must often be allowed to stand, to breathe and be given life. This provides the time to reflect upon it (or let it dry), without which, one is left with a muddy image.

There is much to each chakra and much to clear and balance. Chakras can even be spinning in the wrong direction. The consequences of this are what needs to change, so try to be patient as we work and rework areas of the canvas.

MIASMS

Miasms are energies of destiny. The core of their energy is shaped by consequence – the decisions that one makes in previous, present and future incarnations. They are the results of living on Earth and have formed through the separation between Self and the Divine. Miasms are forces of a negative amalgamation of space, time, matter and spirit. They manifest from the illusion of this separation, from being here on Earth, which masquerades as reality. Homœopathy does not rely on the notion that the world is out to attack the human constitution through an onslaught of bacteria or contagious viruses. It does not believe disease can be 'caught' but is propagated within, given the right circumstances, though this is not to deny the existence of bacteria. These 'right circumstances' are the forces that pull Self down into a state of ill health. These forces will determine Self's disposition to any given disease, depending on Self's own relationship with them, their mix and activity. This process is also true of the group as well as the individual, for these circumstances can also be induced collectively through fear. Fear in itself is tremendously powerful and is both created by miasms and used by them to further their cause.

In homœopathy, the understanding of energy gravitates to a central philosophy that differentiates between the forces that lie behind disease. These different forces are called miasms and the pursuit of their understanding establishes further insight into the nature of the human kingdom in relation to the other kingdoms and the purpose to life. Essentially this is humanity's relationship with the Divine and how this relationship is played out on planet Earth. This knowledge of the workings of the miasms leads to further understanding of homœopathic remedies, including the nosodes (remedies made directly from the disease state of each of the miasms), for they resonate somewhere on the periphery as the vibration of the miasms moves outwards. In the centre of this vortex is the syphilitic miasm from which the other miasms resonate. This is why most remedies have an action upon all the miasms. How close a particular part of this vibration is to the central core of the human constitution at any particular moment will reveal the need for the equivalent remedy – the 'like' or similimum in vibrational energy terms. It will partly or completely contain the solution to counter the metamorphosis of miasmatic energy, which if Self allows, will help to unlock the constraints of what is essentially the result of karma.

All of us as guardians of the human race need to constantly remind ourselves that within this world it is wrong to blame natural physical responses such as disease on bacteria for example, when it is the soil of the soul that is the garden in which miasms are planted and cultivated.

Miasms have traditionally been taught within the context of the time line of human history. Their development has been associated with the way in which the human condition has evolved and as it has become more conscious of the physical function of its body. This approach places the Psoric miasm as the forerunner, it being primarily, in physical pathological terms, to do with the elimination of toxins through the skin, the first alternative to the bowels and thus the first negative physical alternate state. The skin also marks the boundary, again in physiological terms, from which Self can be sure where it stops and starts. Therefore this boundary can be considered the initial point that denotes our awareness of being Self and so the subsequent fear of separation, which is too much to bear, leads to its suppression. If we explore a little more of this physiological point of view, the sycotic miasm is then born from the storing of toxins that the bowels and the skin fail to clear, creating lumps and tumors within the physical body. It's thought that from this internalised energy the soul compensates by gorging upon inner desires as a means to tolerate its newfound freedom. According to this premise, the syphilitic miasm evolved as a result of the inadequacy of excess to provide a suitable solution to the torture that the soul feels from the fear of separation. The next physical solution manifested by driving the problem so deep within the tissues that it could no longer be detected, and being so well hidden the soul could convince itself that it has disappeared. In the human quest to understand its function within the universe and thus combat its fears, it utilizes the reactionary force to separation that when unleashed is primarily destructive – the syphilitic miasm.

Within this historical perspective it is thus considered that this destruction led to the formation of the next miasm in which all the boundaries have been demolished through perversity (essentially the improper means to reconnect). This state enables the amalgamation of all the previous miasms by flowing into one another and by doing so creates the Tubercular miasm. This nebulous, uncontainable energy, finds expression in the tissues by having been buried deep inside, leaving hollow spaces behind as it tries to find an exit route. Once it is discovered that this does not equate to a genuine exit strategy, usually when the energy starts to run out, one compensates for having no boundaries by pushing oneself up a tight alleyway where all can be eventually condensed into the falsification of boundaries – the Cancer miasm. These unreal boundaries are the most dangerous to the physical part of the constitution as cells proliferate under their pressure.

This physical miasmatic development that has just been outlined can be plotted against the seven chakras, starting with Psora at the base represented by the element earth. They continue upwards until they amalgamate to form the Tubercular miasm. Some place this miasm at the heart chakra and others at the throat, but once again this is only a physical slant and so only a small piece in the jigsaw puzzle that indicates how the miasms work together within each of the seven chakras. This is not a true representation of how the miasms evolved, just as the traditional western historical representation of the evolution of humanity is not correct, but a manipulation of time and space that is solely interested in the fitting of physical events. Even scientists are beginning to realise the inadequacies of relying on the assumption of material evidence. It is true that due to the expansion of matter, physical life has adjusted accordingly. However, this reveals very little on how the miasms interact as a collective, as energies of the seven chakras and of the Seven Principles of Man. This book explores this relationship, for it is the study of the interaction of the seven essential life vortexes that are the seven chakras, which reveals miasmatic activity as they are meant to be perceived as the result of human karma.

The spiritual nature of human evolution has been ignored by historians, glossed over by academics and controlled by religions. This evolution will manifest as miasmatic disease when mankind chooses to ignore it, as miasms in themselves are able to influence consciousness. This also includes Divine consciousness or to be conscious of the Divine as opposed to Self. All the other lower kingdoms therefore, do not manifest disease in the same way, for they do not have the capacity to question Divine Will. However, with such consciousness humanity does have this ability, as co-creator, to place its influence over these lower kingdoms. It is only through humanity that disease can be introduced to the other kingdoms here on Earth.

This rationale places the forces of destiny that manifest miasmatically in a different context to that which can be obtained and be perceived by the five senses. The Psoric miasm may be the least cruel of the miasms to the physical body, perhaps because it is in direct cognition with the earthly element that in its creative sense is the making of the soil of the Earth. Therefore at present it is easiest for the human form to find harmony and unravel the secrets of its home, but the consequences of the Psoric miasm can be detected more deeply within the human psyche on the higher planes and if unresolved will flow over and affect both the next generation and of course the next life after reincarnation. This can hinder much in the way of possibility for the purpose of a life. When the Psoric miasm is looked at within its consequence upon the higher planes, the true extent of its pain can be ascertained.

Miasms therefore do not simply pass their way through the bloodline and along the ancestral stream. The consequence of one life also feeds into the next as essentially this dictates the necessity for rebirth. The energy of past events bleeds through the time barrier in the form of miasmatic inheritance and is thus contained within more than just the physical and etheric bodies. Therefore, if miasms pertain to the other bodies, they have the means to draw on energy resources that go back a long way. The drawing of such energy happens simultaneously, as essentially in evolutionary terms there is only what we know to be the present. Therefore when treating using homœopathic philosophy one can only deal with what is presented but one has also to be aware that it is only the tip of the iceberg. Miasmatic energy is fed parasitically by past patterns on which they gorge and it is thus within their interest to maintain these patterns as it is from these that miasms are kept alive.

It is because miasmatic damage manifests in the 'here and now' that much can be done to free the soul of its constraints. This is why we are only a meditation away from our past lives, from one's history, from healing the past, as all in reality is happening simultaneously. This is what we are as a whole. It is only when miasmatic energy transcends on the spiritual plane that spirit, through the soul, is no longer limited by their bounds.

In this book, the syphilitic miasm is presented as expressing itself through the other miasms. This is a different way of looking at the evolution of the miasms and questions the more traditional point of view with regard to their function and growth. Central to this is the notion that miasmatic activity is safer on the human constitution when acting on the physical end of the chakra line and much more devastating when acting on the spiritual. All the miasms are the product of the separation of Self from the Divine. It is the varying ways the different energy centres that we call chakras inter-relate, which not only differentiate the miasms from one another but also explains how they coexist and thus pertain to a particular chakra. Like the chakras, we only differentiate the miasms so that we can access them to further human consciousness using the limitations of the human brain.

Miasms fascinate us even though they are the result of negative karma. We need to enter their dark world to understand them, for they are a means to healing and by healing we enter the light. We gain from them much insight that is innate to the human individual purpose. This purpose uses the mechanism of reincarnation in which spirit has its part in the evolution of all the planets and not just Earth. Miasms test our understanding and thus the structures that humanity places on the cause of disease and therefore the subsequent treatment. They place the responsibility of this not simply on the actions of Self but also on the group. Both are of miasmatic making and the greatest cause of miasms are actions created out of fear.

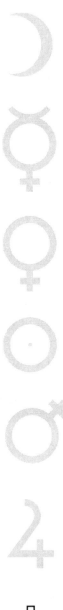

 Chapter 1
The Base Chakra

THE BASE CHAKRA

There is a process to life, which evolves one's spirit working through each chakra in reverse order to when they were first visited by spirit during the act of incarnation. So in effect, we re-climb the ladder, exploring what was once known but then forgotten by the conscious mind. This enables Self to replace that of the old with the new. All ladders need a firm footing and the purpose of the base chakra is to provide this for the child and later the adult. A good base chakra provides the opportunity to explore life in all its diversity, in short, to take a firm grip of the reins and take it on. The importance of this footing cannot be stressed enough, and when taking the patient's case an assessment in relation to the quality of the childhood should be carefully addressed. How is the level of trust, as opposed to fear, learnt through the patient's construction of their base chakra as a child, and subsequently how does this now reflect in the conduct of their everyday needs?

The base chakra marks the beginning of a spiritual quest: to rise from material limitations of physical life. To do so means the lessons of Saturn (the governing planet of this centre) must be thoroughly mastered, for it will not allow the student to pass through its gates until it feels that the definition of physical truth, as opposed to illusion, has been imbedded in the personality. There are many adults who have yet to master this initiation. We know in homœopathy that the more the patient is present and integrated, the easier it is for them to evolve through their treatment. This is the cut and dry of this centre; it either works for you or it doesn't. There is no room to haggle here, no maybes or loose loitering around its periphery, for it requires full

Chapter 1 ~ The Base Chakra

attention if Self is to progress. It is fairly easy to ascertain the connection between the development of the formative years and the way they play out in the habits of later life. Poor development or function of the base manifests in two different ways: the soul either hides within the base chakra or the spirit has a problem accessing it. In either situation, there is a fear of allowing Saturn to participate naturally in life. Avoidance does not push the will of Saturn away and thus it is applied over and over again until its lessons have been learnt and the gate opens on Self's voyage to the next chakra. The repercussions from Saturn's relentless pursuit, if ignored, lead to devastation, as all that is held dear is lost. By the time that Saturn has outmanoeuvred the avoidance of Self by removing each obstacle placed in its path, Self, if having relied solely on material gain, can then find itself ill prepared and incapable of change. Saturn's lesson is that of flexibility. It forces Self to make the decisions that are necessary, those that Self is reluctant or feels incapable of taking. In challenging personal rules it removes the need for excuses – the false gods that Self accumulates in order to justify its reluctance towards the new.

To be stuck in the base centre results in the action of holding on to what one's got, be it a little or a lot. This is to be a slave to the material world and indicates a lack of trust in the process of life. It does not mean that the material world is not important, as it sustains our purpose for being here. However, there is a point to this relationship and that is to loosen its solidity in order that Self may shine brightly through it and not have it govern its shine. Or to put it another way, it is the sunlight that makes our planet so green, not the green that makes the sunlight. Material possessions should be gained to assist Self, but instead they have become the means by which to express power and to reflect status. Status is the primary mover in material dominance and is motivated by the fear of loss. There is a universal law that states: change can only happen for the better. It has no other motivation and the energy of the base is the preparation for such changes, of which there will be many during life. Those who cling to the material world like a life raft find it impossible to locate dry land on which they can explore the challenges that life presents. It is only through letting go that one can correct the old, pointless cycles of the personality, which is part of what Self is here to undo. The more materialistic humanity is, the further it will be from its purpose, and this will sadly be reflected in the wishes of Self. However, within such a materialistic world the child may be born into or attract great wealth to support its purpose for being here. This can bring about great change, for which this wealth will be needed. The test of Saturn will be to prevent this wealth from becoming the motivation. The material world and Self should operate in harmony, otherwise nothing of note will be achieved. In the West this has become more of a challenge, for society has placed great importance on possessions. Saturn has only one outcome in mind, to teach Self trust, so that it may pursue its purpose. Some of the remedies required when facing difficulties here are *Lycopodium, Silica, Clay, Earth* and *Yellow*.

The inability to get into one's base chakra makes the physical manifestations of life's natural needs difficult to cultivate. It is impossible to catch the bus if you haven't made it to the bus stop. The stability that this centre provides is simply not available for construction if the spirit is not around to benefit. This also makes homœopathic remedies very difficult to use on a person who is not in their body and therefore not present to receive them. Often in this case base remedies, especially *Sulphur*, will be needed to re-establish the connection of body and spirit, often before other remedies will work. These will root the person to their base, enabling them at last to make an assessment as to the state of their lives, which have been continuing whilst they have not been around to make any purposeful decisions. It is fairly common these days to hinder a child's development by throwing them out of their body and away from their base chakra. One major cause of this is vaccinations. Can the spirit of a child really be expected to hang around during an attack of insidious, negative karmic material that directly bypasses the immune system and thus besieges its home? In this way we could say that the energy of the crusades is still among us. Violence on TV will also do this, as of course will fear instilled by their trustees. We can now begin to see how much the base chakra has influence over the yet to be developed emotions. There is much in this modern world to which the child has to be wise and not overly open. But then sometimes a new child enters the family with its own karmic quest for protection in mind, unconsciously making demands, one of which may be to not be vaccinated. This throws the family into turmoil, for on a conscious level they don't know or can't see what is motivating this new form of questioning within them. The child will thus change the dynamic of the family by reminding it that things need to be different.

It may also be said that part of this inability to touch base can be a

Chapter 1 ~ The Base Chakra

reluctance to temper the excesses of the Jupiter centre. The base centre is supposed to instil limitations in order to balance out this excess, the brake with the throttle. But alas some people get addicted to the pleasure the personality desires. In this day and age much prescribing is required at this junction. In a sense, a good base creates the confidence to say yes and a good sacral centre provides the judgement to say no. So, often to activate the function of the base chakra, remedies of the sacral centre will be required. *Tiger's Eye* and other remedies more tuned to the sacral centre may be needed to release the patient from their procrastination and into the stability of their own direction, which is the function of the base centre. The ladder's footing supports the balance and provides the foundation of all the other chakras, so it will often require attention before any other changes can be tackled. If the patient is not at one with Saturn's energy, fear will inhibit the prescription. Fear is the reaction to Self-preservation and will stimulate the secretion of adrenaline from the adrenal glands, which are related to the sacral centre. As the base centre has no glands of its own, it relies on this secretion in order to protect the life of the body in times of danger. With a poor base centre the person will feel more danger than there is in reality. This is the illusion already spoken of and it leads to the depletion of adrenal energy. Without a good base, the message of never-ending caution drains the kidneys and over stimulates the nervous system. The base chakra teaches the rules of safety and without these there will be a lot of fear and a lack of trust. This centre therefore is in need of constant redress in homœopathic prescribing in order to create stability, and this should not be overlooked.

The body's reaction to fear and anger, which is controlled by the sympathetic nervous system, is to flood the heart and muscles with blood (energy). This is instinctual, governed by the secretion of the hormone adrenaline. If the body feels under stress then the adrenals will compensate for this. But if the extra energy is not utilised, be it not a true "fight or flight" situation, then this boost leads to an overload of the nervous system, creating nervous shock. If left to continue, this constant stimulation leads to a manic disposition and the erosion of the base chakra and subsequent overactive sacral centre activity. Danger motivates adrenal flow either directly in the individual or through group consciousness. Politicians and social leaders have been aware of this for some time. The group in which Self lives provides much in the way of a base as does its home. When either of these change, this has an uprooting effect on the base chakra. In order to keep a grip on power, group leaders have used this to their advantage by maintaining their people in a state of fear through making policies that make it appear that the group's security is under threat. One of the most effective forms of this manipulation of fear is through public health. In America, for example, one does not own one's health; it is a matter of national security. The level of resultant resistance to this is dependent on the quality of the base chakra. The same applies for any form of shock, which is equally debasing and can knock the spirit right out of its body, and may result in being comatose. When Self is not in contact with its base, there is much paranoia. Such an individual is easily riled and the result is a jumpy, nervous personality.

INCARNATION

To be born on this planet is an initiation. No matter how much science likes to see it as simply a seed growing in a pot, there is of course, much more to this process. Incarnation in its full sense does not happen in a split second. Contained in the philosophy of the Kabbalah, is an illustration of how each chakra is visited before spirit settles in the physicality of the base centre. Here the base acts as a huge mirror, attracting light downwards so that each chakra is explored and is then reflected back up as consciousness. The unconscious experience, which is gained through such exploration, is available to spirit to serve in the process of developing each chakra during life, as it makes its way through its spiritual unfolding. Fear cuts off this connection, denying its innate communication, rendering it stagnant.

The timing of conception and subsequently of birth has a relationship with the planets of our universe coinciding with the destiny of one's own karma, or the chosen path of spirit, which is guided by Divine Will. The desire to reincarnate from a state of bliss must be a powerful yearning, for the incarnating Ego is possessed with a passion to improve in the pursuit of Self's own spiritual destiny here on Earth. When an astrologer maps a birth chart, it is the influences of the universe that may determine this improvement that is revealed. Where each planet lies in a particular sign under the influence of its house, indicates the manner in which the collective energy of destiny will be played out. We are all here for a reason or a purpose and part of the homœopathic practitioner's purpose may be to help others to find theirs. The function of Saturn, the

Chapter 1 ~ The Base Chakra

ruling planet of the base chakra, is to aid that purpose by helping to keep the candidate on their true path.

The female pelvic bone acts as a doorkeeper from one world into the next. During birth, the baby is compressed through this cavity, which is the birth canal. From the realm of the mother's protection (female energy) the door is opened leading to the first stage of independence in the newborn's challenge of purpose. The base chakra is where the instructions to life's survival kit are learnt during the course of the child's first seven years. It will provide the tools and the foundation to assist in creating the best opportunity to achieve its purpose, which is inevitably to lighten the karmic load. This is why the formative years are so important and where true trust as opposed to fear is developed. After the compression of the birth canal, there is the reactionary expansion when the child is introduced to his new physical world as part of this initiation. In this world he will cherish the daylight, the warmth of the sun, breathe the air, drink water and eat food, absorbing the solar energy that he needs to survive. He will expel toxins, search for shelter and gain the love that makes him feel more at peace within his world.

Birth is a bridge from one existence into another. Interference at this stage can result in birth trauma. Part of the expansion from the contraction of the birth canal, is to allow the body to activate its centre line in order that all the chakras can line up and allow spirit to dip in and out of them, enabling the child to reach out and embrace their new surroundings. This process is triggered by the first vocal expression of the throat chakra. If this is hindered or interrupted, then this expansion may never be achieved and will be reflected in the child by the contradictory behaviour of clinging fears, compensated by bouts of egotism and self-obsession. Consequently lots of remedies will be required, especially the base remedies already mentioned and *Psorinum*. *Dolphin* is also extremely useful here and will balance the cerebrospinal fluids, lifting their intake into the nervous system and thus promoting calmness. If *Dolphin* is given during pregnancy it will connect the mother and child more closely, resulting in a more harmonic birth. It is also useful to give to the mother if she is dithering between whether or not to vaccinate, or if she is under pressure from the father to vaccinate the child. The father tends to be the most fearful on this subject and the least connected to the maternal communication. The centre line expands from and is marked by the activity of the heart chakra, it being the pivot of chakra activity. *Dolphin* and other heart remedies will release the heart at any age if this expansion is hindered.

Amethyst and *Ayahuasca* will be required if the heart is too burdened to fully incarnate, however, this will be explored more fully later. Remedies such as *Purple* and *Ayahuasca* will be required during pregnancy and possibly during labour to lighten the karma of the baby and the mother. They will also help to turn the baby into the correct position if her natural path is hindered by her own history, usually caused by a resistance to incarnate. It can however work the other way: babies with heavy karmic loads can be born under impossible circumstances and at great pace. Birth, if looked at in reverse, is the junction between the first seven unconscious chakras joining the seven conscious ones. So it will be the energy of the unconscious Jupiter chakra releasing the child from all that is ethereal and into the material, which is the base centre, where physical life begins. Like Moses in the basket, the pact that is made in being physical is to trust in the flow of life. And thus, once having collected a body, the lessons, limitations, paradoxes and dualities of life are explored in a pact from this starting point.

Since the symbolic notion of the parting of the waves, life has been about the separation of the one into the two. This can also be seen as the yin and yang, male and female, the body and the mind, joy and sadness, the physical and the spiritual, the Ida and Pingala. It is through the symbol of the Star of David or the hexagram that we get a representation of the unification of the two sacred opposite energies.

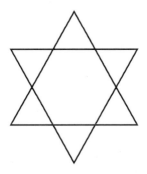

Figure 1. The Star of David.

It represents the "cosmic dance" of Shiva and Shakti, where all the descending energy of the cosmos meets the already manifested physical

Chapter 1 ~ The Base Chakra

consciousness ascending from this planet. This is represented by the top three chakras forming a downward pointed triangle, which then infuses with the bottom three, an upward pointed triangle, both of which are balanced at the heart: as above, then so below.

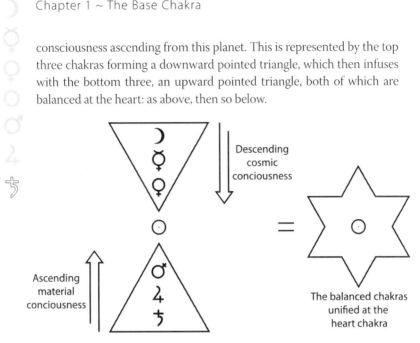

Figure 2. The Forming of the Star of David.

When balanced in this way, the chakra system exhibits much protection and, with its ability to clear Earthly karma, acts as a portal into other worlds permitting safe passage so that each world, realm, space or time can become one. Such travel expands the mind, tapping into ageless wisdom and bringing peace.

The existence of humanity on Earth has been presented esoterically as having five stages of development called 'root-races.' We are presently in the fifth – the Aryan. How the root-races fit into evolution will be explained more fully in the brow chapter, but briefly, they represent a specific time in Earth's planetary cycle that has come about by the human race undertaking a significant change. This change is not only established within knowledge, wisdom and perception but also within the human physical form.

Before the end of the third root-race, there was not this pull from one dominating force to another, as with division, only the harmony of the whole. As homoeopaths, it is these dualities that we try to heal in the pursuit of balance through wholeness. As it stands in our part of evolution, the fifth root-race, this separation can never be eliminated but the challenges, the ups and the downs of life, can be made smoother and more easily integrated. During the majority of the Age of Lemuria (the third root-race) which subsequently bore the Atlantian Age, the psoric miasm did not exist. There was no division within Self as such and neither between Self and the group. In fact there was no division between anything that had celestial communication. Beings acted as a single unit glued together by love, such was the open heartedness of existence and such was the level of telepathic communication that they did not require the limitations of the brain and certainly not of the physical body. Then developed the wish to divide and thus the individual became the keeper of a different kind of consciousness. Self's consciousness became the bastion of the individual's mind. A new structure in which the role of the individual could be played out was required. This became Atlantis, which represented the lowest point of humanity's descent into matter on the planet Earth. The material struggles of Atlantis led to its destruction, for the huge knowledge of spiritual power became the source of personal gain. Great strides had to be made when civilisation found that matter was all with which it had to work. Physical desire became so dominant that it developed the determination to be stronger then any other power. What was an opportunity to once again follow the path of the Divine Will, failed quite literally in misery. Dark forces fought with light ones and their karmic consequences are still with us today in the form of miasms.

To house the individual self, an individual body was evolved. The spirit and the soul became bound in the restrictions of the human anatomy. Bones were formed to create structure and a framework to protect those precious elements of life now manifested in the material world. An organ formed a single barrier between this new inner and outer world, this is the skin, the layer that covers fibrous tissues and which in the physical world denotes that which Self is and that which it is not. Existence had crystallised and with it came the significance of gravity, the pull of the planet into the matter of the Earth, from which it and Self could contain and retain atoms. This has a direct correspondence with the conscious mind, "for these things do matter." So what was not physical before had become so in thought. Physical form had to evolve if the desire to be individual was to succeed. The psoric miasm came to be like a chess piece making a move against an invisible opponent. Its relationship is intrinsic to that of Saturn and the base chakra. Psora is the compromised communication between the guidance of divine instruction

Chapter 1 ~ The Base Chakra

and this new awakened "free will" of the individual Self or mind. It is the abandonment felt by such a division. It is not, however the cause of the division: the answer to that lies at the heart chakra. Telepathy, which had previously been bestowed on the group collectively, was now for individual use. The brain grew inside the body and the third eye, the portal for collective consciousness, receded to what is now the pineal gland.

The conscious mind thus took precedence over what was innately connected before separation and subsequently much was lost. In the psoric miasm we pine for this re-connection: to go back to that from which we were banished. Independence has come at a price that each one of us has to pay in the pursuit of security. We know, however, that Saturn is on our side and this makes the psoric miasm the healthiest and easiest of all the miasms with which to work. This is because presently we are so deeply instilled in matter that the element earth is the easiest to relate to. However, this can also make earth the most difficult element to work with on the higher planes. To be on the outside looking in is Saturn's way of reminding us of what we have forsaken – if only we could control the base chakra. Greek mythology shows us that this is not possible, for apart from Jupiter, Saturn consumed all of his sons. It has been suggested that this was through envy, for he feared they would dispose of him, but the myth relates more to the ultimate sacrifice made to the gods. The essential nature of the base chakra is about the changes we are reluctant to make because they appear to threaten our very survival.

All the failings of Atlantis have been passed on in the form of life atoms leading from one nation to the next and are designed to inspire the next evolutionary step. It was during the downfall of the Egyptian era that the balance between spirit over matter was lost, for the time being. During its flourishing years the predominance of the higher worlds over that of the material one was in great evidence. The fact that the pyramids were built using levitation reveals that the power base of Atlantis was still master over the physical world, however this was to change. The Pharaohs who channelled the vision that guided their nation were replaced by the leaders of armies who were bent on greed and destruction, and graded their power over another through their material wealth. Many people died in the pursuits that ensued. Civilisation turned its back on its spiritual purpose and strived for the level of materialism that we have today.

We can no longer ignore this and if we do, it will be at our own peril.

This does not, however, mean materialism has to dictate our purpose. That which was deemed to be spiritual (powerful) from then on became wrapped in the materialism of religion and so owned by the state rather than by the individual. Instead of the inner contemplation coming through the third eye, the physical eyes became open and were directed upwards for all to see. The same is happening to homœopathy for it is a spiritual pursuit with its own science and at the time of writing it faces its biggest threat in Britain, to be owned by the state rather than the individual, which perhaps was inevitable once people became determined to prove it works. The security of the individual is held in Common law in this country: to suppose we need another structure or more structure suggests we are not safe. In Europe this "more" was created by Napoleon and through his laws it would be him that the individual answered to. As a more Napoleonic system encroaches upon Britain, the individual's right to practice, prescribe and have access to homœopathy faces an unclear future. If you wish to see an example of inspired homœopathy being stifled and driven out then look no further than its use in the rest of Europe. We must guard against that which has seen freedom wiped out in country upon country. Fear is the failure of spiritual belief.

Incarnation takes time and involves the coming together of many functions. To become fully in-tune with a new environment in which every faculty is interwoven with the here and now and readily accessible, is in fact a process of natural acceptance. This is the truth of trust, the crown chakra united with the base chakra. The birth of the cosmos described in Greek mythology relates exactly to the process of incarnation. To be fully incarnated means to be in full possession of the seven vehicles, which have been revealed by Madam Blavatski. It could be said that all Virgos at present struggle with this concept, as while their ruling planet continues to go undiscovered, to a certain extent within themselves, so do they. However, in evolutionary astrology one considers more karma than is normally dictated by the stars in one lifetime. Karma is speeded up by the use of homœopathy, meditation etc so as to bypass the stars and place the responsibility on Self.

A lack of acceptance can prevent the spirit from fully incarnating, a condition we know as autism. This condition is like having one foot in and one foot out of the world. This can arise before, during or after birth but it differs from the description of autism given to vaccine dam-

Chapter 1 ~ The Base Chakra

aged children who have been knocked out from their base by these innoculations. Being not fully in their body, they are hindered from accessing faculties that in truth they do possess but may never be able to use in this lifetime. The official criteria for diagnosing autism seem to widen year by year, a reflection of the breadth of faculty being eroded by the actions of ever increasing fear. The circumstances of incarnation are influenced by the events of previous lifetimes and the bloodline. Being part of an ancestral chain means that there is a karmic relationship which is so deeply interwoven that each action in life will have a consequential effect on the spirit of each ancestor involved. Subsequently, when great strides have to be made to find, act on and follow our purpose in life, then the ripples of change that are required to make such a leap, vibrate down the whole ancestral vine. Some or perhaps all of our ancestors may welcome what effect this will have on them, but others may resist, having been unable to make similar changes through fear or inertia when the opportunity beckoned. Remedies such as *Ayahuasca*, which is the vegetable equivalent of a species that best pertains to this interwoven ancestral vine growing on Earth, will help loosen this bondage, allowing the person to transcend. Other new remedies may also be required as well as also kidney remedies such as *Natrum Mur*, along with kidney supports.

It is impossible to separate the karma of previous incarnations with that of the bloodline; together they make up our karmic load. In reality, we are in the here and now, without a future or a past, for they are all wrapped up together: they only exist in the present. Self lives in the past through the future and in the future through the past, which can only manifest through the here and now. So in a sense the future and the past only exist in Self's imagination. The more we contain ourselves in the moment, then the greater connection we have with what is possible. Children do this – by way of the Moon they use their connection with the cosmos or instinct to steer themselves around the pitfalls of learning to build through the base chakra. This is beauty in motion when the duality of the opposite chakras attract in harmony. The openness of this process in children needs to be protected by the means of the thymus gland at the heart centre.

The only way we can truly grasp the reality of an event, whether it be in the past or in the future, is to bring it into the here and now by visiting it. This can be done by the means of astral travel, which is also the way parallel time is explored and goes someway to describe the space in which the actions of the here and now resonate and influence the consequences of the ancestral psyche. The karma that Self changes will open up new pathways for when its associated ancestors reincarnate. Does one surprise oneself or everyone who came before, who doubted one? This load is contained in the kidneys and at this point it is important to be reminded of the difficulty in separating the base chakra from the function of the sacral chakra. The interaction of their energy works so very closely together, jumping in and out of one another. The kidneys often need much support when working on the base, for ancestral energy will undoubtedly add to any resistance to change.

KUNDALINI

Located at the sacrum, which in Latin means 'holy place', rests the vantra of the lingam or kundalini. It is visualised as a snake. Coiled, it rests on a downward pointing triangular bone which assists in pulling together the inverted union of its three elements, the Ida, Pingala and Sushumna, with one's own spirit. Kundalini is said to resonate at a higher level than light, as absolute pure love. The union of body with spirit allows this creative fire to run along the column of spirit, the spine or the pole of Paracelsus. The kundalini remains dormant until called upon in order to awaken higher consciousness in a quest for absolute knowledge. This is a quest to once again reunite with the Divine and in doing so each chakra must be purified in order to develop perception, psychic powers and spiritual emergence. This transformation is the greatest challenge of all and thus is fraught with much danger and psychological upheaval. It should never be rushed or undertaken without the help of wise advice born out of experience. Previously, kundalini was only awoken after much spiritual work was undertaken, usually in sacred places and under strict guidance. The action of this aroused force can create all things, including death.

Today in the West, many choose to use kundalini to further their personal development. However, spiritual emergence can also occur out of the blue, as part of fate, and what a gift this can be. This experience needs to be recognised, but unfortunately in the West these mental and emotional upheavals are often confused with depression, panic and anxiety. As these are often accompanied by moments of pure joy, this opportunity for greater enlightenment is misdiagnosed and suppressed

Chapter 1 ~ The Base Chakra

by allopathic drugging, often in institutions. This attack on the psyche can be intense, for it challenges the truth around our separation of Self and the Divine. The most difficult junction to this separation and the subsequent pursuit of reunification is at the heart centre, in the abyss.

With the onset of the Aquarian Age, many more will be faced with the desire to pursue the secrets of the kundalini. More guidance will be required and thus the present knowledge of its relevance will become more widely disseminated. This is to be expected, for the astrological sign of Aquarius rules the house of vision. This sign, the original ruler of the pineal gland, which is also the third eye, is the point of focus required by the kundalini after its three parts, the Ida, Pingala and Sushumna, separate at the pituitary gland. Their differing directions form a cross: that of the second crucifixion.

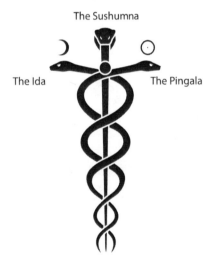

Figure 3. The Second Crucifixion.

This symbolic image refers to the act of transcendence from all Earthly constraints. To the left goes Ida, representing the moon and to the right Pingala, the sun. The unconscious is said to be the lunar self, whereas the conscious is the solar self. In the centre lies the Holy Spirit or Christ's consciousness. From this, Jesus became a representation of the Sushumna energy by means of humanity pulling down this light to manifest physically here on Earth, in order that it too could understand the process. This central column continues upward to the pineal gland and on to the Eighth chakra. This will be detailed more precisely later in the chapter on the Brow. The start of the Aquarian Age signals the need for the continued development of the third eye, which like a dish that's been simmering through the Piscean Age, now needs the spice to be added to further the function necessary for humanity to move out of its material enslavement. Homoeopathy, in its pursuit to heal under increasingly difficult circumstances, in order to understand and maintain a footing with what the word health implies, will need to call upon this extra perception more during the next age.

Many adjectives have been used to describe the power of Kundalini over the years. But to truly understand the forces at work, one needs to fathom the direction of its source. Like a wooden henge, whose centre is formed by an upside down oak tree, it has its roots firmly in the sky. This is exactly the same for the kabbalist diagram of the Tree of Life and is reflected in its shape like an upside down tree.

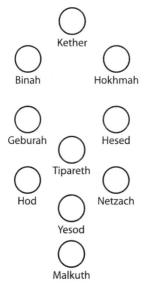

Figure 4. The Tree of Life.

Hindu mythology describes this beautifully as kundalini power manifesting from the heavens, which of course represents the Divine source Sada-Shiva. His power and also his spouse or female counterpart, Adi Shakti (meaning primordial power) is that which does all things. One works

Chapter 1 ~ The Base Chakra

through the other. She is the supreme mother goddess who represents the driving force of the active, dynamic principles of feminine power. She gave birth to the universe, all the gods that attend over it, and all deities and celestial beings. Her presence in humans manifests as kundalini. Its pure (virgin), feminine energy removes the sins of all children, working through the human auric egg and delivering consciousness to the Higher Triad. Each and every one of us has this source within.

Not one ounce of enlightenment is possible if the process of raising the kundalini is not firmly rooted in the Base centre. As human beings we choose to be incarnated here on Earth and therefore kundalini and Self need to manifest firmly on the ground to be earthed, or else Self's faculties will float off into the realm of fantasy. For this part, Kundalini is housed in the stability of the dense bone of the base centre, where earthquakes are said to be few and far between, only every twenty-eight years or so. Here there should be little to disturb its sleep. This is considered to be of such importance that this area of the pelvis is the last part of the skeleton to be destroyed when the body is burnt. The life force of kundalini is in all living things, it being a necessity for existence on each level and its mystical import can be found throughout religions symbolically as the snake.

In the West it is mostly those who have studied Eastern philosophy that are aware of this knowledge. Western culture is evolving differently and has subsequently lost much in the way of spiritual connection in the pursuit of material gain and the development of the intellect. On a superficial level knowledge of the power of kundalini is nowhere to be found in Western consciousness and consequently, on the whole it has not acquired the respect or knowledge to safely raise its huge potential. Beneath the surface however, its knowledge has been taught by groups in the pursuit of spiritual development for as long as in the East. Its meaning and all that is attributed to its wisdom can be found in the scriptures of the West if you know how to read them properly. The importance of the Bible is not just found in what is written but in the way that it is read. The wisdom of the occultist goes hand in hand with the development of kundalini, be it during meditation, ritual or by other means of self-development. This is why those who want the information, the wisdom, without doing any of the work, fail. It is the same in homoeopathy, for you may well be given examples of when to use remedies and presented with lots of cases in which there are many answers, none of which may work when confronted by one's own patients.

Much work has to be done on the base chakra before the kundalini feels able to make its journey upwards, for without this work all that it sets out to achieve will come crumbling down. Once again Saturn positions itself as doorkeeper, preventing anything from entering or leaving until it feels the time is right. Like the three pillars of the Kabbalah, the kundalini has three psychic meridian lines but remains as a single serpent when dormant. In this state, it remains coiled around the bottom of the Svayambhu Lingam, which is the invisible pillar of light with its visible foundation stone. This stone denotes the division between form and the formless or Absolute, between that which is real and unreal. This is what Self in existence is being spontaneously asked to explore. The head of the dormant serpent rests on this foundation stone, facing downwards with its tail in its mouth directing cosmic energy in an inverted direction until called upon. Then kundalini readies itself by moving its open mouthed head upwards in preparation to rise up the pillar and at last meet the gods. The central meridian is called the Sushumna, which flows straight upward through the etheric channel of the spine. The other two counterpart nerve energies weave around this central column, reuniting at each chakra until finally dividing at the point of enlightenment. As the energy rises, it works its way through etheric webs that cover the portals of each chakra, laid down during the formation of the body by the spirit as it left each chakra in its pursuit to incarnate. Through the ascension of kundalini, each chakra is cleared of karmic discharges usually from many lifetimes, stored as fears, forms, memories or external beings. This of course will take many opportunities to achieve. The purge should begin at the base, for it is here that one will not only achieve more stability, but in the process of correct progression, each chakra will be cleansed starting with the one immediately below it. This action also allows the protective web to be broken by the new energy reaching up from below. This is not, however, the same for homoeopathic prescribing using the chakras as guides, for blocks and balances require treatment in a far less regimented structure. If each chakra is insufficiently cleared, this will weaken the overall effect of the cleanse on the next chakra, or worse still, the next chakra will fail to be called upon at all. Because kundalini is also awoken through having sex, in the more promiscuous West this tends to be where it will be used, exhausted and thus extinguished. It very rarely gets beyond the sacral centre and subsequently is used for the sexual high as opposed to, in part, the intimate embrace of the male and the female in pursuit of wholeness.

ASPIRATION

Aspiration has an undivided connection with growth. It is the rings on a tree that has been fed by the sun and watered by the rain, with its roots planted firmly in the soul. Its ability to flourish is dependent on the formative years, the quality of the base chakra and that of the parents and group influences. In homoeopathy we use the energy of the plant's essence that when picked contains not only the experiences of its present existence but also that throughout its gene pool, as one seed becomes the next. In humanity, aspiration is reflected through soul consciousness, the place where the lower part of spirit unites with the higher level of matter. In the personality, aspiration manifests at a lower level in the form of ambition, which is governed by the spleen. On a higher level it requires the guidance of Divine Spirit and so the past experiences of aspiration are passed on through the soul and built upon by means of spiritual love.

During the development of the base centre the child is not conscious of this process, but nevertheless is guided by her soul through the group she has entered. Aspiration is the desire to do good on behalf of humanity: it is brotherly love, including all its moral judgements. The group must take the responsibility of teaching the child the importance of his own physical interaction, for any of his actions will inevitably affect them all. The group guides the child by the way its members interact with their own souls until the child has learnt to integrate with his own soul. The fitting is of course made easier, for the child attracted the group and thus already has the love for it. Even though the child's needs are of a priority to the group, the child learns that to make unreasonable demands on them is selfish, for there are also higher considerations and thus the base lays down its connection with the heart. The aspiration of the group or parent is imparted to the child but of course it is already innate within the child as the two are connected. So the base chakra helps to prepare aspiration for conscious use.

Aspiration is different to our purpose, for it is much more individual to Self's karma. The purpose of life is the manifestation of Divine will. What we aspire to do is the mechanism by which purpose radiates. To gain insight into a person's aspiration, then look no further than the aspiration of the parents. It is a baton passed on through the bloodline, the glue that binds a family, group or tribe together. This energy is awoken in the child through the responsibility of those around them, providing a sense of belonging. It influences the aura and goes some way to explain why so many adopted children become disappointed when they finally meet their birth parents: they were meant to be with their adopted parents. This is the connection in which the child is or should be encouraged to flourish and how they will gain the framework that channels direction through their desire.

Part of learning the lessons of the base chakra is to sow the seed of aspiration and balance it against the Saturn energies of patience, perseverance and endurance. Due to the fact that the next generation will always pick up from where the previous one has left off, in our homoeopathic cases it is always good to make a note of what the parents strived to achieve. This is not a question of what car they drove or even what job they kept: the answer lies in what position or relationship is taken in the group in order to give back to it. It is a spiritual question and not simply about the vehicle that was used to achieve it.

That which the parents reach out for has a considerable influence on the moral conduct of the child. This is part of the bargaining that comes with the child's selfish demands and necessary, as he has to develop from a stage of vulnerability to one of cooperation within the group. This does not necessarily mean the higher the aspiration the easier it is for the child: it can be equally difficult to take on high expectations in a changing world. However, due to karma, this should be a natural task. If it is not, there will be blockages in the base chakra. It is as if there is an innate commitment between parent and child, but problems arise when a parent has broken this trust, for this forms part of the security in which the child needs to feel it belongs. Aspiration is very powerful and when taken away or stifled, it will leave the child severely compromised. The parent must not misuse this power, as the resulting manifestation may have consequences for many generations to come. It is the child's responsibility to achieve that which the parent left incomplete. This does not mean the child will mimic what its parents have done, but he will be linked to them by what they deem appropriate for the group.

If the group abuses its trust, then belief turns into abandonment. If Self feels abandoned by the group, the base centre will be hindered. Aspiration is thus muted and if the subsequent trauma is not resolved it often results in patterns that are played out over generations, for trauma feeds trauma. In this situation a child will be confronted by a pathway which more closely resembles a hotel corridor, along which there are many doors, some open, some closed, but all leading nowhere. There are no connections and therefore no bridges or pathways being created. With no flow, Self gets the feeling of being halted when everything tried has a beginning but no conclusion. Like a concertina, one generation hinders the next, resulting in the backing up of stagnant, unfinished energy. Inevitably, and as the result of karma, a child will be born whose purpose is to overcome this stagnation.

This is by no means as easy as it sounds and will require not simply determination, insight, vision and focus but the wisdom to gain that which is necessary to assist in these changes. This will be a spiritual conquest, mapped out in the child's purpose often arising from what seems the most improbable of circumstances. From such experiences, tales and fables are passed on so that they in turn help to lighten the karma and inspire future generations. These are the stories that our patients often relay to us when we enquire into their family tree. The reason for the visit of such an individual may well be for assistance in continuing the hard work that has already begun earlier down the line. Psychics will often see a long line of ancestors extending backwards behind such people. These people are often open to trying, and will need, homœopathy.

SATURN

Saturn forms a bridge between the old and the new, and as such represents the process of preparation and patience needed in achieving transformation. Therefore, he can never be the finished product, but he is one of the most potent of the four Lords of Karma, bringing on the process of redemption whether Self likes it or not. As Self is subject to karma, so it is subject to Saturn. As Old Father Time, Saturn forces Self to face up to the past, whilst preparing for the future. This is the flow of time, which is both destructive and constructive: the pathway to redemption is much dependent on having faith in this process.

The course of time here relates to the Earth and the span of human life upon it. Saturn offers both the strength and opportunity to formulate a plan, whilst recognising that Self is bound by the constant challenge of nebulous karma. This plan will be a combination of experience and experiment. The responsibility of trying to maintain the direction of one's pathway falls on Self's ability to be flexible in its plan so that its purpose can be worked through. In a sense, without Saturn instilling this responsibility, none of the other centres can function in harmony. Inevitably the plan will be a balance between Saturn and one's own free will, in which the possibility of creating new karma exists.

The strength of Saturn is that he possesses great powers of persuasion used in maintaining what he perceives as the only path. His sternness has been much called upon since the separation of Self from Divine. It is precisely for this reason that he has had bestowed upon him all the alarming rhetoric that has given him the reputation of being a difficult and strict taskmaster. This negative portrayal of Saturn is a reflection of Self's inability to deal with the past, for in reality he has only the welfare of all the other centres in mind. This is the contract of truth that was made with each individual and is played out in his or her karma. This reputation for ruthless determination is frightening to Self, for Saturn's influence requires the utmost truthfulness in order for the purpose of Self to function at all. There is no room for delusion here. What is – is. This unequivocal eye is expressed through the slow, heavy and dense presence of its energy. It takes a long time to shift and thus it is through Saturn that all the wisdom of the dead saints is expressed. This collective power incites the soul to do what is right. We are all aware of the incredible healing energy of a young child, this is Saturn energy, that of survival or movement towards the light.

Saturn is the initiator and therefore its defiant energy is present in abundance during the process of birth and of course during incarnation. These two processes were once spiritually respected and thus birth was not the messy high tech conveyer belt system that it is today. Interference in the process of gestation and birth can be damaging, like the use of unnecessary scans, which are not only a shock to the foetus but also create tissue changes, linked to defects such as brain dysfunction and dyslexia. With a lack of respect born out of fear, the wise insights passed on by Saturn's teachings are lost, those of the surrender to love applied by the means of the gravitational pull on the incoming child. A natural birth and Saturn energy are synonymous in this process. The consequence of meddling results in negative birth patterns, which hinder the development of the base centre during early childhood. We as practitioners have a duty to ascertain the problems associated with new techniques, as their results will often end up at our door.

Chapter 1 ~ The Base Chakra

The further the spiritual growth, the greater the demand for a robust base chakra. Saturn tests the child and continues to do so throughout life, in order that she can discriminate between truth and illusion. During the development of the base chakra and through the security of the family, the child looks to her guardians in the belief that they have mastered the lessons of the base chakra. However, if the security of the parents is threatened in any way, often as a result of their own poor base function, then the repercussions leave the child shocked by what she deems impossible. There is much that links to the heart when a child is developing her base chakra and such shocks will close the heart leading to caution and inertia, which as a result will be played out in the physical body and stored in the kidneys.

Green will be needed for the child and adult who is still suffering from the memory of such an event, or who may have forgotten the source of the shock, but which you as the practitioner will perceive. Base remedies will also be needed to re-establish the sense of security. When the child loses the trust of her parents or fails to receive any, this is the ultimate up-rooting experience. Saturn will of course help the child express her dissatisfaction with her parents, which is often expressed in the form of physical symptoms. These are a warning to her family to pay more attention to their own behaviour and thus the care of the child. This lack of regard will be the result of the past and thus the miasmatic dispositions that follow may have been passed on to the child and reflect as physical pathology, further evidence of consequence that the parents all too often would prefer to ignore. The responsibility of these dynamics is thus handed over to the allopathic doctors. A lack of responsibility in the family, and there is plenty of it, will also burden the child with having to find responsibility, which is in itself too big a task at such an early age.

As well as the psoric miasm, the others associated with the base chakra also include the cancer, tubercular and syphilitic miasms. As a result of miasmatic activity, fear and grief from the parents is transferable at the auric level. The child is mostly blind to this, but being so open, will formulate consequential behaviour. It may only be through the behaviour of other members of the wider group that the child learns that there is another way. The development of the base centre is a powerful urge and if the child is hindered in any of the ways that attract its progress, then this can produce conflict and lead to deep resentment in later life.

The cancer miasm reveals itself often in cases where in the formative years and subsequently thereafter, the child has to seek help or a surrogate parent in order to construct its base. This in itself does not create cancer; as the cancer miasm is already at play in the child's karma, hence the fitting of the child to the situation and the great task that lies ahead in changing it. Cancer is not born of this lifetime: its roots stem back to where the seed has been buried and part of Saturn's task is to offer the opportunity to change this, which manifests as the child's determination to develop her base chakra. This pattern is seen far too often and its demand on Saturn energy is a reflection of the carcinogenic society in which we live, for inertia is its energy, which is contrary to Saturn's requirement. Saturn rules the process of crystallisation, a warning to us all that if ignored, then rigidity will surely follow.

Physical life begins in this centre and it is important to grasp that the faculty that preoccupies the child during its first seven years of life is its physical development. Now, each seven years can also be subdivided into individual years and each relate to a corresponding chakra being developed on a yearly cycle. But this is a 'sub' structure used in order to support the whole, which in this case is the development of the base chakra through a seven yearly cycle. This sub-development is required, for each chakra needs an essence of all the others in order to evolve. Nowhere else in life will the demand to grow a body at such pace and transform from immobilised dependency to young explorer, warrant such energy. Therefore, the child, not having yet developed an adequate emotional sphere, will manifest trauma in a physical manner, this being the child's only conscious outlet. If this wounding is not resolved, it will subsequently evolve into the emotional sphere, that of the sacral centre but as a physical response. Any such trauma will, however, have consequence on the stability of the sacral centre and it can be observed that quite a number of patients have experienced traumatic issues around the age of eight or nine years of age as a result of base chakra shocks coming to light during this transition. The aetiology of these traumas will have been forgotten but energetically they have been instilled in the body. This is also a means by which to protect the insufficiently matured mind during this time. Later when the child is reminded of this trauma or is placed in a situation that reflects the insecurity around it, the pattern will wake up the physical memory of the response. This then becomes a habitual reaction to a given traumatic feeling.

If allowed, this cycle will continue throughout life. An allergy for instance, or a stomach upset that reoccurs before a job interview is a

Chapter 1 ~ The Base Chakra

natural response to past insecurities and a sign that they are yet to be resolved. The physical response does not have to be just a sneezing bout or diarrhoea; it can be physical deformity, septic states and also ritualistic behaviour. Obsessive repetition of gestures, movements, those things that children have to do ten times out of compulsion, will be a physical response to emotional trauma. An aspect of self-harm can be placed here, revealing that the syphilitic miasm also has influence over the function of the base chakra. Each homoeopathic remedy proving contains the duality of the physical and the emotional body. The physical manifestation of symptoms of the personality, similar to that of the physical symptoms of the remedy proving, will have an effect on the base chakra but will not necessarily contain the cause. In other words, as well as having hidden aetiologies in the base chakra, there will be aetiologies in other chakras that look like base chakra problems, for the mind locks them away in the physical. Changes in the higher levels may have to be addressed first before health works its way down to the physical body. This may not be achieved in a single lifetime but strides can be made that will also help future generations via the gene pool and thus lighten Self for the rest of its journey. In respect to these changes, much in the way of a positive response may not happen until the base chakra starts working for the patient, in effect, making it more comfortable to be here.

The Eastern symbolic animal that corresponds to the base chakra is the elephant, it being solid, stable and dependable. It is precisely these qualities that determine what is possible. Such stability is reflected in the fact that the base has no governing gland, for through their reactionary processes of stimulating hormone production, glands swing. It is the function of the endocrine system to regulate and balance energy. If needed, each centre will use the energy of a centre directly above or below it to support itself in times of weakness. So if the base is floundering, it will be the kidneys that have to carry the can. The distribution of kidney energy is very much shared by both the base and the sacral centre. When the sacral centre is weak, then kidney energy being directed towards the spleen and the liver is decreased and the reserves of the solar plexus are also compromised. If the kidneys are conserving energy, this will further weaken a base chakra if already under pressure. Supporting remedies to use in this situation include amongst others: *Apis, Berberis, Kali Phos, Nat Phos, Blue, Calc Carb, Tiger's Eye,*

Hornbeam, Jet, Goldfish, Rhus Tox and *Phosphorus*.

When Self is not grounded, it is in a state of flux and the sympathetic nervous system is then stimulated by the subsequent fear via the adrenal glands. Saturn is aware that a constant feed of adrenaline can become addictive and some people do crave it like a stimulant hit. Constant adrenal release also drains the kidneys, so Saturn applies constraint wherever possible by reminding Self of the laborious tasks of everyday functions that help keep the feet on the ground. Although people can feel excited by running around like headless chickens, invariably not much is achieved and their physical structures, both of body and of the world, cave in as they begin to burn out. The most severe examples can find themselves admitted to psychiatric hospitals, when in truth they have simply just repeatedly over stimulated their nervous system. Base chakra remedies such as *Causticum, Lycopodium, Black Obsidium, Copper Beech, Yellow, Jet, Oak* and *Mimosa* will be needed in these cases along with other remedies to calm this system like *Buddleia* and *Blue*. In addition, remedies to counter that which originally created the need for such adrenal addiction will be needed to target what really lies at the heart of the matter, which will of course include *Syphilinum*. Here there is often a marked history of tuberculosis close by in the family history and also a disruptive childhood, inhibiting the formation of a good base. This will be reflected in the throat chakra and thus an unbalanced thyroid gland, which will become apparent as the case unfolds. Two of the best remedies for grounding people and moving them away from their adrenal fix are *Sulphur* and *Oak*. *Oak* when repeated low over many months can run along side other remedies, for it will not interfere with them.

The elephant is known for its long memory. Saturn's purpose is not only to act as judge in the academy of spiritual preparation, but also to remind each student of his or her spiritual past – the memories of a brighter tomorrow. The cosmological energy of Saturn's role is what we all are connected to through the function of our own base centre. Its energy creates changes that are designed to steer Self back to its rightful and preordained path, so the further Self has wandered away from it, the greater the expected change. These new directions are lessons that eventually have to be adhered to, but the manner in which they manifest, be it smoothly or with difficulty, depends much on the individual's relationship to their own base centre. The feelings of fear, anxiety and a

Chapter 1 ~ The Base Chakra

sense of abandonment here can be great; one of the reasons *Psorinum* is often indicated in cases of suicidal thoughts. These feelings seem to go to the core of our being, for Saturn is not interested in hitch-hikers – there are no free rides here. Where Saturn lies in the birth chart will produce an insight as to how it will make its influence known on the individual's life. For example, when placed opposite the Sun, one's native astrological sign, then this denotes personal struggles in the search of one's identity, as each of them squabble over the rule of Self's ambitions.

Historically, Saturn has been depicted as a tall, cloaked figure with a beard and sunken eyes holding a scythe. To the Romans he was the god of agriculture, but in truth the sharp blade of the scythe represents the directness of his action. He also has a relationship with the seasons, for the scythe casts the shape of the Moon, the ruler of cycles. This indicates change is always upon us, like the recovery of the winter soil from the summer bounty. But it is after harvest that Self can reflect on its entirety, Saturn/Moon and all that is in between. No wonder the motto to this Karmic Lord is 'we reap what we sow.' Saturn wields the scythe in sharp defiance – the field will be cut in order to enable new growth. With the utmost determination, he makes sure that change is carried out. Woe betides anybody who stands in Saturn's way and he has precisely this in mind with his relationship to the candidate. Being one half of unification with the Moon, he is aware that there is a long way to go and therefore establishes the kind of discipline required in order to succeed. To the Aztecs, the relationship between Saturn and the Moon was reflected in their worship of bird's feathers, for they symbolised the animal that both walks on the earth and flies in the heavens.

Saturn is also known as the 'examiner.' Every structure will be tested and if that structure is weak (a false truth) then it will break. The journey of life could be seen as two railway lines running from the station and into the distance. The task of Saturn is to keep Self on track. Some early Renaissance astrologers compared Saturn to Pluto but this is not easily justified. Its energy does not have to be that frightening, for its instruction should be seen as that of the teachings of a wise one – just and unwavering. He is a friend that has only Self's best interest at heart and it is nothing more than Self's mistrust that prevents it believing this, causing panic.

According to Vedic astrology, because Saturn is said to be the son of the Sun, then through him the integrity of life is dramatically improved for the benefit of all. If Self can work with Saturn, it could not wish for a better companion. The drama of its "all or nothing", coupled with its dark cloak and scythe has long associated this planet as the figure of death, of physical finality. The meaning here is no different in Greek Mythology as Uranus was the first father or the father of all fathers and Saturn (Cronus) was his son. Therefore, we can trace all our Earthly ancestral and personal karma back to Saturn in the cycle of life and death, not only from what we are made but where we are going. This is what it took for humanity to gain physicality and enter the Earthly realm in order that this planet could pursue its cycle of conscious development.

This illustrates how intrinsic a strongly established base chakra is within all of our endeavours. If Saturn is the first son, a reaction to the two or separation, then Uranus represents the sun in the sky that impregnated Mother Earth. This may also explain why the Egyptians worshiped the sun god Ra as creator, forming humanity from his tears, the blood of division, and like Uranus he evolved from chaos so wasn't alone. There is much more in the universe being developed, of which Earth is a reflection.

Whilst meditating on Saturn, much in the way of deep insecurities can arise as a result of this Earthly journey. This is felt tenfold if there was a sense of abandonment during the formative years. As a child, the result of a deep loss of security can lead to a compensatory castle being built in which all these fears are locked deeply within its vaults, being too painful to leave out in the light of the sun. The pursuit of transforming this illusion through healing can be a very frightening experience due to this long history of a lack of trust. But an illusion it is and will prevent the possibility of living one's purpose, which in itself is a process of extinguishing fear with light. A lack of base will be the result of deep wounding and base remedies will be required repeatedly here, interwoven with constitutional and miasmatic remedies.

Saturn in retrograde during our earthly calendar year, along with other planets make the individual's and global events occur in a much more intense manner. Saturn's influence during Self's first seven years of life is due to him moving through the first three signs of the birth chart, each of which lasts two and half years. Although it has a marked influence every seven years on each of the four quarters, Saturn officially re-enters the chart at around the age of twenty-eight. Saturn being judge of direction here on Earth provides a major opportunity for Self to reconnect with its purpose if it has been led astray or found wanting. Being

Chapter 1 ~ The Base Chakra

the father of Jupiter, even the King of the Gods bows his head in respect to such authority but usually when confronted alone. He represents payback and further re-enters the chart at the age of fifty-six. As a result to this build-up, a mid life crisis can accompany his return. This will occur in circumstances where achievement does not collate with purpose and so at this age the desire to correct this and the dreaded emotion of regret that comes with it can be very strong indeed. It is frightening when Self realises that a well-trodden path is not the true one. It can feel like having the rug pulled from under your feet. When *Sulphur* is given, these insecurities can be revealed or relived but it can also resurrect the psoric miasm: if given with *Yellow* this miasm will be calmed and the transformation can be made more smoothly.

In the play "A Man For All Seasons" by Robert Bolt; William Roper, who has not only an eye for Parliament but also for the hand of Thomas Moore's astute daughter Margaret, calls for Richard Rich to be arrested. It would appear that Rich has been scheming against Moore on behalf of Cromwell. This is amongst a political climate derived from those who lacked integrity and so were open to deception in order to further their personal standing as the religious and political circumstances in Britain changed. Previously, Moore had recommended Rich to teach in order to serve society, a thought that could not have been further from Rich's mind. Rich pleads with Thomas for help, for he knows his conscience will forsake him and that he will betray his friend Thomas's inability to sanction his support over King Henry's desire to divorce Catherine of Aragon. Rich's soul has its price and he is prepared to trade aspiration for that of its younger brother ambition. It is Rich's eventual perjury in exchange for wealth and position that finally seals the fate of Thomas Moore. Within the following quotation from the play, is an extraordinary definition as to the importance of the role of Saturn in providing a good base chakra. We pick up the scene just after Thomas has rejected Rich's plea for employment, for in light of his scheming, Thomas is aware that the only action he can take against it is to maintain the integrity of his office. This is why when Rich is called to be arrested by members of Moore's household, Moore explains that he cannot arrest Rich for being 'bad', for that is for God to do.

Margaret	Father, that man's bad.
Moore	There is no law against that.
Roper	There is! God's law!
Moore	Then God can arrest him.
Roper	Sophistication upon sophistication!
Moore	No, sheer simplicity. The law, Roper, the law. I know what's legal not what's right. And I'll stick to what's legal.
Roper	Then you set Man's law above God's!
Moore	No, far below; but let me draw your attention to a fact – I'm not God. The currents and eddies of right and wrong, which you find such plain sailing, I can't navigate, I'm no voyager. But in the thickets of the law, oh there I'm a forester. I doubt if there's a man alive who could follow me there, thank God... (*He says this last to himself.*)
Alice	(*Exasperated, pointing after Rich*) While you talk, he's gone!
Moore	And go he should, if he was the Devil himself, until he broke the law!
Roper	So now you'd give the Devil benefit of law!
Moore	Yes. What would you do? Cut a great road through the law to get after the Devil?
Roper	I'd cut down every law in England to do that!
Moore	(*Roused and excited*) Oh? (*Advances on Roper*) And when the last law was down, and the Devil turned round on you – where would you hide, Roper, the laws all being flat? (*He leaves him*) This country's planted thick with laws from coast to coast – man's laws, not God's – and if you cut them down – and you are just the man to do it – d'you really think you could stand upright in the winds that would blow then? (*Quietly*) Yes I'd give the Devil benefit of law, for my own safety's sake.

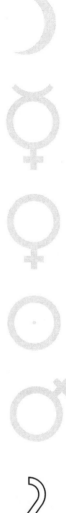

Chapter 2
The Sacral Centre

THE SACRAL CENTRE

Out of the physical constraints of Saturn comes the emotional development under the majesty of expansive Jupiter. However unlikely as it may seem, these opposites do attract. Saturn applies constraints to the runaway Jupiter and Jupiter prevents Saturn from becoming too crusty. These two energies may be seen as the first duality embodied within the personality; whether to expand or contract, to make a move or retreat, to be in the past or the future. If this duality is perceived to be unbalanced in a patient, this can be enough on which to prescribe. The process of this integration from the base to the sacral chakra can be manifested in a volatile emotional state, that if suppressed or not handled well, may reveal scars later during adulthood.

The child develops the energy of the sacral centre between seven and fourteen years, when Self can be observed trying to discover its identity within the group. Identity is part of the little ego: it is that which maintains positive thought and determines whether our interactions are good and protects against negative points of view. The child comes to terms not only with the circumstances of his own incarnation but also the integration of his own personality in his quest to become an adult. The emotional interaction with his fellow contemporaries is uppermost and is directed by the force of reason. The child is no longer standing alone among the lessons of survival, but is now immersed in a fluid cloak, which should be lovingly encouraged to fit by those closest to him. This

Chapter 2 ~ The Sacral Centre

will enable the child to interact so that he may discover who he is within the etheric framework of the group.

The child explores these new feelings through the intimate and physical interactions of personal relationships with friends and family. In effect, they explore themselves through others. It is with the use of reason that the child understands these feelings and fathoms her response. This is achieved not only under the guidance of the brow but also unconsciously with the heart and the crown centre, for the sacral centre's true creative force is that of the stars. This is the first place where one truly comes under their influence, as the soul yearns to reach for the heavens. Thus, the sacral centre is often regarded as the first centre on the step to spiritual growth. Exploration here requires the tools of Divine guidance through judgement. Much is formed through this creative source under the protection of divine purity, allowing in-born authority to play innocently until it has grown into the power of thought. It is then that reason becomes master to the emotions and spirit is ready to venture forward to the next centre. It is also equipped with the guidance and structure provided for the means of safety by the base chakra. The child should already have secured that which is good for them and that which is not. The opposite chakra to the sacral centre, its mirror image but on a higher plane, is the brow centre. They both look out for one another and will reflect the others mood. The sacral centre develops the young shoots of judgement so that they can mature in the form of wisdom to be focused at the brow chakra. The Shakespeare play, *A Midsummer Night's Dream* is about this connection.

For the child, the second set of seven years should be a stimulating exploration, for they are blessed with the abundance of Jupiter energy. Jupiter is the great maintainer, so emotional knocks here should only help to give the child the impetus to widen its exploration and gain the experience it requires to tune its emotional responses to the environment in which it lives. This responsibility is to grant the opportunity to gain emotional stability through fun. This is the adventure playground of life. If there is excessive physical or emotional trauma at this stage, extending beyond what can be sustained by both Jupiter and Saturn working together, the subsequent shock will severely restrict this influence, reversing an outward expression to an internal one and placing the child's potential on hold. This stage in the child's development is important in determining the future of its emotional balance.

Positive interaction with others is crucial in fulfilling the potential of one's purpose. Failure to conquer this centre results in its stagnation and the corresponding immaturity will have repercussions that run throughout close relationships until this trauma is released and the gate is reopened. Jupiter's association with the development of the emotional body reaches deeply into creative thought. Positive thoughts create the conditions around Self in which it can expand and grow. The image that reflects the individual self should radiate one's love and not be buried in the superficial details of appearance. Negative thoughts create conditions ripe for procrastination. They build up so that their subsequent physical manifestations tie down any means of emotional growth. The expansive Jupiter energy inverts to create worry and poor self-image. If this is allowed to continue, this energy can be powerful enough to produce entities that will remain present throughout several incarnations, attaching themselves to the soul and thus trapping its potential with cycles of morbidity. Such is the positive creative potential here that its opposite, which is the result of misuse, is to be perpetually stuck.

A lack of confidence in this centre, which is created by segregation from the group against the child's desires, will manifest as conceit. The ego overcompensates for the insecurities in the emotional development and will present itself as vanity, which is the sacral chakra's form of aggression. To have an over exaggerated opinion of oneself is to have pent-up resentment, which is negative Jupiter energy. This is often said to be the result of suppressed sexual energy, but it is more than that. It is an inability to give and to share. Vanity refers to the inner thought of 'look but don't touch.' Any abuse of this centre will shut down its flow and be reflected emotionally as Self places its emphasis on the qualities and attributes of the kidneys and not the priorities of the higher chakras. In effect it refuses to raise its aspiration above the lower desires of the personality.

Disease enters the bloodline here through sexual contact in the form of miasms. As the blood feeds the brain, it is obvious that the brow centre has a vested interest in the activity of the sacral centre and will use all its influence to call upon the crown chakra in guiding integrity upon any union. The brow centre uses love to watch over its naive friend, for it knows that emotional development feeds the heart. However, amongst all the expansion, Jupiter's influence provides a clear direction. If we picture this scenario as a ship sailing across an ever-expanding sea, although the waves pound against its sides, it is being

Chapter 2 ~ The Sacral Centre

guided by the hand of Jupiter, a beautiful, peaceful, flowing path of pale blue light created by moonlight in the night sky; its course having already been plotted by the Moon through the stars. There is, thus, a link from the base up through all the chakras to the Moon, for this path is of Divine guidance or the divinity of starlight. This represents Jupiter's role within the collective of the seven chakras, the power of his lightening bolt gently supported by a healthy sacral centre.

The sacral centre's unlimited creative potential is channelled through the element of water, that mysterious transparent material upon which life is dependent and which is solid when frozen and vapour when heated. This is perhaps the reason why the element sits between the chakras of the base and the solar plexus. It is not surprising that the sacral centre controls all the fluid activity of the body, for the spiritual purpose here is to evolve unconscious thought through the depth of emotion in the watery realm. The primary purpose of this connection is to understand how we feel about ourselves in comparison to others. In this centre this manifests as service.

During the fall of Atlantis, and as an attempt to cleanse the self-centredness that humanity had come to represent, the land mass was pulled into the sea in a last ditch attempt at purification. Purification or blessing is always an attempt to once again serve the Divine, through how Self treats itself, and thus others. Our bodily fluids represent this quality and their clarity is an indication as to the emotions of the past, of the present and therefore what is to come. This is why the sacral chakra acts as a vessel in which true ideals and principles can be prophesised, inspired unconsciously by the emotions that pertain closest to the welfare of the group and supported by the preparation learnt at the base chakra. Water will always try to find its true level and with Jupiter as guide (the monarch of the planets who watches over this process with unquestionable authority) it will aim to fill the cup that was perhaps not quite so full in a previous incarnation or drain a little when overflowing in this lifetime. If you are sensitive enough, you may just perceive an old tidemark.

Ancient fluids connect us all, not only with each other but also to those that have come before. The whirlpool of life does not start with birth or end with death, for it acts as the vortex of direct connection from what was (Saturn), to what will be (Jupiter). We know it as the gene pool. It is the logic of the etheric world. Contained within all creation is its energetic equivalent, the design from which it was built. In the human body, this is passed on through the male sperm. The mother applies physical form to this etheric double, which through its flexibility incorporates the means to change its shape whilst expanding under the influences of Earthly life. The body's blueprint, the father's contribution, waits in the etheric sphere for the incoming soul to fill it with spirit. Much like a conductor in an orchestra, this blueprint is responsible for the precise physical interaction, so that the movement played out has all the right notes (atoms) in all the right places. This etheric double remains and will even replace the function of a minor organ or a limb if its physical counterpart has been lost. If there was sufficient energy to do so, as there once was during foetal development, or a time when humanity relied less on its physical constraints, then the missing tissue would even grow back. The etheric body remains connected to the physical body for a further three days after death, therefore care should be taken of the physical body before this process of separation has completed. Once released the pranic energy returns to the natural reserves of the planet Earth, from whence it came and so belongs.

The etheric equivalent of everything created here on Earth will also include thoughts and ideas. When a wavelength is measured in conventional science, a tiny percentage has to be subtracted from the finding that represents the energy of the intention of the person who is doing the measuring. Within quantum physics, this relates to the problem of predictability, for nothing can be observed in its true context if the very nature of observation changes the result. Even our thoughts contain energy and are already registered in the astral field to be manifested. Therefore if we direct energy into something, it will always be reflected back. This is because the karmic lesson here is to expand consciousness using all the gifts that have been made available to us. It is the energy of these intentions that enable one generation to lay down the gauntlet for the next. This shapes our evolution. It is where the collective unconscious acts directly on the influences of our everyday choices, creating understanding of the unconscious through the fluidity of water, the substance of life and the vehicle of our emotions. We cannot get to the brow centre without first having developed this earthly faculty, that of understanding our feelings. If the energy of the sacral centre is flowing well it will increase psychic insight for it allows one to float along the stream of consciousness and enter into the etheric world, that of abundant creativity.

Chapter 2 ~ The Sacral Centre

There is a strong relationship between the sacral chakra and the spleen. This is not unlike the relationship between the adrenals and the base chakra in so much as the spleen, being of a higher centre, feeds energy into the kidneys. This is pranic energy, which is siphoned from the sun, synthesised in the spleen and distributed by the kidneys. The spleen changes this male energy into female caring energy, through which vitality organises the physical body. Prana is transmitted through the etheric world. Prana and ether are in fact the same and said to be a reflection of a structure passed down by those doing similar work but on a higher level. Prana feeds the blueprint so that matter can attach itself to it. The spleen provides solar nourishment, a magnetic field, which determines the maintenance and therefore also the destruction of all matter. It is this energy field that charges the blueprint to which all physical bodies of the four kingdoms adhere, together with everything that pertains to them, which includes thoughts and ideas contained in a web of etheric storage in the brain.

Ether is the link between our senses and our emotions. This is why the quality of our emotions is so important in maintaining good health, for negativity pushes prana out of the body. We, as a culture, take holidays and recuperate from depletion by sunning the spleen and resting the nervous system. Prana holds and allows for the expression of atoms, whilst governing function, the environment and all circumstances pertaining to it. Any vitality that is not used by the body radiates outward in the form of auras that can be seen by some emanating from the body, the colours of which can be used to detect ill health. It is important that the field of aura should remain intact, for it is the shield that truly protects us from the world outside, so vitality is integral in maintaining this division. As well as poor health, many things can create holes in auras, such as the misuse of kundalini and the inability to close down and thus re-seal the aura after the practice of meditation. The resultant doorway lets the outside in, enabling things like entities to inhabit the being either by slipping in to the resultant gap or infiltrating one particular chakra or even all of them. This form of infiltration leads to problems associated with free will and conditions varying from dyslexia to schizophrenia. Remedies such as *Green, Blue, Purple, Berlin Wall, Syphilinum, Okoubaka, Medorrhinum, Rose Quartz, Sycamore Seed, Microwave, Peridot* and the combination of *Syphilinum Ayahuasca, Holly Berry* and *Moonstone*, will all encourage Self to restore its boundary. Here if you intuit this scenario with a patient, use the same intuition to discern the appropriate remedy or selection of remedies, for there are many more that can help and so many more to choose from. If this cannot be achieved with remedies an exorcism will be required.

DNA AND GROWTH

DNA is a rainbow from one life into another. It is a rotating field of light, the shadow of which is the rigid, two-dimensional image of the marked strands, used to record it. It is not solid but vibrating. It pertains to Jacobs' Ladder and the pillar of Osiris (the pillar of God). It is known in the bible as Merkaba, the light of the body or precisely the infusion of light, spirit and the body, which then surrounds Self in the form of rotating fields of light and is used by those to resonate with the rest of the universe. The greater the integration of all the subtle bodies, then the more brightly this light will shine, making access to astral travel easier through the portal in the top of the head. Merkaba also assists the kundalini by helping to balance all the chakras, allowing greater movement of energy throughout the body and helping to open blocks and cleanse chakra portals. There is then an unarguable link between DNA and the processes being conducted on the higher realms, leading to questions as to exactly how much of an individual indication it is.

The light known as DNA penetrates every cell so that its information can be passed on in the process of growth, which never stops. The production of hormones stimulate growth by reaching an individual cell's specific receptor, which responds only to a set hormone. With the addition of phosphates, this instigates a chemical reaction from which with the guidance of light (information), utilises building proteins to establish a DNA replica. It is the genes that produce proteins, the information (light) of which is passed on by the parents from the ancestral bloodline. These proteins determine what the cell will look like, what its role will be and how it will be arranged; in short the appearance of Self, even down to the colour of the eyes.

DNA has twenty-two strands of paired chromosomes and twenty-two amino acids, which help build the proteins. The Hebrew alphabet has twenty-two letters in which it is said contain all the answers to the universe. DNA is therefore a record of reality within Self. It is the seed or the centre of the higher triad. Its point of creation reaches back far beyond the separation of the Self, to the place of reality which is the

Chapter 2 ~ The Sacral Centre

first expression of spirit in the universe. This is our genesis, the record of spirit's progression within the subtle bodies and the reflection of its free will and the free will of its group. This reality, which is DNA, enters this world via the Incarnating Ego and is rewritten during the pursuit of consciousness, which is not reality but a reflective process of humanity's evolution through which to clear Earthly karma. It has already been proved that genes can be altered through words and different sounds alone. This is of course intention. The consequence of these changes will also be laid down in the personality. When one incarnates, this new combination that is created, when added to the genes of the parents, contains the conclusion of all of Self's previous lifetimes in form and in spirit up to this point. This will be alongside that of the bloodline that is deemed ancestry and is the only means by which it can do this journey. It is unlikely that this life will be an end to it. This signature of existence is that which an iridologist or palmist uses to read, for it is reflected in form, being part of the whole. This record cannot simply be cut away or removed on the physical level by the use of gene manipulation or therapy, for within is contained the genesis of Self. Much more has to change to correct a faulty gene, which homoeopathy, being a vibrational medicine, is said to be able to achieve. The two parallel strands of DNA are the duality of light and dark and only in the light of the Merkaba can the dark be cleared. Many of the new remedies have the power to instigate this process but it will be light that will ultimately alter it.

The twenty-two pairing chromosomes are able to intersperse genes through the generations, mixing in the pursuit of harmony, during a natural quest for balance. These pairings of chromosomes are exactly that, the same on either side of each strand. The twenty-third chromosome of the male is a mismatch of X and Y. In the female, they are both X so form an equal pair. The Y chromosome remains very similar if there is a long line of male descendants from fathers to sons. Historically, this has always determined a strong desire for succession, for the Y chromosome can only be passed down the male bloodline. Unlike the autosomes, the term given to the other twenty-two sets of chromosomes, they do not exchange as frequently throughout the generations, hence the Y swaps only a small amount of DNA with its X pairing, rejecting the advancements of X infiltrating its central core by only trading a few of its outer genes. By its very nature of being male energy, any further seepage is deemed to be a relinquishment of domination. These genes that have attempted to join, fall to the wayside, incapable of any lasting effect. Therefore the X and the Y chromosomes swap very little information between each other and so the Y chromosome in the male will be almost the same as that which is in his sperm. Thus the son will inherit an almost exact chromosomal replica that will be passed on to his son if he has one. Ancestry can be linked using these similarities. This link provides a further comparison when investigating disease patterns through the male bloodline, which of course are the repetition of ancestral karmic patterns.

If the comparison between the structure of DNA and the Hebrew alphabet is not to remain a coincidence, then the reason why the sex chromosomes have been emitted from the count has to be understood. This has much to do with division. To divide is to separate that which has been complete. We know that the sex chromosomes are not an equal match and therefore there is something at odds with them. Civilisation could never have left the Garden of Eden without having such a subdivision of Self. Because of this, the Y aspect is considered an extension or evolution from a non-sex chromosome, which has been necessary for the physical exploration of humanity. It is, in fact, a question of ownership and that which would eventually be played out in Atlantis. It is the male aspect, once having been only internalised, but is now on the outside, in need of the reconciliation of physical form. The Y chromosome is an exact copy of the X but due to the creative forces at play in the expression of material nature, it underwent changes in order to evoke the true meaning of the notion opposite.

Hence from having the balance of both male and female within, humanity extended this mould in order to adapt to its new environment, as its presence became more physical. The sex chromosomes are the resultant structural record. They denote the physical manifestation of the two halves, male and female. The creative force behind this change is the X or the female. This explains why the female goddess, or world mother, or to the Hindus, the origin of all matter – the goddess Kali/Shakti/Parvati – and so on, have been the centre of worship for at least the length of this current root-race. The origin of all life is female.

Put more directly, there is only female, for in reality there is no male; it is a bluff. In the grand cycle, humanity has already begun its evolutionary return back towards its source. This will reveal the truth around the illusion of the male being something separate, which the male ego will have to come to accept. So in the light of this, there are only twenty-two pairs of chromosomes and one mimicking pair, for although they can be recorded and thus detected in the physical world, the physical is simply an illusory reflection of the higher planes. This is the same as the means by which Self gathers its consciousness. The twenty-third pairing chromosomes are the way in which humanity can sustain this illusion and be here, a reflection and not reality. Much of this relationship will be revealed when the cycad plants are eventually given a sufficient proving, and surely reveal secrets of a time when female energy was self-productive and thus hopefully have a profound effect on healing the genome. Even though individuality has subsequently moved on under the influence of greater information or focused light, links that hinder this perpetuation still need to be solved but will be provided for. What is required always readdresses the illusion and in doing so brings genes up to date.

SEX

The awareness of Self's gender is a primary force undertaken during the development of the sacral centre, which is also explored long before the awakening of the sex glands by both the male and the female in preparation for puberty. These glands are the only endocrine glands that do not operate immediately from birth for obvious reasons of development, and are held back by the function of the pineal gland under the guidance of the Moon in relation to Jupiter. Jupiter and the Moon are the two watery planets, and Jupiter re-enters the astrological chart every twelve years, the first time of which signals the start of puberty. In partnership with the light of this watery realm, the reproductive cycle is regulated, the Moon being that which governs the tides. This is the cycle that places practicality on Jupiter's lustful ways. Historically, cultures have paid great credence to the number twelve. To some, three times four was a way of balancing the odd with the even, or the yin with the yang. It is the same for puberty, Jupiter balancing the male and the female through intimacy.

At puberty, the child begins to feel more equal within the group, allowing more deeper interaction as she wrestles with the morality of her new feelings. As to how this is expressed while the personality expands depends more or less on a combination of the child's karma, miasmatic inheritance through the bloodline and the responsibility of the group to integrate these changes through the heart. This need to connect, interact and be shaped by her race, within the group's morality, ethics, protocol, customs and etiquette, is for the benefit of the whole group. The child's wish is to be a part of this love, without which the isolating effect is felt like cold water. If the child does not express these qualities then there is a problem. This sacral energy is expanding and collaborative. It should be directed, but if inhibited will lead to intimacy problems in the future. This is energy that requires expression, as already mentioned. This force fuels the entire creative being. The sacral centre is the powerhouse and so is the link into the energy provided for the will of Self, that of the solar plexus chakra directly above it. When this energy is halted, then it will back up and over stimulate the sexual function. The internalisation of excessive sexual energy fuelled by miasmatic inheritance in this centre can lead to sexual perversity. A similar expression can happen to a person if they raise kundalini into this centre too quickly or inappropriately. No manner of sexual activity will suffice the hunger of this centre when it is excessively powered up.

The sacral chakra contains much karmic activity and potentially, for women, is the centre that receives and retains the consequence of a great deal of abuse. Let me explain this. In previous incarnations Self has either been male or female. If healing is performed on this centre and if Self is presently female, then inhibited creative energy formed over many lifetimes will manifest as deep emotional blocks. The reason being that this is the centre of creativity, which is feminine. The emotional connection and the opportunity to cleanse it is not the same for the male. Work here often means to awaken deep karmic blocks, which can lead to much emotional instability. For women, the clearing of these energies can lead to the freeing of some of the hardest forces by which to manage, for they relate to celibacy, miscarriage, abortions, sex for the sake of sex, undesired sex, sex for survival or money and even rape. These energies bring about the deepest of remorse and despair as they rise to the surface in order to heal. There may also be the grief from a hindered desire to give birth stored in this centre. This could be due to a loveless marriage or many other reasons. Of course one does not have to have children, however this is not the point: the resultant block will manifest only when the desire to do so is prevented. It is the qualities of female energy that produces new life through maternal love and that on a higher level produces universal creativity. If this centre is closed, the full extent of this fails to happen.

Chapter 2 ~ The Sacral Centre

Male energy as the partner has historically often played a part in preventing these blocks from healing, but this seems to be changing as the balance of power shifts much more towards the female. In recognising this need to heal, especially from this centre, the feminine energy is still the driving force, which explains why the majority of people that frequent homœopathic clinics are women. This too is slowly changing. The sensitivity of the genders is slowly amalgamating, as it should. This centre, when charged with much negative karma, is physically revealed in the symptoms of the menstrual cycle, such as dysmenorrhoea, amenorrhoea, polyps, cysts, fibroids and abnormal cells. It should also be recognised that the menstrual cycle clears the negative karma of both male and female in a partnership. For a female, meditation on this centre will do the same.

Negative karma in this centre obviously has miasmatic consequences and it is here that the majority of this is passed on. When one has sex, all the sexual karma of all the previous sexual partners on both sides is exchanged. In the past, as it still is today, groups like the African San People used plant medicine for the means of purification with the same premise as we use homœopathy. The tribe was aware as to how disease could be passed on in this way, so they were very strict about sexual activity, especially so for the young who were the means of survival for the tribe, for it will be the quality of their blood that nourishes the growing foetus for nine months. If the sexual partners did change, then the karma of the previous sexual partner was cleared using plants and rituals. As time moved on and religion replaced tribal wisdom, this protection was replaced by guilt, which only further repressed the beauty of the function of this centre. It was and still is considered by some, that chastity raises spiritual enlightenment. The sacral chakra however is not a centre to be suppressed in its natural expression, for this can lead to perversion and even insanity. Further to this, if one is sensible, little sexual karma is passed on and concern about this should not prevent the making of relationships, for love will clear any obstacle in its path.

Through the heart, sexual expression enlightens the soul and to deny it, is to deny love. Only a few have reached a very high level of enlightenment where the physical pleasures of the body become superfluous. For the rest of us mere mortals, sex can be a profound expression of love and the means by which to pass on aspiration by having children. Loveless sex however closes down the heart centre. What a waste! It ignores the wondrous polarity of the male and female coming together to form the one, the reconnection to the Divine by way of the Kundalini. Through the limitations of our physicality we express the deep love felt for another. Love should take time to grow as two people explore the possibilities of a lasting union: sex is the result of the celebration of that union and not the thing to start it. If it is the starting point, then any long-term relationship runs the risk of being maintained by having little in common other than the sex connecting it.

This centre is a vehicle for physical beauty, which naturally plays on our emotions, for physical attraction fuels desire both in love and in sex. Beauty entices us, drawing us in through desire and the promise of the pleasure of physical touch. We once connected without the division of the skin. But now it is through the skin that our beauty often radiates. Touch is registered at the higher octave of this chakra, the brow, in the frontal lobes, of which our fingertips are an extension. The physical expression of love is very important and it is raised in the brow, differentiating it from the level of animal instinct. If it were to remain purely a function of the sacral centre, animal instinct is all it would be. There is a temptation here to be taken over by animal desires, and karmic blocks in this chakra will be reflected in the person's sexual behaviour. The remedy *Thuja* will often reveal and clear such blocks. Indeed, the history of sexual guilt is a major factor in the picture of *Thuja*.

Society, families and the group use the energy of the sacral centre to maintain much control over a person. While I was at College, a young woman patient came to see me and told me she had been sharing a flat belonging to her family with the sister of her brother-in-law. The patient and the in-law had fallen out, resulting in the other girl moving out. Then her sister's marriage broke up and the blame for this was put on my patient, as the problems in the flat had caused much argument between the two families. Her now separated sister had nowhere else to go, so came to live with my patient in the flat. The patient was being repeatedly reminded of this blame by her sister and by her mother. She was very close to her mother and it was making her life intolerable. She cried constantly throughout the consultation, so I gave her *Thuja*.

The patient returned a month later unable to explain why everything had changed. They were all getting on famously, having fun and laughing as if nothing had happened, as if, she said, they had also been given a remedy. *Thuja* had released the ancestral guilt locked away in her

Chapter 2 ~ The Sacral Centre

past that was making her a victim. The block was in her sacral chakra but the shame was preventing her from exerting her will (solar plexus). Once this block had cleared the family was forced to look elsewhere for blame, and hopefully to themselves at last for answers. The patient's creativity could now express itself. A further development was concerning her childhood sweetheart, who was still living in the West Indies, where my patient had grown up, and even though she had been having relationships here in the UK, she always felt he was the one. The family had been strictly against her moving back, but at last ignoring their wishes, she did. I received a postcard about six months later thanking me and saying all was going well in the relationship. I was so grateful for this case at the time, for it took me away from the academia of college homœopathy and gave me an insight into the real beauty of what homœopathy can heal.

It could be said that the flowering of guilt through this centre was inevitable as its seeds were sown during the development of the two sexes. When the female reproductive organs evolved to accommodate the act of copulation, a sheath was formed which remains intact during virginity. This is only found in the human female and not in any other animal. Its tearing may be seen as a reminder from divine spirit as to the sanctification of true love and a painful reminder of its separation. It may also, however, act as a cosmic web, formed at this portal to protect the inside, the energy of divine mother's creative potential, Shakti, from the corruption of outside forces. It is, in effect, a sheath of pure selection and as it is only broken once, evokes the meaning of the correct decision or true connection, which has emotional consequence for females. This is for women to know instinctively and the male to learn. The heart and the head should work as one, so that the openness of the heart through sex can purify the mind. This also works the other way round, for the purity of thought should reflect through physical action. During the act of copulation, water is the element of purification, cleansing the sacral chakra before the genes are passed on to the next generation.

The two miasms that manifest as syphilis and gonorrhoea use the sacral centre to jump from one body to another and from one generation to the next. One is the yin to the other's yang, so both find the other highly attractive. They are both woken up and spread through sexual intercourse. Part of their insidious or manipulative behaviour is to evoke sexual attraction, often in the form of lust between a syphilitic dominated person and a sycotic one. This is how they evolve, it being their means of survival. Through bodily fluids they make their presence known physically, using the fact that the personality is vulnerable under the temptations of Jupiter. This presence then progresses throughout the body and because like attracts like, promiscuous people tend to attract one another, thus doubling the weight of miasmatic influence on all of the chakras. It is the nature of failings in the sacral centre that evolved miasmatic disease in the first place, this being precisely their favourite root of proliferation. The syphilitic and the sycotic miasms exploit the fact that the flesh grows weak under their activities, and for them this centre is the vehicle for perpetual life, for it produces offspring. The syphilitic miasm is particularly advanced in its ability to survive and is capable of disguising itself within any given ignoble characteristics in order to remain hidden. Part of this includes the impulse to be undetected, and even results in it masquerading as the sycotic miasm, for the sycotic miasm is only an extension of the syphilitic miasm. So for the practitioner it may look like a sycotic case, when it is in fact a syphilitic smoke screen – something to hide what is going on underneath, hence the lumps.

The syphilitic miasm corrupts the energy of the patient so that the disease process will know when you are on to it and act accordingly. This also means energetically that the activated miasm will be aware of the dose of the syphilitic nosode coming its way. Remember here, just as discovered in quantum physics, the boundaries of communication are different in the etheric world. Remedies may be needed to tease out the miasm-influenced behaviour of the patient before a dose of *Syphilinum* can be landed at its door. The best method for this is confusion. *Plutonium* is very effective at doing this, so a dose given before the *Syphilinum* will stall its ability to hide, providing time for the nosode to in fact do a deal with Self.

Because the syphilitic miasm renders the tissue to rot, it has devised, over many generations, a mutated form of disguised beauty, an illusion of health, designed to attract many potential mates. For the very flesh that it has weakened, is that in which it expects its survival to rest through reproduction. This of course, is reflected by the remedies used for such a circumstance, which glisten on the outside but are brittle in their centre, such as *Amethyst, Rose Quartz, Chalcancite* and *Rhodocrosite*.

Chapter 2 ~ The Sacral Centre

Historically, being in this condition means that many attempts would have been needed to succeed in a pregnancy and also many children if one of them is going to survive. The syphilitic miasm may well lay behind the case of a repeated miscarriage even if it initially looks sycotic in nature.

Sycosis is the miasm of sexual excess and is enticed by beauty in the knowledge that its desires will be fulfilled. It uses its innate magnetic powers, that of the snake charmer, to seduce its catch. This works on its opposite, the syphilitic miasm by inevitably making it feel better about itself. Bearing in mind that the syphilitic miasm represents the pain of separation, for this to happen the sycotic miasm is considered to be a manifestation of the syphilitic miasm designed to keep it company. This need for company is a natural phenomenon that arises from ancestry, so there are no surprises that the syphilitic miasm is attracted to it and innate throughout its character. Although an extension of the syphilitic miasm, the sycotic miasm does exist in its own right. This is a bit like how a single cell divides after being impregnated by the sperm containing the anomaly of the X and Y chromosome. The syphilitic form of seduction works through fear and the sycotic miasm will do anything not to feel scared. These are the dilemmas confronting Self in clearing negative ancestral inheritance. Contained inside ancestry is the great well of this irregularity, and within it the sycotic miasm proliferates, while the syphilitic miasm drinks.

Magnetism is of the most powerful physical energy in the universe and it is produced by the attraction of opposites. The sycotic miasm will suspend this fairy-tale fantasy that enables the syphilitic miasm to feel whole again just as long as it can revel in lust. When this is over it will start to panic. Its rampant, lustful desires lack integrity in its excessive pursuit of pleasure, the consequence of which fill the flesh with pus and mucus as the body finds no other outlet for this revengeful cocktail of toxins. Neither of these miasms produces pleasant bedtime reading. It is in the sacral chakra that we find the true home to the sycotic miasm which is only used by the syphilitic miasm, like an unwanted guest, as a means to an end. The sycotic miasm is misused Jupiter energy. It is the desire to gain but with no regard as to the consequence. Gluttony will inevitably bring down all the rest of the other chakras as reflected in the way the sycotic miasm attacks the heart.

GENDER AND GENERATION

The separation of Self, which developed out of the desire to be god within, was also motivated by pleasure. Self wanted control over pleasure instead of having to acknowledge it as part of Divine grace. Self had gained knowledge of the plants that bore fruit and now wanted to taste the fruit. Divine knowledge was no longer enough. Self wanted to pull the strings in order to partake directly in the richness of sensation. This was granted. Self was soon to discover that pleasure is rooted in creativity. Pleasure has to be nurtured and developed, before it can be put into practice, for it has consequence. Out of a single sexed, self-reproducing, egg laying being, came the desire to love another in the same way that had previously been felt with the Divine. The previously highly developed heart had changed to one in which the soul could remain private under the confinement of Self. The heart was no longer an open casket for communication and the soul pined for company. The being needed to pull this connection down into the physical world and so searched for its equivalent. The single division into Self was not enough, it needed an opposite in order to reflect and practice with love. Soul searched for and found harmony and balance. Self now belonged to a group within a group, within a group. This new group was gender, and the love for another brought more desires, one of which was its expression through sex. Sex fulfilled the ultimate feelings of pleasure reflected down on Earth that humans wanted, but it was the celebration of the creative force, Kundalini, that bore children. The creative consequence of this force in this centre is reproduction be it in any form, not simply from offspring.

Creativity is not possible without all four of the elements but it is water that is most closely connected to the Earth, for it nourishes the soil and makes it fertile. One's creativity always addresses the quality of the base chakra, for what is possible has to be rooted in its correct existence otherwise there is no nourishment in order for it to take form. Therefore, within the four elements, for one to express and develop one's purpose on Earth, the elements of earth and water must be interlinked. In order for this to happen their role has to be mastered by Self to create flow. If there is a propensity towards water, the proliferation of the sycotic miasm will result.

If water is the element most directly connected with the Earth, then air is the element that could be considered to be the bridge between fire

Chapter 2 ~ The Sacral Centre

and water, even though fire is traditionally placed between water and air in the evolution of the chakras. But fire pertains to both worlds for it is essentially only spiritual in its essence. Therefore air can be seen as the link between the earth/water balance and fire, be it cosmic fire or any other form. If we extend this insight to the nature of the syphilitic miasm and how it connects to the higher realms through the ether, it reveals that it does not simply pertain to the element of fire but also the resolution to our separation. Until unification, there is a balancing to all things. The relationship between the sycotic miasm and the syphilitic miasm, fire and water, produces steam in the physical realm, which is carried by air. The balancing of the four elements can be interpreted, metaphorically, as the revealing of the first four seals. The four horses are ridden on the road to one's own resurrection: this is what is meant by the apocalypse.

The sacral centre is the coming together of the male and female through their differences. The sex of the child is determined at conception and from then on the hormones secreted from the gonads (ovary or testes) determine our nature and our outlook, be it positive or negative. When the child evolves into the energy of this centre around the age of seven, the first true understanding of one's gender and the effect it has on the other gender is explored. Puberty states categorically, "I am of this sex" and brings with it an awareness the child has not faced consciously before. This energy needs spiritual guidance and for this reason puberty can be seen as an initiation. Becoming sexually active is the potential to manifest power here on Earth. When this power or creativity is not used for sexual gratification, it can be utilised for spiritual growth, it being a physical link to divine power. In a loving relationship the creative opportunity of intimacy allows much of the pain of the past to heal in both partners. Both have aspects of male and female within, enabling them to bond, to join, to immerse, and to grow. Growth is never that simple and the resultant friction it produces energises the life of the relationship. When there is no friction left then there is not usually any relationship left. The discharge, which is the result of the female monthly cycle, is the vehicle for cleansing much of this friction. This is the discharge of the couple, for the male as well as the female. This lends further weight to the dangers of the contraceptive pill, for it suppresses this clearance. The elimination of these bodies is so important in combating disease, that in many cultures it is thought to be dangerous to have intercourse during the time of menstruation, as energy that should be eliminated is retained. In older cultures, this has been open to manipulation, extending to menstrual blood being put in food to act as a poison on every level. Conversely, as is in the nature of balance, it is also used in medicine as a form of cure. It will be the etheric webbing of the discharge that holds the result of the eliminated energy and those who understand its significance have exploited these properties.

The role of karma regarding the attraction of one to another is great. We attract another by means of an understanding that one will support the other. This is a fusion, which again lies in aspiration, in a sense one bloodline intertwining itself in another to create something better. However, relationships that are formed due to the memory of their marriage in a previous incarnation can be very difficult, because invariably when the two fall in love once again, the previous work had not been resolved. These relationships have an air of being stuck in destiny whilst the preceding karma has to be unravelled first. Eventually, if this is achieved, there may be little left to the purpose of the relationship. Part of the healing process in a partnership can be to have children as this can clear much in the thymus gland and change ancestral habits. Many children are born in order to change ancestral karma. The connection to all these factors has a bearing on one's ability to attract the right person or amalgamate through a blood opportunity. Abuse of the sacral centre weakens this ability. Miasmatically speaking, it is not better to sow the wild oats first. It is far better to assess the level of consciousness in a prospective partner long before sex has a role to play, for it is not appearance that is of importance to your ultimate wellbeing but the inner quality that radiates. If the relationship is right, it grows on a level that feeds its way down to the etheric, stirring the emotions and irradiating the aura. This radiation connects to the other, transferring itself from each partner and creating an aura of the relationship. This auric connection deepens as their actions together grow. Inertia will be the thing that breaks it – one or both partners not wanting to change or the purpose of the relationship coming to an end. This aura can expand over thousand of miles so that the two can still be in communication, such is the desire for Self to share with another.

The coming together of one gender with another brings with it the potential of much change and much healing. However, the knowledge

Chapter 2 ~ The Sacral Centre

of miasmatic behaviour and its relationship to disease has been known for some time, leaving it open to abuse. As part of the slave trade during the last millennium, African virgins were brought to the West because they carried the malaria parasite, although due to reasons of immunity showed no signs of illness. Men who were suffering from latent syphilis, it having progressed to its third stage, subsequently acquired these women. By having sex with them they transferred the syphilis by swapping it with the malaria, having already made sure that there was a bottle of quinine close at hand. The malaria could thus be treated whilst the female slave was condemned to a slow and painful death. The behaviour of miasmatic disease is far easier to understand on its physical level. On the etheric level it becomes that of the invisible obstacles to Self's progression in the world.

The negative side of the sacral centre arrives in the form of temptation. This centre has much to offer, for it is the driving force of potential. We have a simple choice; to use it for spiritual or personal gain, that of fame and fortune. Expansion is a very seductive force. It suggests that all is possible, but if the understanding of duality has been properly adhered to, then awareness of the karmic consequences of giving in to temptation is the safety barrier in this centre. The two opposing genders often balance out excess in each other as one contracts while the other expands, which is also reflected in how the base and sacral centre have come to work hand in hand. Saturn restricts, contracts and crystallises, whereas Jupiter is fluid, watery and expansive. To move forward is to exert the balance of the two. They should in effect be working as one, which might be perceived as more prevalent in the male, for it could be said that in men these centres combine more thoroughly and in women they remain more separate; their creative sphere is much more focussed on creating and having the means to rear children.

However, this is changing and the responsibilities are not only evolving from one generation to the next, but are part of a process which will eventually see men relinquishing the power and women working much more with Mars energy through Jupiter. Reincarnation also redresses this balance, for the ability to master a gender comes with practice and understanding and requires having struggled with the opposite gender. Male and female is a push and pull, a battleground in progression. Gender enables Self to wrestle with these balances of energies that are polarised within the division of the male and female. This is pursued during past lives and also played out constantly within the ancestral pool as is the nature of the differing qualities of these energies. In order to achieve balance the amalgamation requires the struggle of opposites which goes on simultaneously to Self's present incarnation. This means that the male and the female ancestry are quite often at odds as to their influence within Self's actions and this energetic struggle is part of what Self also has to work through. Their opposing stances generate, in part, Self's development. They result in the balance of the forces of nature that help Self evolve.

The ability of humans to survive as a species has depended on entering the world from a womb, being able to use her own womb if female, and fertilise it if male, all in twelve short years of development. This rapid development has been exploited in times of disease outbreak, or when the tribe required rapid growth. In the West there are strict age limits that allow sexual contact only after the solar plexus chakra has been sufficiently explored in order that Self is deemed to be in command of its own decision-making. Western society does, however, encourage its children to operate from the sacral centre in other ways, for reasons say of economics, without any guidance for spiritual growth. This only encourages the negative side of Jupiter, that of desire for personal gain. Advertising agencies exploit this by constantly bombarding children with images designed specifically with them in mind, the information of which is to awaken the consumer within rather than the creator.

During the Second World War many young soldiers moved through Europe and with them the spread of gonorrhoea, which reflected the greed that had instigated the war in the first place. Each war has its own motivation and subsequent disease. The stirrings of the sycotic miasm coincided with and was necessary in the establishment of the beginning of the hippy movement during the early nineteen sixties, the polarised opposite and thus balance to this greed. To be a hippy meant that one had something to lose, to give up and not have the financial means to support oneself. The process of dropping out was in order that things could truly be explored in a different way. Those who had nothing to lose then filled the hole that subsequently opened up and they masqueraded as hippies. It was they who exploited the use of drugs in order to imitate the dislocation from the constraints of the planet that was

Chapter 2 ~ The Sacral Centre

being undertaken naturally by the true hippies as part of the exploration, although some also explored the use of hallucinogens. The problem with using drugs is that they never enable the user to integrate the actions required to create change – they not reconnecting to the planet, their base chakra, in order to follow through with the consequence. In other words all they manifest is delusion. Those who survivied the loss and learnt from the experience were plucked by others, either born before the movement or already advanced out of it, and placed back into prominent areas of society in order to further the important lessons. This was to take humanity into the next realm of its development, a greater integration between East and West, creating a new way of seeing that is continuing today as the Age of Aquarius beckons.

There are always two sides to each miasm. After the Second World War and during the following decades the function of the sacral centre rose to great prominence in the cultures that had been involved with this war, providing the impetus for the era of "sex, drugs and rock and roll". The restless, adrenal driven beats of rock music resulted from the effects of the sycotic miasm on the nervous system. The young generation were becoming pumped up, which could be seen in their clothes, lifestyles and attitudes. The positive side to this pumped up sacral centre was a creative outpouring, a reaction to the misery of the war. The disaffected American teenager of the nineteen-fifties movies was just the beginning. During the sixties, under the influence of Uranus in Virgo, this expansion developed into rule breaking. Conventional structures had to change and the method for this was to 'drop out' in order to explore the new. After years of social repression, relationships also became part of this exploration, hence the sexual exploration and baby boom of the sixties. As a young generation struggled with new ideas, the excitement of the times also exaggerated the desire for a mate and for 'mating'. Image became emphasised, that which was popular or "cool". The terms 'pop' and 'cool' took on a new status represented by the pop idol, a new teenage phenomenon of the times. These idols had projected onto them the feelings and desires of a new generation, which for the first time had the power, the lightening bolt of Jupiter to hand and pointed at the impotence of the older generations. This was a karmic outbreak from the kind of aspiration that had led previous generations to war and the positive side to the proliferation of a miasm. Of course this became lost in image, which in order to maintain its material myth, constantly expanded. Idols had to be replaced by those who, for that brief period of time, reflected the new ideas before they in turn became associated with the older generation. In effect, each subsequent generation was able to materialise in the form of a number of individuals, its own aspiration.

The rejection of parental values also brought about an increase in the subsequent divorce rate. The nineteen-seventies found one-parent families becoming the norm, as was a diet of American-influenced television. During the eighties self-centred ethics encapsulated in the phrase 'make hay while the sun shines' burgeoned on both sides of the Atlantic. This finally crashed when Saturn tested it beyond its limits and its message went out to all. British society has been nervously plodding on with this lesson ever since and America has entered a phase of extreme neo-conservatism. As a result, British society has had to keep a watchful yet mistrustful eye on Europe whilst it attempts to unite, for here lies the dilemma. If America is an amalgamated system of European and British social freedoms, which have blatantly failed, then what system is going to be adopted by an amalgamated Europe that is going to work? It will have to be one in which Europe has to fit into Britain, with Britain being more advanced as Britain is esoteric to the European exoteric. These too are the dilemmas of the sacral chakra.

THE KIDNEYS

The kidneys are responsible for the filtration and therefore the concentration of the blood. They regulate all the elements and transport any excesses away from the body, collecting them during filtration within purified water known as urine. This function is governed by response to the secretion of the hormone ADH from the pituitary gland, which maintains a healthy balance of bodily fluid volume. Within the sphere of the kidneys the sodium balance controls the pressure of the blood and the mineral composite and cell PH are regulated, all of which are very important to life. The kidneys also synthesise and maintain the material that constitutes the reproductive fluids, the etheric connection between ancestral blood, purified water and the potential for new life.

Nutrient filled blood passes through the liver where the toxins are removed, ready to be secreted as solid waste. The kidneys then filter the clean blood, for their function governs fluidity and not waste. According to Traditional Chinese Medicine, the kidneys store the essence of life

Chapter 2 ~ The Sacral Centre

– Jing. This power is required for growth, maintenance and emotional development and is unique to every individual as it is bestowed at the point of conception by the parents. It is the expansive force of Jupiter, which is the reason why this planet is known as the "Generator".

The closest we have come to measuring this essence is through DNA. This essence maintains the fluid levels in the body and nourishes the bone marrow and the brain cells. It is passed on in the newly electrolysed blood from the kidneys, having also been mixed with pranic energy arriving from the spleen. The kidneys (service) are the mother to the son, the liver (will) and relate to the physical quality of one's memory at the Brow centre. Many liver and gallbladder problems can be traced back to pathology of the kidneys, not supplying what is required from the essence of life. An under functioning liver overburdens the kidneys with toxins and the cycle continues. The quality of life essence is also depleted in the kidneys through ancestral karma and therefore through miasmic activity. The kidneys are paired in order that they may find a balance. They are the marriage, the harmony of the possibility of the past to that which is possible now.

The Seventh Commandment – thou shalt not commit adultery – offers much more wisdom to this relationship between the function of the kidneys and Self's desire to change, than simply guidance on sexual activity. It truly refers to the working through of the darkness within. It is by means of the bloodline that we are offered the chance to follow in our father's footsteps, but not to copy his mistakes. The 'essence of life', the energy of sustaining existence, is the power to unify, to make whole. On the seventh day of creation, God rested. The Seventh Commandment refers to this complete manifestation and how this can be destroyed through karmic energies exchanged not just during intercourse but also through thoughts, emotions and ideas, which inevitably take on form and result in actions. The ancestors are the first link into the spiritual world and what is being asked here is to raise the stakes for the benefit of all. Completeness is the creative desire that, at this centre, connects the higher self through the heart and the crown. This desire and subsequent rest on the seventh day is the reason why it is possible for a child to be born prematurely and yet still survive unaided by high-tech intervention only after the seventh month of pregnancy. This is Libran time where the soul has sufficiently infused with the body, enabling it to access all of its functions and most importantly, the life supply contained in the kidneys.

Chakra Prescribing and Homœopathy

The seventh sign of the zodiac is Libra, which rules the kidneys. One kidney in the body is slightly higher than the other, an illustration of the Libran necessity for discrimination. Its scales are finely balanced between light and dark forces, maintaining equilibrium in the pursuit of balance and harmony. These scales play judge to ancestral karma, indicating whether an action will contribute towards or deplete kidney energy – the essence of life. They are supported by a chain of love that pivots from the heart chakra and balanced through the justice of the solar plexus chakra. This kidney energy represents the joy of uncharted potential that motivates Self to explore the higher centres. The marriage referred to in the seventh commandment is the commitment to the harmony of the seven churches, the seven chakras, balanced by Libra through the life energy of the kidneys. To ignore the prime purpose of this centre, that of service, inhibits the desire for unification, and is represented as adultery. The true beauty here is seen when Self relates to another with concern and consideration.

The kidneys are not contained by any fibrous ligaments but are held in place by the energetic presence of the organs around them. They are very sensitive to any change in these pressures and behave like emotional receptors, feeding the brow centre with the unconscious impulses of these feelings. When spirit fuses with the physical body, it unifies the communication between all by means of etheric threads that attach one organ to another. Energy is fed to each organ by the blood and is further distributed by means of these threads to maintain an even balance. Generally the kidneys will support any depletion, especially in the liver and spleen. As well as receiving impulses from other organs, the kidneys hold the cellular memories of childhood emotional trauma, which will inhibit energy flow. They act like two batteries in which the energy required by the constitution is stored and therefore a lack of Jing will produce poor physical growth. Being so sensitive to shock, the stability of the emotional development during the second seven years is important to their strength and subsequent vitality of the body. This is also dependent on ancestral inheritance: one's ancestors can hold back the progression of Self, if they in turn feel threatened, which then leads to over sensitivity to change. This congests the kidneys, including the formation of stones, which are the calcification of fear.

From such an ancestral background, fear of change will be innate and for this reason fear forms the conditioning that Self relies on in order

Chapter 2 ~ The Sacral Centre

to stay exactly where it is. So it is Self that is scared to change. Self's fear here is not just that it cannot cope with the pain of its conditioning but that further change represents the probability of more pain. Homœopathy's task is to show this is not so. Physiologically, the kidneys create more space as the ancestral hold is loosened, increasing vitality that brings about growth. Congestion stagnates the free flow of energy, hindering the power of Self and its creative potential, all because of this innate ancestral fear of change. Such stuck energy in the kidneys can even lead to death as the body shuts down when the lights either slowly or suddenly go out. When the practitioner perceives such stuck ancestral energy, kidney support remedies will be required. The kidneys are the containers of fear, most of which will be from the past. Jing will also be depleted through excessive or improper sexual activity, the symptoms of which lead to impotency and excessive urination.

Shame weakens the kidneys. Anything that puts Self at odds with the moral conduct of the group, including the ancestors, will undermine the sacral centre through guilt. This is an emotion in which Self can drown. It's a river that runs back through the ancestry and surfaces as pools of negativity when Self least expects it, often being completely unaware of its origin. Through change Self can prevent itself from becoming an ancestral scapegoat. Water of the kidneys is said to be Yin and because it is distributed throughout the body, it relies on its quality. Yin is also depleted through excessive sexual habits or poor kidney function. Poor kidney Yin leads to the deterioration of vision, dizziness, tinnitus and sweating during sleep. Water of the bladder is said to be Yang and a deficiency of kidney yang results in the depletion in the fire of spirit, leading to susceptibility from the cold. If Prana energy, the vital energy that circulates around the body feeding each organ, is low in the kidneys it will cause hearing problems and a shortness of energy.

The kidneys are highly sensitive to the emotions, the etheric currents that act on the nerve centres of the body. Any kind of shock will affect their function and can lead to problems with the circulatory system, bladder and the flexibility of joints. HRT also inhibits flow, the natural need of the wisdom of the matriarch within the group. The spiritual lesson of the sacral centre is service – for the benefit of the group, and kidney problems are often the emotional response to the hindrance of this desire to serve, which is of paramount importance within the bloodline. As such, the loss through adoption will also be felt in the kidneys by both parent and child. Blood transfusions however, do not break the family bond in the same way, as its link will still remain within the etheric double, regardless of what happens to the blood. However, transfusions will mix the karma of the two tribes, which may lead to much confusion and hence the need for *Carcinosin*. This can of course work both ways. I once had a patient who in her late twenties presented with symptoms of having had meningitis. She had been given a blood transfusion at birth. Within the first month of a repeated dose of *Carcinosin* she changed her job, partner and put her house on the market. She may well have stopped acting upon the karma of the transfused blood, replacing it at last with that of her own desires. On the other hand however, she might have had the blood transfusion to enable her to get the *Carcinosin*. Without ancestral clarity, the fluidity of the emotions stagnate, producing silt, which then hardens through crystallisation, just like the rocks of the Earth. Therefore, mineral remedies and those of precious stones, like *Sapphire*, will be needed to readdress the flow. Of course, as grit is the product of the kidneys, all the sea remedies should be looked at, along with *Buddelia*, *Nettle* and *Silver Birch*. It is the emotional body that produces the greater troubles in the lower nature of the human kingdom.

The kidneys are where group energy is held. This is ancestral karma. However, some individual karma may also find itself stored here if it pertains strongly to the group. We can understand this by picturing the kidneys as two large houses crammed with relatives, although a more accurate representation links them with fluidity. The kidneys have a constant exchange of fluids running in and out of them. This tide is like the embryonic fluid passed from one mother to the next. Each new generation has been baptised by this magical blessing. Water is imperative to life; this clear blood cleanses, purifies and filters the information that has manifested through the sweat and toil of many hands. This sap of information sustains life and life gravitates to it. The flow of fluid is the emotional vehicle of loved ones and, through their genes, they pass on to their offspring that which has been shaped by the evolution of the race. It represents the love and compassion that has been invested in the individual and with it comes the gift of life, the opportunity. Deep water represents the depth of emotion created through high stakes and aspirations. Water is of course very powerful, for it can wear away the

Chapter 2 ~ The Sacral Centre

earth. Deep emotions have a profound effect on the purification of the karma of the individual. This happens through reproduction, for it is deemed right to provide the opportunity to integrate with one's own tribe through love. The universe is not one for waste. Kidney function is under the influence of the habits of the race that have preceded and attracted Self. Remember each chakra has its own individual way of working on the physical, emotional and spiritual levels. Therefore, the "fitting" to a group, the responsibility of the sacral centre, will not only give a sense of belonging to one's past but will also present the opportunity to transform the world with the individual's vision.

Each person has the potential to make a difference. The connection to the bloodline is chosen by the soul. It is the duty of the ancestral line to maintain a healthy soil so that the seed planted will grow for the benefit of future generations and with the avoidance of disease. Negative thoughts, sexual partners or suppressions, be they either of the truth or a disease state maintained by allopathic drugging, will all influence not only the body that the incoming soul inherits but also the climate and the atmosphere. This terrain will either help or hinder the level of difficulty faced in maintaining the direction in which spirit believes things should go. How many people as they get older find themselves acting out the patterns of their parents, even after rebelling against them, due to an inner fear that things are not going to change? Much work has to be done on the kidneys to clear the shackles of ancestral habits, which contribute to what homœopaths often call 'maintaining causes'. Mother Earth provides water, not only to sustain but also to cleanse and purify ancestral karma. The act of drinking water blesses the kidneys with this magic and so each day lived lightens the ancestral load.

THE ADRENALS

The kidneys also function as endocrine glands, secreting hormones to regulate the loss of urine and also to regulate the flow of blood to the adrenal glands. Even in normal function this is a vast blood supply in relation to the size of each gland but it is increased significantly more when the adrenals demand action. Each adrenal gland sits on top of a kidney, with each gland being made up of two parts; an inner medulla, which is not essential to life but synthesises amine hormones, the main being adrenaline; and an outer cortex that secretes steroid hormones, mainly interrenalin, upon which life is dependant. Interrenalin is responsible for the healthy growth of brain cells, maintaining concentration and vigour. Again the function of the sacral centre is reflected in its opposite chakra, the brow. Insufficient cortex function means poor development of the brain and voluntary nervous system, to which it is also closely associated.

Adrenaline is held in great quantities of reserve in the endocrine glands, ready for use if required. Its secretion is markedly increased through fear, rage and excitement, causing vasoconstriction of the blood vessels so that the heart, brain and muscles may benefit from the increased flow of blood (energy). This reaction is instinctual as part of the "fight or flight" mechanism of the sympathetic nervous system. However, problems arise if the adrenal glands are stimulated more frequently than the one-off emergency for which they are designed. This is the result of poor base function or an over excessive sacral centre, including an indulgence in negative thoughts. There is a two-way relationship between the liver and spleen – the sacral centre supports them both, so their function of regulating anger means that anger will also stimulate adrenal secretion. In the case of these false 'fight or flight' alarms, the body has no outlet in which to utilise the subsequent boost of energy created by an increase of glucose from the liver, which is added to an already enriched supply of red blood corpuscles from reserves waiting in the liver and spleen. This unused energy is dissipated through the nervous system leading to nervous shock. If this is repeated continually, it results in panic attacks or even mania. The reserves of adrenaline become depleted, coldness and exhaustion set in as does worry and the involuntary need to cry.

This often leads to a complete breakdown, in which the nervous system is unable to cope with the smallest of demands and can include deep depression and even suicide. Negative thoughts are so very destructive, not least because the cycle they create swallows its own tail, so the patient has no knowledge of its beginning or end. At this stage a negative thought presents itself as a natural response. The over stimulation of adrenaline has to be put right before the patient's natural response can become a positive one. Jupiter energy acts directly on the adrenal glands as they are the volume switches to the kidney energy. Optimism and joy empower the adrenals and therefore positive thoughts that influence the emotions create a healthy balance of secretion.

Chapter 2 ~ The Sacral Centre

Women who exhibit a greater distribution of male energy or who have been forced into an exclusively male group have found that the secretion of the adrenal cortex neutralises that of ovary secretion, for adrenal power is masculine. To rebalance these secretions the women may require the remedy *Oak*. *Oak* is the best remedy we have at present for grounding and it will calm over-stimulated adrenal activity. If the adrenal glands of the baby are damaged during labour, excessive amounts of secretion can result in mixed genitalia: whereas if these glands become diseased prior to birth then premature puberty can result. Adrenaline, like all other hormones are living cells that circulate by means of the body's fluids, reaching far from their origin and working by either stimulating or inhibiting other cells. No organ of the body goes untouched; such is the importance of a proper balance. The harmony of the adrenal glands is an important factor in the nature of our outlook, be it either positive or negative. The adrenal type of personality is an action led person with a seemingly limitless bound of energy and great stamina. The face of such a type often has a brownish tint and large freckles. It is rugged and clothed with a low hairline. The age at which this type usually burns out is around thirty-six, when Jupiter re-enters the chart for the third time. In numerological thought, the number three represents Jupiter, so it may be considered that three times twelve is the limit or opportunity in which Self has to resolve its sacral centre.

THE SACRAL CENTRE, TRANSMUTATION AND THE THROAT CENTRE

Transmutation of the sacral centre's endless creative potential is the result of the alchemical relationship it has with the throat chakra. When this creative energy is raised to its highest resonance it is expressed at the throat by the means of sound. The level of creativity within the sacral centre ranges from that of the earth to the sky. At the throat chakra, this creative energy is the same but its significance has intensified tremendously. For Self, it is far easier to wrestle with its emotions within the material world than to develop the focus required to deal with them in the spiritual world. The sacral and throat centre sharing the same energy simply means that Self, in order to progress, needs to master its emotions on these differing levels. Both are associated with the creative function, the sexual organs and the voice. Weakened kidneys will also constrict the throat and airways.

Alchemy is achieved when the transmuted force of creative energy becomes the tool for divine purpose. So the quality in the sacral centre will be that which later manifests itself in the throat, hence the importance of developing a healthy sacral centre within the group. Abuse, especially of power felt in this centre, closes down the voice or hinders its quality. This also explains why bad language mainly has reference to the sexual act or organs. Language will indicate the quality of the personality, the expression of which will transpire around both chakras. If the child or adult has problems vocalising, standing up for itself or speaking in public then the problem may lie in an ineffective sacral centre. Too much sexual emphasis or stuck sacral energy will also manifest in language. In view of the energy of the two centres, which in essence are the same, symptoms that pertain to poor creativity will filter up or down or be indicated in both at once. At the throat, creativity is spoken in the form of intention, a wish that expects to be fulfilled. At the sacral centre this energy is much more located towards the physical end of the chakra line, so concentrates on providing a space, a context in which physical form can manifest. So before the wish can be instigated, the context in which it will eventually be required needs to be explored first. This is what is meant by the word reproduction. In short, the conditions need to be provided in which matter can manifest. In the sacral centre reproduction requires both a male and female counterpart. Without exploring what is possible, one lacks the instinct to expand upon what is already there. Patients who are not prepared to venture into the possibilities but only dream from afar have poor sacral function and will find it very difficult to express their wishes from the throat chakra.

The failure to raise kundalini energy up out of the sacral centre results in immaturity, the childish foibles of a weak Jupiter. Those who get stuck in their sacral centre find it hard to take on the process of intimacy that comes with this energy as it moves Self through life. This also includes the inability to extend the throat chakra, which prevents growth from happening. It will be at the throat that doorways to development will fail to open due to poor energy and it will be at the sacral centre that these doorways even fail to manifest if the energy is stuck. Such characters may spend a lifetime naively exploring the differing possibilities of life, but never having the maturity to commit and work up a platform for real growth. They make excuses or find distractions that for a short

Chapter 2 ~ The Sacral Centre

time captivate their wonder, just as children do but then being only equipped with curiosity, they lack the confidence to make something happen. Those vaccinated against TB may not even have that; it denying curiosity, so their creativity may not even extend beyond the armchair. Confidence is an important trait and the result of a healthy sacral centre. Adults who remain children do not develop confidence, having not mastered the emotions. This chakra is expansion, that when lacking confidence resurrects itself in the land of fantasy. Trauma, such as parental separation, is one cause of such under active maturation.

JUPITER

The planet Jupiter is surrounded by two major force fields, one being radiation and the other being a magnetic field that if visible to the human eye would make up the largest structure in our solar system. It serves the universe by acting as a vacuum cleaner, attracting all the unwanted debris, dust and meteors that would otherwise engulf the other planets. It thus protects humanity from that which would otherwise besiege its existence. Because Jupiter has no density of its own it would appear that from this debris, its satellites have been formed. Jupiter's magnetism is that which pulls Self into situation after situation: a magnet to Desire. Miasmatically speaking, sycotically driven people become governed by this energy, for they worship its fortitude and reflect its obsessive nature. Once having been pulled in, this energy rubs off on them, producing magnetic characters that seem to love life and share in its generosity. This magnetism has a relationship with ether, for when it is mixed with solar energy it has the ability to permeate the entire universe – the universal wisdom of Jupiter. This gives him his rightful place as king over the gods.

Although Jupiter is made up of a ball of two swirling gases, hydrogen and helium, and has no solid surfaces, its atoms don't behave like a gas when compressed but more like a 'supercritical fluid'. Where the planet Mercury is concerned with the focus and communication of ideas, Jupiter is involved with the creation of ideas: formative prophecy. Water, the element of this centre is the universal memory, which contains the secrets of nature's way, that of creativity. Water is a powerful element, but is lighter than earth, and capable of changing its molecular structure, finding its way into all aspects of physical life. It represents the fluid connection between the conscious and unconscious mind. It is an energy receptor as well as purifier, a receiver of the electrical spark, the lightening bolt of Zeus. Within its depths we contact the emotional realm, deep feelings, intuition and psychic spheres that facilitate the gift of cleansing the past. Water sources have long been cherished for their spiritual purification, such as that of Tunbridge Wells and Chalice Well at Glastonbury. Meditating on this centre provides insight into nature's fluidity and it is in the sacral centre that we find a link to the vegetable kingdom. That which is life is fluid, and this lifeline is reflected in the sap. Plants have no choice as to their position once rooted in the ground and this is much the same as human ancestors. This is one reason why the selflessness of the vegetable kingdom resonates within the human kingdom and why so many plants are used in homœopathy to clear the blood and raise vitality. Visualise all the sensations of being in a beautiful garden or on a country walk in the height of summer and let this engulf all the senses. One can imagine the effect of this in creating positive emotions.

The vegetable kingdom is home to many light beings that require no physical body and these can be called upon to help the sacral centre and to assist in exploring its wonder. They are often met in dreams, as this centre allows the spirit to join the unconscious world by way of sleep. Plants provide much in the way of support for Self as it struggles in undertaking its tasks. They do this unreservedly, tuned in to the functional limitations of Self's own physicality. The lack of choice the plant experiences reflects its openness to serve and the selfless desire to provide for the greater plan. The vegetable kingdom intertwines itself with humanity in many ways, as the sycotic miasm is synonymous with the sap. Plant life depends on a fine balance of nourishment which lies somewhere between flood and drought, as does the human cell.

The two great planetary gas giants are Saturn and Jupiter. Jupiter is the largest planet in the universe, being three times the size of all the other planets put together, placing its reputation as monarch of the solar system. Its red spot alone is three times the size of the Earth. Because its magnetic field emits radio waves (communication), its force field is known as a "magnetosphere", just like that of the Earth's but a great deal stronger. Jupiter gives out two times more energy, the source of which is heat from its very hot central core, than it receives from the sun and this equation means it is depleting the planet's resources. For this reason some astronomers have likened its behaviour to that of a star rather than a planet but this trade off should be truly linked to creativity, for to give

Chapter 2 ~ The Sacral Centre

is greater than to receive. As king of the planets, or to the Greeks king of the gods, Jupiter, together with its satellites who are lucky enough to grace the royal court, acts as a mini powerhouse of creation, like a small universe within the universe. Jupiter acts as the universal womb for the incubation of new life, pulling on the essence of or harnessing the four elements of its many moons that orbit as it slowly spins. The rhythm of this is precisely in tune with that which goes out and that which comes in, which is what it means to be king. Amongst the subjects are the Galilean moons; the four largest of which each represents an element of latent potential and they too have their followers. Together they create the possibility for new life, for without somewhere to mix the ingredients and a framework in which to place them, there is no life. This is the same for the four elements when perceived in the teachings of the kabbala, as they represent the four worlds. As already mentioned these can be interpreted as the four horses that are ridden from one life to the next in the pursuit of transcendence.

The first of the Galilean moons is Io, which is more geologically active than the Earth. Its volcanic eruptions create a cloud-based climate that is blue in appearance and creates snow in colours of red, yellow and orange. The element here is air and represents spiritual purity, to be crowned, born or initiated – to have trust. Ganymede, the second moon, scrapes against Jupiter's magnetic field, creating 3 million amps and vast electrical storms that run wild on the surface of Jupiter. This is fire, power, the desire and experience. The next is Europa, which although covered with ice, contains within oceans of warm water that are thousands of miles deep. The element here is water, the balance of growth that leads to maturity. This moon alone is more vast than the planet mercury. The fourth moon, Callisto, has throughout its life been violently pounded, hit by meteorites that have left it scarred and marked very much like our own planet. Its element thus is earth – death, the vehicle for transformation. These moons together with Jupiter present a beautiful picture of inner creativity, a gyroscope of balanced input that is the elements rotating around a central pod of swirling gas-like fluid energy that is gently caressing the inner fertilised potential – a womb of the cosmos. When this visualisation is meditated upon, it supplies much in the way of insight as to the creative force within one's own being. A womb cannot exist without the presence of all the four elements, a fact yet to be understood amongst archaeologists when considering the construction of the Egyptian pyramids.

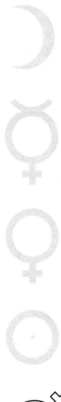

Chapter 3
The Solar Plexus

THE SOLAR PLEXUS

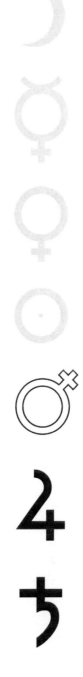

This centre encourages the exploration of individualism. Around the age of fourteen to twenty-one years, the young adult is under the instruction of Mars and thus has to learn to act for himself through the development of his will, in order that he can make decisions that suit him best. Fire, the element of this centre, will rise from the liver in order to direct will into action and enable Self to steer through the many choices it faces. It is important to put this passion into context here. The will of this chakra is still associated with the personality: it still being closer to the earth rather than to the heavens. This is why it is considered to be the little will and not that of Divine will.

Armed with the undeniable truth of its group, Self feels compelled into action in order to explore the truth within. In the male this urge is much more forceful and reactionary due to physical strength and the present balance of nature. The method by which desire is met can be quite different in the female: in the female, passion is much more reflective and is centred on inner strength, the energy behind creative force. The lessons of early childhood, the exploration of feelings and emotions within the guidance and structure of the group are now called upon in the development of independence. Very much like an un-licensed pilot taking to the skies for the fist time, initially the instructor is still present in the aircraft, but the pilot knows that the time is right not to call upon help but to take the opportunity for the benefit of growth. Some teenagers are not even happy with the presence of the

Chapter 3 ~ The Solar Plexus

instructor; such is the pull to achieve independence. The development of identity within the guidance of the group now diverts away from a focus on the role within the group, towards the individual, though the wishes of the group continue to need to be understood.

To name the will of the personality the 'little will', in no way belittles its power source. While this centre is being developed the flames of passion will rage in the pursuit of possession, or that which is attached to Self. This force of determination can gather what we perceive down here in the physical word as tremendous strength. It is the love learnt from the group, and the love of it, that guides such energy. Such power can be volatile and in certain circumstances the balance between support and hindrance can be a very tricky line to tread, especially for parents. This power, when directed outward, forms action. It is spontaneous, reactive and decisive. Like fire it is all consuming and therefore change creating. Once this power has started, the response will surely follow. However, if the flames are doused at any age, say as a result of poor parenting, the law or of society, the consequent feelings of compromised individualism manifest as injustice. This can feel intolerable and the resultant wrath is either delivered to those closest who are offering support or internalised as the reactionary destructive force of pride. This is the centre of anger, the power of the will if hindered. Internalised anger ultimately breaks down the will and leads to the destruction of the ability to flow with the laws of nature. These laws are written and adhered to by the higher self and, when crossed, formulate diseases such as cancer. These laws are abused when anything interferes with the soul's true path and should not be overlooked by the practitioner. Hindrance at this centre is so often the result of past life patterning, and homœopathy will be needed to free the will and enable the patient to change habits that inhibit its rightful action to manifest.

This stage of youth, between the ages of fourteen and twenty-one, is a right of passage. It is the right to grow up, the right to take a place in the world. It is equality, the right for each to be of value. No one is judged differently as everyone has their rightful place within the group, otherwise they would not be here. This centre concentrates on justice and, coupled with the security of base energy and the service aspect of the sacral centre, it will strive to conquer what is deemed to be just. This is the justice sought when the individual Self was created, that of the right to independence. The fire that such passion creates in the solar plexus is so powerful it will feed into the next two centres above, but due to their differing natures this fire will be expressed in differing qualities. Therefore this alchemy is dependent on the achievement of the solar plexus in providing decisiveness. Mars, the fiery planet that insists upon separation, places much dilemma on the teenager who is suddenly under its forceful influence. This is an energy that demands selection, the judgement of Self in order to make a decision. Development is fraught with many obstacles and challenges from the choices that Self makes during the construction of confidence. This development should be encouraged. It is never a good idea to suppress another's will. We have learnt through remedies such as Anacardium, the problems that are brought upon the group through the resultant resentment from a downtrodden will. This does not have to be caused by physical violence but will result from the reciprocation of a controlling force, which in turn is handed on through a chain of behaviour and thus the cycle continues. Mars is the planet of war in which the actions of revenge are played out by the personality. If one's will is strong, it requires direction and not suppression.

The opportunity to utilise the power of Mars at this point of development is generally missed or not understood by Western societies. Modern educational methods often incarcerate what is, or should be, a burst of activity and they care little about how to direct what this potential can accomplish. In schools where pupils are seen only as a group and not as a set of individuals, separate aspirations get clogged together in a manageable, affordable clump – mindless, direction-less and nameless. At the solar plexus each individual has their reason, their level, their action, which needs to be encouraged and most will find that it has little, if anything, to do with information in a text book. If society ignores these desires then it fails to bring the best out of its young adults by not spotting their best attributes. As it stands, the scope for exploring these is shrunk into a homogenised structure that wouldn't stimulate a tea bag. The place for schooling is at the development of the sacral centre. It is here that the child is ready to explore the rules of its environment. This includes reading and writing, which are the lower forms of creative communication and thus should only take seven years to develop, providing the child is in his body. At the age of fourteen, the child should be bursting to be free of such constraints. It is here that the young adult should be encouraged to work on her uniqueness, this being in regard to

Chapter 3 ~ The Solar Plexus

weaknesses as well as strengths for they are equally, if not more, important in producing a balanced personality and one that is adaptable to change as the group and Self develop. These desires will be the driving forces at work throughout life, so it makes sense at this stage to encourage the young adult to explore the activities that they truly want to do in life in accordance with their aspiration.

There are other ways in which the will can be suppressed and many ways that the result of this manifests itself. Mostly anger internalises and switches off the outward beam of light leaving behind a tiny flicker of a single flame, that of the victim. Shyness, introversion, avoidance, depression and even suicide can result when one's fire goes out and new remedies such as *Bay Leaf* will be required here. The ego is aware of this suppression, creating more anger towards Self and a diminished self-opinion. Repressed anger can also build and build, sowing the seeds of destruction in the digestive organs until it finally snaps at the place of the nervous system which can lead to a breakdown, as in the case of a *Veratrum* picture.

Allopathic drugging always plays havoc on the solar plexus centre, especially on its key organ the liver, by inhibiting its healthy function and therefore creating repercussions throughout the body. This is most commonly due to the excessive prescribing of antibiotics, especially at an early age at a time when the establishment of growth is so important. Drug suppression keeps the organs of this centre clogged up with putrefying pus, so when this chakra is called upon in the development of consciousness, it just spits and spurts like an old car trying to start on a damp morning. There will be a trace of circumstance that will run right back through the child's life in which this congestion will express itself as inadequacies and inhibitions. By eliminating childhood illness, we have eradicated great opportunities in which the child is able to throw-off much of the past and gain strength for the future. If we continue to administer poisons that render our children incapable of coping with these illnesses we then store away a problem that will return tomorrow in the form of more serious diseases. Hence the relationship between the growing number of adult problems like arthritis, diabetes, and cancer. Do we want our children to become an incubator for mutating bacteria, a culture dish in a vast governmental experiment? When the smallpox vaccine was introduced during the eighteenth century the incidence of cancer cases subsequently rose dramatically within the corresponding years and was noted by the physicians at the time, both allopathic and homœopathic. Obviously these increases did not seem dramatic enough for the government at the time to act, probably because, like all governments, they look towards the short-term gain. Such has been the same in the management of antibiotics, which have increasingly gained strength while their action on ever-mutating bacteria has diminished. This means the bacteria have been given a nice home, being provided with the correct environment in which to thrive. This ludicrous battle between freedom and containment of even the slightest of inflammations has resulted in the administering of what is little more than paint-stripper. Only recently a women lost not only the outer layer of her skin but also the first protective layer around her organs after having received such medication.

A colleague of the Author was challenged at a dinner party once a fellow guest became aware that his children were unvaccinated. He, or rather the children, were accused of bringing the potential for disease into the playground. In fact it is already there, bubbling away in a never ending cycle of mutation and reproduction that will bring new strains to the compromised immune system of the vaccinated child and threaten the unvaccinated child who may thus also have to deal with them. The positive action of this chakra should result in informed choice, whether to take it or leave it. This is freedom, or the right to be a citizen. It is the power to question what is deemed to be the truth as opposed to your own truth. It is that which is bestowed upon the parent as guardian through love to protect the child and explains why many of the so-called academic experts armed with the facts are not in possession of the truth, as witnessed by parents. Congestion of the organs is by no means only the result of vaccinations. I have treated un-inoculated children who have problems of elimination due to their miasmatic load, but it must be remembered because they are not vaccinated they still have intact their innate vitality to heal, and still have the opportunity through childhood illnesses to restore strength. But it should also not be forgotten that their miasmatic inheritance is part of a vaccination program that has now been passed on through generations via the genes. We may never become miasmaticaly free but we can still have the freedom of our individualism by avoiding the dark shadow that attacks the bastion of faith. Self-belief should be cultivated here. for this is motivation. It will be with this help that Self can become miasmatically free.

Chapter 3 ~ The Solar Plexus

Vaccinations are the product of city dwellers. It is here that disease became rife amongst a dense population that was malnourished and had no means to sustain basic hygiene within the depth of poverty. This environment only became sanitised after water diseases such as cholera got into the ruling classes' water supply. Vaccinations were seen as a way of keeping disease away from the greedy so that they could continue to hold power and wallow in their excesses. They were never motivated by the greater good of humanity and are still not today. Disease is the ultimate fear for those in power and much effort is spent in controlling it without having to make the kind of financial commitment that would address its cause. Vaccinations fit this remit exactly.

Because the constitutions of those living in the country are stronger and the fear of disease lighter as a result of a greater contact with nature, a different mentality has been passed on, in which vaccinations are not deemed such a necessity. How ironic it is that it was on these strong constitutions that they were first devised, or was that deliberate?

It is from constitutions closer to the earth that much of the anti-vaccination lobby has stemmed. This mentality is completely different when compared to the generalised term 'the working classes' living in the cities today. Mentality is laid down over generations, it is boundary forming, containing both positive and negative information that binds a group. Aspects of mentality go back so far that their roots can be lost in time, requiring the instinctual mind to fathom them. Vaccinations were developed for the more vulnerable city dwellers who were involved in the next evolutionary steps and of course, the creation of a new economy. They bought these people time during both the advancements in their activities and the conditions in which they lived and worked, but at a price – further vulnerability to deeper disease states. It was a price that the ruling classes were prepared to pay and without doubt they were privy to this fact. It was not, however, vaccinations that removed the threat of disease but the improved condition of the cities. Ninety percent of deadly diseases were eradicated through better hygiene, which was forced upon the ruling classes, not only by their own susceptibility to disease but also by a growing skilled workforce that had in itself become a commodity. This message that it was hygiene and not inoculations that eradicated most disease is yet to be universally understood. Although times have changed, the memory associated with the fear of those times has not: this is inexplicably linked to poverty and the class system within cities. It is passed on from patterns of belief by one generation to the next and is part of the education system, one which is not interested in promoting individualism. Ask yourself this, when was the last time a so-called working class mother entered your practice with an unvaccinated offspring? Here lies the challenge.

To be an individual requires the support of the other charkas, especially the opposite of the sacral centre, the throat centre, which is ruled by Venus. Venus is the compassion to the passion of Mars, without which Mars would just march through any opposition. However we know this would not achieve much. Each centre has and requires its counterbalance in order to even out its role through the system of the seven. With so much potentially destructive energy Venus, the voice of beauty, whispers softly to the raging animal that has been let loose inside: gently advising its spirit as to the true necessity in the given situation. Without this balance, this centre is prone to over reacting and will manifest as violent, aggressive behaviour. Even when balanced, this does not mean that this great source of power has to be diminished, for this is a requirement of a proficient solar plexus and will often be needed to pursue one's purpose. This character will exhibit bounds of energy that will evoke much determination. Such people can be very forthright and difficult to deal with without being swept along in their wake or hindered from maintaining one's own cause. The manifestation of such energy will not only be revealed in the decanate of both the sun sign and the ascendant sign in the birth chart but also where Mars sits in each sign and house. A person with high Mars energy will still have to learn to tame it and this is precisely what many angry teenagers are also trying to achieve whilst bringing into consciousness the energies of this chakra.

The level of combustion that is at hand here should not be underestimated. When positive, this power makes action possible and when negative it becomes destructive. It can drive Self towards unlimited joy and the deepest of despair, being equally as stubborn in both domains. Rebellion here will be greatly influenced by one's karma. To discover oneself through the exploration of the ego, inevitably comes up against the restriction of the past, which is formed by passion or the result of an extinguished flame. Either way, the use or misuse of one's power in a previous existence will figure in the battle between light and dark forces today. Even if repressed, as long as Mars maintains influence within the stars, this energy will be present: but perhaps only by the means of rebel-

Chapter 3 ~ The Solar Plexus

lion, being the only course of action left open to the solar plexus chakra, will Self direct its fire to create the confrontation required. The problem is that anger can be such a destructive force and if it is allowed to persist throughout life, it will do much damage to all of the subtle bodies. Anger often needs to be expressed to reveal that Self is in opposition but the better place to be is one where the confrontation is under control. Again the events of the past will have much influence on this. Change is the result of action and it needs to be recognised that only when the power of this centre is utilised can the new be instigated. To create change Self needs to make space for it. For this to be successful, certain factors need to be put into place to safeguard its stability. Old Father Time will assist by putting the correct signs on the right doors in order to bring about the circumstances that will achieve its permanence. This is how negative karma is cleared. *Moldavite*, being a piece of a meteorite, will assist in this process by speeding up one's own karma. Because it is not from this planet, its energy will loosen the constrictions put upon the work being done here. One can wear it, but this can be quite a brutal way of releasing karma, and not the easiest of rides. It is by far gentler and less pushy to take *Moldavite* in potency along with other new remedies that are specific to clearing the trauma of the past.

'Can't' is the word that disengages this centre. There are powerful effects that surround this word and it is the one that is often repeated to the child in an attempt to establish boundaries. The teenage years are an opportunity to find one's own boundaries and also a chance to free oneself from the constraints of the guardians. This is a natural transition into adulthood and should, though with support, be encouraged. 'Can't' establishes the rules in a society and its counter – 'can', is the questioning of authority, of knowing oneself as opposed to one's place. All the limitations that instigate the use of the word 'can't' do so for material gain and in the West that usually manifests as privilege. In effect it is 'can' which is the driving force of this centre, and it is karma that is the instrument by which true worth is justified and recorded. Within the action of 'can', astral light makes an exact representation of the desire of Self, which opens the door to possibility and perhaps later to achievement. It is the nature of the karma that will inhibit this and much change will be required to counter it if there is difficult karma. One action that results in change may be induced by the taking of homœopathic remedies, which will help to free that which has a stranglehold on the possibilities of today. These constraints will have remained unresolved and pertain to unconscious memories like the manner in which Self previously died, how it was understood, what harm befell it, or how its conscience was steered through previous incarnations. These things will all have consequences on the will of Self and as to what is possible. It is as if on the astral plane, there is a battle being fought between what has been and what is going to be done, creating confusion as one side and then the other gets the upper hand. Inevitably Self pays the price one way or another for its actions. Those who are visionaries will have often had the greatest of battles between these two worlds and in Western societies they find it the hardest to instigate their actions. More and more in the West, one's worth is measured by the progression of material gain, hence the spirit is eroded, for support is applied only to those who can guarantee a financial return. This is now apparent in all walks of life as a means to control investment. Self's obligation to fire is to work within these systems of spiritual constraints, in order to change this.

THE SPLEEN: GATEWAY TO THE VITAL BODY

Prior to the heart, it was the spleen that was the central organ upon which the development of humanity relied during its formation. At this point the heart had not sufficiently evolved to cater for what was later to influence it. This changed as evolutionary actions shaped its structure through consequence. These actions would force the heart to change its role as the soul retreated within it. Each change coincided with major transformations that marked the period of each root-race, the changing circumstances of humanity. It was the choice of humanity to place the heart as the central organ, the sustainment of life, for individualism dictated that true love could only start with oneself and thus sacrifice could only be achieved at the heart centre. The spleen had sustained early evolution, for the absorption and sharing of solar light was sufficiently within its remit when existence was not so laden with karmic weight. Most of that which was interchangeable did not require the significance of matter. The burdens that were to come overpowered the spleen and thus the heart became the temple for the throne, where the light of spirit was to sit.

Ambition falls under the ability of the spleen to create a structure, guided by the soul, in which one can put forward one's actions.

Chapter 3 ~ The Solar Plexus

Ambition, because it is the energetic, physical counterpart to aspiration, can bring to life one's desires through the power of the spleen. The spleen is the organ of frustration. It likes to express and share ambition and will swell if this is suppressed. The array of hindered ideas will clog the blood, burdening the liver, and stifling the brain. This can result in fevers or an emotional outburst that represents a spleen that is too full of stagnant impulses and unable to accept any more, so will vent. Ambition generated in the spleen promotes the will of the liver, which in turn governs individualism. If the motives of such ambition are compensating for perceived weakness, remedies will be required to strengthen the spleen in order to carry out desire. Such remedies include *Ceanothus, Amber, Ruby, Bay leaf. Caesium, Goldfish, Ash, Apple Tree, Cotton, Thymus Gland, Orange* (colour) and *Sandalwood*.

Ambition, being linked to aspiration, will have its own alliance with achievement, that of purpose in this lifetime. Achievement can be greatly enhanced through speeding up one's karma, or in effect releasing more karma than one would otherwise be destined to achieve in one lifetime. This is what homœopathy does. To those more enlightened, this will be motivation in itself. Such motivation may be induced by the psychic function of the spleen, for this is an organ for receiving instruction and here the choice is whether to use it or ignore it. To further develop psychic reception from the spleen may involve quite a test, for Self becomes more sensitive to the interaction of sensation. It is important to stress that as with all psychic skills, if they are not used for the benefit of the group, they will be taken away and this is especially so when they are misused in the pursuit of financial gain.

Contained in the spleen, is the balance between ambition and mediumship. Mediumship is of a lower psychic quality but one which is very important in the development of the soul. Because the spleen is the gateway here, mediumship will manifest in some way within all humans, for it is the feeding of etheric energy into that which needs to be achieved. Truly developed mediums can also feed pranic energy into a visiting entity in order that it can manifest a form and communicate in our sphere. This experience will require a great deal of energy, which will deplete the medium or instrument, especially if the messenger has travelled far and has much of significance to say. Remember, fluidity has to do with information. The visitor arrives via the astral plane and because the division between the physical and etheric bodies of the medium are not so rigidly defined, this enables energy to be diverted much more freely. The vision of the medium determines whether this connection is a safe one. This discrimination should also be supported by information received from guides. Some mediums have no control over this selection process, which prevents them from having any choice over that which they receive. This is distressing for the medium and creates the need for stimulants, which either anaesthetise their visions, creating a break from them, or boost pranic energy needed to compensate for the drainage that occurs. The medium can gain control over what is received, for this is part of the initiation into psychic ability and from which training provides the choice.

A child who possesses the ability of being psychic is vulnerable to being misunderstood, which in itself will be a difficult burden to carry through life. The child may face misinterpretation of his feelings through his actions and his speech. In order to compensate for this or in an attempt to fit in, the child may develop characteristics of manipulation, for their heightened level of sensitivity can be far too much for others to bear, especially when these others feel that too much of themselves is being revealed. These children even resort to lies and deceit to try and win favour in order to hide their level of sensitivity. *Medorrhinum* may be prescribed in order to ground them. They are, however, in a world where much more is felt than usual and this makes it doubly important for their guardians to help them find a connection, a role, a position on the planet where they can be loved and protected and feel useful.

Poor spleen function lowers vitality and renders the fluids of the body unbalanced. This also includes that which is required by the sexual organs and will manifest as a lack of sexual energy and desire. In addition to a lack of daylight, Self's negative thought process also weakens the spleen. Dark emotions, fear and anger hinder ambition and the flow of prana energy, that which sustains form, and when lacking manifests as melancholy in the human psyche. The spleen is more developed in the human being than in the animal as the demands of creation are greater and thus the quantity of prana energy required is also greater. When Self and Divine separated, Self, through the nature of desire, became co-creator of the universe. This is the consequence of our actions already mentioned. For the future, Divine has offered guidance through the Holy Spirit so that our endeavours match that of purpose. Thus it would seem that Divine no longer has ultimate power over all things but Self in possession of its

Chapter 3 ~ The Solar Plexus

own ego, its own free will and the responsibility of judgement, now has influence on all the various levels of creation. This is action governed by thought and the spleen puts structure to realisation, so it may get stored as ideas in the mind. The greater the demand on the mind, the more the spleen will deplete, which is what happens when pressurised by over-studying. A weak spleen inhibits the absorption of information. High desires vitalise thoughts akin to the sun shining. If a robust liver supports the power of the will then this and the spleen energy create a vibrant mind and the capacity for pure thought.

Ultimately and purposefully, the spleen directs prana to the mouth to perform the important functions of speech, taste and breath. Once we have gathered our ideas and have blessed them with sound, the spleen enables the portal to open so that we may place back, via the ether, that which we have now made conscious and call into manifestation. Through this portal, the waste of negative emotions can be eliminated from the blood within the expelled breath. The colour, quality, shape and size of the lips will indicate spleen activity. The coating of the tongue will also aid information as to the quality of both the spleen and the liver.

BLOOD AND THE EGO

Blood's only concern is with the preservation of life. It is magnetised with prana energy as already spoken of in Chapter Two and its movement and containment is determined by this energy. Without the structure of these etheric energy lines blood would not follow its path but seep into the tissues of the body. It and all the liquids of the body are of the same source. When spilt blood is seen, say in a news report, the vision of its pool still has the capacity to shock us. This fluid of life symbolises our own mortality and the image of its spilling from such a vulnerable container, during this present time in which strength is counted in mass, seems such a fragile way of maintaining physical existence. In reality, Self should be aware that true protection is fate. This shock of the sight of blood stimulates the animal instinct, which is endlessly exploited by filmmakers. It is one of the few shocks that still remain in the name of entertainment but even this is waning. Spilt blood represents the pain and the suffering of those circumstances thought to be under the domain of the devil. The war in the angelic realm over who was to reign supreme in heaven, mentioned in the book of Revelations, was won by the archangel Michael over the once archangel Lucifer. It was the use of 'the blood of the Lamb', the blood of Christ or blood mixed with Holy Spirit that transcended from Earth, which proved to be the deciding factor. Only this blood bore witness to truth gained during its journey through the seven chakras. Infused with consciousness that provided the fire from which radiates the vibrant red colour, Lucifer found he had no defence against this power and fled to Earth in order to obtain it. The story is an indication as to the material from which this battle will be fought, the blood of mankind. So far it shows no sign of abating. It is for this reason that blood frightens Self. It warns us of impending doom, of the battlefield, of the dark, macabre world that we may well have indulged in during the past. It constitutes the result of our actions. Whilst in the body it remains hidden, clear, content, vibrant. Once out, it represents the colour of the devil, as well it may, for this indicates the actions of wrong doing which have caused it to spill in the first place. Blood reminds Self that it is not God.

If we indulge in desires that evoke harm then the blood will require purging, which generally happens through fevers. Myths and legends have been made based on this power struggle over blood. Souls filled with rampant desires need to replenish, renew, purify with fresh, clean, pure blood and this is the reason why vampire stories illustrate aspects of both the sycotic and syphilitic miasms. The term 'to be written in blood' means to hold a mirror up to oneself so that all that is reflected cannot be denied by the ego. It contains, undeniably, the weight of the whole of Self, a true commitment. This has a connection with the astral world via the Akashic records, for it is here that everything that has ever happened, and will happen, is recorded. The liver receives information from the astral world and is the storehouse for blood. Blood thus feeds the mind with images. These images are information maintained in the records of the Akashic scrolls and manifest down here as astral thought forms. Out of Akasha, everything is formed. It is here that these images are received and presented via astral light, which is collected in the blood and sent to the brain in order that Self can make sense of them. These images are thus an amalgamation of transcending and descending factors. The eyes also absorb images, a similar process to achieving sight. Pictures are gained by washing blood over the nerves in which information is gathered through sensation. All, in fact, is seen from within. Not all these thought forms are appropriate and some may be threatening.

Chapter 3 ~ The Solar Plexus

We have the ability to absorb both that which is self-building and that which is degrading, which will clog the blood and weaken the cell. It is the element of fire that enables the sludge of waste thoughts in the form of images in the blood to be incinerated and eliminated through exhalation. This is also why exercise is important, as it oxygenates the fire and releases more of the dross.

Every soul within the universe, including things like rocks, stones and trees is an author of the Akashic scrolls since earliest creation. You yourself are also an author. It is the filing system of the astral plane and where every action, which is the mark of an event, every thought or feeling is systematically placed in the book of life. The very thought that this can be denied is filed under 'denial' and will reflect in experiences here on Earth. Psychics can access these scrolls revealing answers as to why a particular life experience is happening. With many past lives one's own file can be very full, thus forming a complicated set of circumstances, structures or maintaining causes to which present life will adhere. For instance, the actions of a life in the first century Roman army will have a bearing on the actions and thus perceptions of present day activities as decreed by one's own record.

The astral plane is a meeting point for the descending unconscious energies as well as ascending consciousness from Earth. The angelic re-writing of these scrolls will also benefit from redemption and the transcendence of negative karma. We know that our activities down here are a reflection of work underway on the higher planes. 'As above then so below', meaning that what the soul has managed to clear in the past, as part of the progression of the higher Self, will also be recorded and reflected in present actions. The quality of actions here will also help in reverse, having a positive effect on those higher planes. This is what differentiates the Akashic records from the collective unconsciousness, which constitutes a part of the scrolls, but the sensitivity of the scrolls extends much further to include every vibration in the cosmos.

As we explore the function of what is considered to be these outer planes of energy, it is also good to grasp that every plane contains seven sub planes. It is far easier to receive information from a plane that is denser and thus has more energy around it, and harder if a great deal of energy is required to reach into it. This is because the farther planes are closer to the gods and have to travel a long way in order to be brought into manifestation.

As time does not have the same significance in the astral plane as that divided up mathematically by humanity here on Earth, it is also possible to obtain information on future events. For actions to have consequence they must be reflected back in order to become conscious. These actions are awaiting our fate but can be seen by those who can read. Reading from a book is not reading in its purist form: it is bringing into one's own consciousness that which is already known and is simply a method used to disseminate information. True reading pre-empts this process and is similar to the energy exchange that is made between the practitioner and patient. We perceive time as linear but in the astral plane its true essence is innate. On our plane we see events that have been taken out of context in order to be given the structure of time, a form from which they can be perceived. So the boundaries that we force on our own existence are very different in the astral plane. In fact here is contained all the possible combinations of spatial constructions including the fracturing of time, its retrograde and its sideways layering, that of parallel time scenes. These scenes are interrelated, for they influence separate events that are going on simultaneously but of differing genres, which we perceive in evolutionary terms, but are in fact feeding energy into each other as they exist side by side.

The connection between blood and the Devil is the result of blood being the vehicle of sin. Throughout time groups have used blood in rituals to remove sin in order to appease the gods. Taking the wrong path reveals blood's connection to the karmic lord, Saturn, who has been mistaken for Satan. The determination and courage of Mars helps to take on the Devil within Self. It is the quality of the blood that determines the pathway into the heart chakra. This is the first battle between dark and light that will inevitably be pursued at the heart centre. The solar plexus is the place where the heart hedges its bets. It is the first charge of the cavalry, designed to weaken the opposition long before the knights and eventually the king enters the fight. This is where the true might of each army tests the strengths and weaknesses of the opposition and where the decision to retreat or to march on is decided.

Blood is influenced by the energies of all the charkas, for it flows through each one of them except the base, however even here it will have a direct influence on its quality because the base chakra is responsible for keeping things on track. The base centre also maintains a strong foundation in which the great power of the solar plexus is able to make

Chapter 3 ~ The Solar Plexus

its will known. Through the connection between blood flow and chakra, disease is able to enter from any centre of the body and spread within it. It is the quality of prana energy and thus the function of the spleen that maintains the aura and thus protects against disease. Prana exists in a balance that maintains the fire of the blood. With an abundance of prana energy there will be much fire but, if lacking, stagnation of blood and of all bodily fluids will result. So we can say prana maintains the heat in the body and blood maintains the humidity. Fire fights disease by incinerating toxic dross and at these times the liver may require extra energy. This is provided by major etheric lines that connect the liver to the kidneys, a bit like jump leads.

Similarly, when the liver cannot cope with the removal of toxins then the lungs take up the work. Asthma is often the result of poor energy transference between liver and kidney function. Blood fuelled by fire is that of the realm of the animal kingdom, where the sap of the plant kingdom becomes the fluid of free will. However, before the Age of Atlantis there was not the need for such fire and human blood was clear. When the fire goes out, death will ensue. This is why anaemia is so close to cancer and why it represents being spiritually drained.

It is with blood that the beginning of humanity is marked and we are now some way down its thread. On the level of the individual there is a psychological manifestation of what has shaped oneself as opposed to another and which differentiates one as 'I'. Therefore, the accumulation of actions resonates down the bloodline to form what one believes one can personally achieve. This is ego, the ability to see one's own consciousness and just like looking in a mirror, you become your own identity through reflection and thus it requires the mind to make an assessment. Spirit shines the light as to who you are, ego is the light that you think you are.

The ego, is spelt with a little 'e' here, that of the personality, rather than that of a big 'E', which is the ascending incarnating Ego, that of immortality (of the higher Manas). The ego is home and makes its presence known in the blood. It uses the solar plexus as an information centre, a place where the wishes of Self can be directed to the brain and manifested as decision. The ease by which this is possible depends greatly on the quality of the blood and thus the work of the liver, gallbladder, stomach, spleen and pancreas. Such is the weight of importance of the solar plexus in expressing the wishes of the personality, that such an infrastructure of co-operating organs is required to maintain this healthy activity. Feelings from these organs will resonate through the blood, hence the expression 'that made my blood boil'. Time and time again, homœopaths see patients whose problems stem from this centre and in modern society it is much abused. We should never forget the little miracles in bottles that sit on our shelves, waiting to happen, and the circumstances of karma that enable healing to occur.

Blood, through the organs of the solar plexus, provides life by transporting sustenance for the renewal of the cells. This process began when the first physical body was formed and thus humanity was presented with the notion of life and death. The fact that Self had to face death was a major adjustment, it meant that the soul had consequence and the spirit therefore was to undertake retribution. The will of Self was karmic, producing a battle between right and wrong. At first the lower mind was insufficiently developed to have control over the abundance of will energy. Self had little understanding of consequence and even less judgement as to its meaning with regard to sexual pleasure that had been awakened during the Lemurian Age. As that root-race gave way to the next, that of Atlantis, sexual power mutated into ownership. Most Atlanteans were riddled with deceit. Who were they deceiving? Well, inevitably themselves, but also those who had taken up the responsibility to try and govern the race towards its rightful purpose. These people were the most enlightened and with the deepest developed minds of their time. They achieved a structure and an audience, yet the stealing, manipulation and greed continued behind their backs. These leaders were not blind to such activities but became resigned to the fact of war in a last ditch attempt to try and save the root-race. The weapons of destruction used were those of what we now call magic. The faculties at their disposal were the same as they are today but they had evolved the capacity to direct thought, so their manifestation was subtler. This miss-use of magic was to lay the foundations of what was to follow. Dark forces had a hold on those with little more than animalistic desires and who cared little whether their magic was black or white. Control was of the utmost importance because in the new physical word it meant power.

In the beginning, ego abstained from commitment during the early development of Self, but during the last third of the Lemurian age, under further development and the guidance of the mind, it entered

Chapter 3 ~ The Solar Plexus

the body. From this day ego has felt vulnerable. Once on the inside, ego found itself on its evolutionary path under the authority of a weak mind. The mind was and is forever acting on its own free will, weighing up the decisions and the compromises as to where to direct energy in its pursuits in the physical world. This frustrated the over-powered ego and it found itself in situations that it would normally avoid. The mind was determined to understand more through experience and the ego's interpretation of this was to compete for ownership. The notion of ownership in the body is sensed within the blood. The bloodstream is the river in which the ego identifies every cell as its own and every atom with that of individuality. From birth this has not always been so, as the blood of the child is not at first able to access a sufficient supply of red blood cells from an under developed skeleton by the way of bone marrow, and so relies on the source contained in the thymus gland. These cells have been supplied by the mother's blood and are in part, a link between the child and the ancestral bloodline, a reflection of the child's dependence on it. This is the way in which these connections are instilled until the thymus gland atrophies when the 'I', the child's individuality and thus its independence, begins to evolve under the influence of this chakra at around the age of fourteen years. The thymus does not, however, stop producing cells and maintains the bloodline link, which is amalgamated with the function of the spleen. One can lose either the spleen or the thymus but not both without death occurring.

All that the child and later the adult has accumulated in the way of darkness in the thymus will be transported by the blood and reflected in the attitude of the ego. The more toxic the blood is with this stuff, the more the ego will be awash with it and want to hide it. This may not be possible and may be let loose when the young adult starts to apply its will during the ascendancy of kundalini within this chakra. The quality of our blood rests on our thoughts but it is also fed by the thymus gland, so will be vastly effected if this should be damaged, such as through inoculation at an early age. A damaged thymus will not be able to prevent the dark forces from infiltrating the ego, manifesting as pessimism and cynicism. This will inflict much external damage but it will be at the heart centre where the most internal damage will occur. The heart centre offers us the greatest opportunity to change this karma. But, and it's a big but, the work has to first be successfully applied at the solar plexus for the Kundalini to continue its ascent. The spiritual purpose of the solar plexus centre is to be master over one's own desires during the pursuit of independence and the higher manas. Power over blood has power over man.

The rate of blood flow is governed by the emotions. The blood's pressure is maintained by feelings which influence us and because everything is measured and recorded in the astral plane, it will all have influence to a lesser or greater degree. This, in part, is how the energy of the planets interacts with Self. It is actually under the bequest of the throat chakra, the balance to the solar plexus, that blood is distributed. Through the command of the throat centre, the solar plexus strives to maintain all the functions of the body and will divert distribution if required. Energy pertaining to problems in other chakras will be felt at the solar plexus centre, and for this reason it is where cancer enters the physical sphere. Many cancers are digestive in origin as they reflect the failure of Self to utilise the power of Mars to strive through the difficulties that life presents. Spirit, through its link with the mind, is able to live with desires if they are conducive to the pursuit of change.

This is done by transforming emotions into thoughts through action or experience. It is important to grasp the level of sensitivity here amongst all this powerful passion. This centre forms the point at the top of the ascending triangle, which is that of the personality reaching for the heavens and bowing at the gates of the heart in pursuit of the elixir of life.

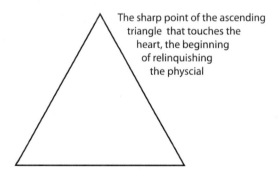

Figure 5. The Ascending Triangle.

This point strives forward and with it must carry all the precious resources that have enabled it to manoeuvre into position, aware that it must keep up its strength to reap the benefit. This is not stubborn but

Chapter 3 ~ The Solar Plexus

sensitive. Not over sensitive, which is a lack of will, but sensitive to the needs of Self's desires. This is fire alive and the reason why, when gazing into its flames, one is mesmerized by the delicacy of such destructive potential.

The ego is where the astral channel meets the inner faculties of Self's soul. Ego can thus be said to separate Self from the soul. It covers up the ever-lurking dark primordial world, which is the shadow that lies beneath. Ego protects Self from this underbelly by managing and moulding it into a form that integrates into the personality so effectively that it may in fact never be detected by chance. It will however, be seen by those people who have that ability and will be revealed to those who are truly within their own inner circle. The solar plexus centre is the upper echelon of the integrated personality. It is an expert in control by hiding that which it does not wish to see. The ego protects against the judgement of others and if this discrimination is broken then humiliation, the repression of one's will, extends throughout the body. This will also hinder all the plans and wishes of Self that are in the process of fruition, as they are already formed on the astral plane. All ideas are first constructed in the astral plane before they can feasibly be created on the physical plane.

All creations will benefit mankind but they can be opposed by the sludge of negative energy that is against change. This scenario is known as dogma and its sole purpose is to hinder the uprising of positive action. In Asian societies, with their intense structures of social positioning, being responsible for creating change and the possibility of failure can be a very undesirable position in which to find oneself in. Failure is not only seen as a weakness but also a reflection of one's bad Karma. Karma lies very heavily on the solar plexus as it is received directly from the Akashic scrolls and so the will of Self communicates directly with it. This is why so many remedies of this centre have issues pertaining to the ego and humiliation strongly within their picture.

The need to exert one's will commencing from this centre can attract much pathology according to circumstance. *Nux Vomica* is the remedy of individualism caught within a constrained society, whereas *Chelidonium* is only impressed by his own individuality and therefore distrusts any hierarchy. *Nux Vomica* strives to be a part of that hierarchy. *Lycopodium* has already accepted her failings as an individual but finds a safe place in order to be reminded of it once again. Many of the new remedies offer much in the way of relief to a soul caught between the group and the desires of the astral plane. *Mimosa* helps steady the fear, *Hornbeam* closes the cycle that creates the trap and so instils harmony between the group and ambition, or the Self and a significant other. *Okoubaka* releases the inertia from physical matter that is inhibiting astral matter and *Black Obsidian* helps one flow in the physical world when one has been haunted by the ghosts of the past that lay within the astral world and thus presently cause Self to compensate with egotistic displays designed to impress.

To a greater or lesser degree, every society holds a mirror up to aspiration in order to maintain the good of the group. In Britain, this has been perverted by an obsession with political correctness, a device which its leaders, be they local or national, have discovered to be a very effective method of silencing the masses. The right for the individual to express his views, however misguided, is ultimately far more important and safer than to have those views forced underground. The light and the dark do exist and to mask them with the ego creates a very dangerous situation.

Blood flows to, receives from and distributes that which is Holy Spirit, and thus connects to every cell, spiritualising our life with that of the source. The residue of our earthly actions combines in this centre with this spirit and the resultant mix is what we nourish our garden with so that it may grow. Those dark aspects must stand next to the spiritualised ones and thus our thoughts, which are these energies that have been through the filter of the brain, determine how we endeavour to enlighten life with this essence. It will inevitably rest on the mind to determine what the will indulges in. Remember, Self wanted to taste that which was in the hands of the Divine and thus feed itself. This is what is digested in order to be absorbed, to be taken in and to become one. On the physical plane, this is material food, which contains stored light. On other planes and equally necessary, it is the absorption of the many vibrations of the cosmos. The Holy Spirit feeds into the blood via the crown chakra and should radiate outward in the world. A metaphorical representation of this is the symbolism of wine as the blood of Christ, drank to purify the fluids in order to maintain the truth, which is always one's own truth, the substance of the blood. The blood of Christ is said to be the love that destroys the negative ego. Wine has been and continues to be used to help open up the portals in which the mind can receive such insight and not be held back by ego.

Chapter 3 ~ The Solar Plexus

THE STOMACH, FEELINGS AND THE WAR OF DIGESTION

When food is taken into the body, war is waged upon it. This battle takes place in the stomach. In order for the great conversion of many chemicals to become of use to the body, an army of combating troops have to disable it, break it down and assimilate it. This is in addition to distributing what is necessary to maintain life and eliminate that which is not. Food is concentrated solar energy. Its conversion in the body requires a fight in which all the organs of the solar plexus centre work in harmony to achieve success. We separate out the organs of the solar plexus for the purpose of study, however, like the chakras, their operation is that of a single unit. The stomach contains the battle and it uses reinforcements in order to gather its spoils of war. This is applicable to the emotions as well as to food. The stomach is the place of absorption of food, thoughts and emotions. It is where thoughts are digested and in turn will initiate action. This place is very sensitive to that taken into Self and will readily reject that which it deems inappropriate. Problems here will indicate an inability of the mind to incorporate thoughts into the personality. These will be the emotional blocks in the patient. The term solar plexus or coeliac plexus refers to a collection of nerves that are located just behind the stomach which link into the sympathetic nervous system and in particular the vagus nerve. These etheric ties enable Self to feel and assimilate in a very physical way that which is not always so obvious. This is often referred to as 'gut reaction'. These reactions are relayed to the mind in order for it to place judgement upon them. This is how the stomach plays its part in determining whether the personality decides if something is right or wrong.

If the stomach were unable to absorb then this would indicate that Self is overburdened with emotion, which would refer to an imbalance in life. The thyroid gland, which is of the throat chakra, works very closely in the regulation of the digestive organs and is the balancer of emotional behaviour. The throat is also the centre from which what we aspire can manifest. So we can say that when the two work in harmony, Self is able to act on its feelings and this will reflect in the nature of a healthy digestive system. If the stomach is unable to absorb then Self is not manifesting its purpose, being particularly sensitive to the division between good and bad energy. Working together, the liver and the stomach act as a portal through which those incoming and outgoing vibrations will be felt throughout the solar plexus and feed into its knot of nerve endings, via the electrical impulses of the nervous system. When Self crosses its arms, this action is an attempt to cover this portal, protecting access to the stomach from energy being thrown out from another and thus preventing such absorption into the soul. It is the same for the quality of the food ingested, for it has great effect on the quality of the cell and so the quality of what is felt. The sun and the cell share the same symbol for their life fuels aspiration and it is the energy of the sun, the soul and the Earth, where food is harvested, that flows through the astral, etheric and physical body.

THE LIVER, THE GALLBLADDER AND THE ASTRAL WORLD

It is not possible to isolate the function of the liver from the spleen. Blood is fed to the liver from the spleen, stomach and intestines as well as via the hepatic artery. The energy of the liver is male to that of the female spleen. The liver acts as a ductless gland helping to maintain the nitrogen and carbohydrate metabolism by breaking down proteins to form amino acids, the building blocks of life. While the spleen manages the blood, the liver is responsible for its quality. This quality creates vitality and the clue is in its name – the liver – which is the ability to achieve much in life. It stands guard against poisons that may enter the body and if its function is poor or such poisons are difficult to eliminate, then congestion will result. Now, more than at any other time in human development, the liver is faced with a sophisticated barrage of toxic material that represents the modern world, placing the liver under much pressure to succeed. All that is foreign to the body will require filtering and depositing from it, including chemicals, metals and dangerous bacteria. Miasms are also a form of poison and they can harm the liver immensely. The liver will try to free not only itself from such dispositions but also the interior of the whole body. The liver has wondrous powers of recovery; the power of Mars, but it often requires the help of an energy conscious therapy, from which it usually thrives.

The quality of the liver feeds the brain creating a cycle, as the quality of thought governs the blood and thus acts on the quality of the liver. The liver forms a portal in which our thoughts connect with those of the astral world via feelings that are made conscious by astral light. These are the universal truths of the cosmos. Depending on the level of

Chapter 3 ~ The Solar Plexus

consciousness, the manifestation of this connection can range from gut reaction to clairvoyance. This is an ancient form of communication that has not disappeared but has been pushed into the background by the lower intellect and ignored. Meditation is a practice that resurrects this channel, along with refining the solar plexus chakra so that its clairvoyant quality may come to life when inhabited by kundalini. In reality the astral world should never be ignored, for it registers with each and every one of our thoughts and thus, because thought determines action, it is also present in all our actions. Our thoughts produce a reflection of reality; we reflect on what is real.

When Self leaves this world, it first sheds its dense body and then the etheric one, which dissolves only a couple of metres away from its physical counterpart. The astral body, along with the soul and spirit, ventures up into the astral plane where awaits an exact replica of the physical vehicle left behind and all the other structures of the cosmos. This replication softens the shock that Self faces during the transcendence from one existence to another. However this replication is not physical, for nothing pertained to the astral plain is, so it is important not to perceive this level with the fears and notions that we carry as part of the experience of existence in the physical world. The purpose of the astral plane is to shed the astral body and with it much negativity that has been gathered by the actions of Self, in order that spirit can venture further. This is a place for adjustment: the greater the quality of consciousness, the less adjustment will be required. In other words, the more refined the astral matter through thought, the easier it is to transform the seven sheaths of the astral body. During incarnation, ancestors help to shape the waiting body in the astral plane before Self enters the physical domain, which begins with the etheric body. So due to the act of reversal that is part of this process, their influence will also be shed at this point of transition.

The astral plane has seven sub levels and according to the laws of enlightenment, the level in which one enters and the degree to which spirit has movement between these levels will be dependent on karma. The first three levels are often depicted as hell, an extremely difficult place to be, for here spirit is confronted by the worst misdemeanours of its lower self and is also surrounded by the results of every other soul's depraved passions. Here we find trapped souls that are unable to leave this constraint for reasons of still being connected to the material desires of the Earth. Again it is important not to view this space through the fear of the physical eyes, for it is a place of great opportunity, which on its lower sphere enables much wrong to be put right and unresolved projects to be finished in order that they may be brought into being on Earth by future generations. Even in these lower levels, spirit will be safe and the picture of pain and suffering perceived through the narrow Earthly experience of physical pain is not the same here. Neither is this experience terrifying, despite it often being depicted by those with a vested interest in perpetuating fear, for the physical and etheric bodies have been resolved. The expressions used by us to describe the limitations of the physical world are not applicable here, but this level does require spiritual growth. Just before death the instinct is open to this release, which may result in the expulsion of hidden truths that Self has been carrying around and too frightened to release. When spoken, this lightens the being in order to ease the process of death.

On the astral plane, as here on Earth, we tend to ask for an answer when what is truly required is an action. We do this out of insecurity, just as intellectuals often do. If a chakra needs clearing then action will promote the understanding that follows. It is the acting out of desires that will form results manifested in the astral plane and then brought to life in the physical world. Many people are faced with the indecision of not knowing what they want or are able to do. Their purpose for being here has been smothered by a succession of confusing experiences and it is only by making an action that they move closer to their task. It is the fear of the consequence of these actions that prevent this. This lack of vision will be a reflection of chaos on the astral plane created by much wrongdoing either by Self or by others towards Self. It should be made clear that on the astral plane, that which pertains to black magic will be registered, active and alive, and thus in need of redemption. Its mark can be seen reflecting physically in the condition of the liver and the workings of the solar plexus. It is upon the lower spheres of the astral plane that one's karma is pondered, the rearrangement of which will then depend on the level of development, if at all, of the soul's progression to the higher divisions. Those with the greater consciousness will spend the longest in these higher sections of the astral plane.

To travel up towards the higher levels of the astral plane is a process of dematerialisation. It is a connection from the Earth to the higher cosmos, a go-between or stop-off point in which one meets, combines and thus transcends into the other. This is why as humans, we never 'let go' of

Chapter 3 ~ The Solar Plexus

anything but only transcend whatever it may be. Self is already complete and to lose something would make it incomplete, which is not possible. Self will manifest in many forms that need change in order to transcend. This is the problem with the blind notion that gene therapy can take something away, for this will only produce a greater problem during this process of transformation and thus further re-incarnations will be required. In the astral plane, thought is change and the resultant actions of Self are all constantly changing in structure, but nothing is lost.

The purpose of the astral plane is to refine the dross of mankind in order that spirit can revitalise its experience of spiritual bliss within the confines of the astral body. Spirit should achieve this before it leaves this plane. In fact, it has to, for this is the plane in which the struggles of light and dark, that of the higher self being liberated from the actions of the ego within the personality, are played out. Illusions, such as glamour and vanity, are thought processes of the lower self and much has to be done to free oneself from these delusions that will otherwise deceive one whilst trying to mark out a life in the physical realm. Powerful emotions and desires that are the nature of the astral world, can blind us from our truth and it is truth that now presents the opportunity to cleanse. If Self enters into opposition to its truth, whilst here on Earth, then these thoughts will rebound back from the astral plain creating confusion. This is how the astral world attempts to raise the attributes of the lower self to resonate with the higher ones. These thoughts may even manifest as shock, thus placing a further burden on the will as to the decision whether to battle or to submit. This state confuses the mind, as it no longer has faith in the choices it makes and thus it loses sight of its direction. The more this is allowed to continue the more this chaos in the astral plane will be reflected in the functioning of the solar plexus and thus in behaviour.

The sympathetic nervous system is governed by this centre: feelings and emotions such as anger are what this system responds to. An excess of these emotions can create inappropriate behaviour, which continues to burden Self with more karma, creating yet more chaos on the astral plane and the cycle deepens further. Therefore, pathology in this centre will not be subtle and as already stated, this is where most cancers can be found, as fire burns regardless of care and through necessity. The fire that rages under chaos can at best be very distressing and at worst ultimately destructive. The purpose of these flames is to burn the stubble, feeding the soil so that the dynamism of positive growth can re-establish a new crop. This fire can turn against Self if the individual lacks control of his desires. To remedy this is a very important stage in one's evolution, for this is a point of refinement in order to sanctify the trials of physical existence. This will require resolution before the heart chakra can be liberated with the refined fire which is aligned to solar light. Many, if not most patients will present problems relating to the need for refinement in this centre.

The gallbladder is required as the liver's assistant by acting as its wise guide, the decision maker. If the liver is the ship then the gallbladder is the helm. A congested liver often blinds the gallbladder, usually with pus. This congestion is either the result of miasmatic activity, rich food, allopathic suppression or resentment and the other things already mentioned. Congestion produces a build-up of heat, as well as anger, by which the pus of the liver is baked, using the gallbladder as a kiln, and from which gallstones are produced. The liver is the seat of the fire element, which is fuelled by solar radiation via the spleen and converted from ingested food, coupled with energy being fed from the kidneys. It is the producer of inner combustion, as is the same in all warm-blooded creatures. Anger results when the astral body pushes into the etheric one, the junction of which is the spleen, and the subsequent outpouring of white blood cells lays a destructive siege throughout the body. Fire is the element of reaction; it does not dither but finds its source and acts upon it. For reasons that relate to the gravity of a given situation, when called upon to further ambition, the gallbladder sustains the necessary strength of courage needed by the solar plexus. When change is required, especially by the group and through the vision of the individual, this courage is not produced but maintained by the gallbladder, as it holds the energy steady that rises up from the liver, helping to channel this force in an appropriate direction.

Courage is the force that counters opposition to the will. If the gallbladder is weak then Self's desire to do what is right cannot sustain the velocity created in the liver and thus there will be energy leakage. If there is a lack of fire in the solar plexus then courage will have been eaten away by past events. This dispersed possibility remains formed in astral light but is not given the light of day. Furthermore, this loss of potential on the physical plane perpetuates the weakness of both gallbladder and liver by the inhibited will. This is a centre of warfare, the powerhouse that

Chapter 3 ~ The Solar Plexus

demands an outlet. A weak gallbladder will instil a lack of confidence and poor communication, for emotions will be stifled as will the development of thought. This will also have a knock-on effect in the opposite chakra, the throat centre, inhibiting the manifestation of ideas. This person will be shy and as already mentioned, lack courage. The gallbladder acts as a gatekeeper to the manifestation of personal desires, it ascertains the quality of what will be needed to expand conscious thought arriving via the astral plane and also governs the means by which it can make its presence known. What we thought we wanted is not necessarily what is best for us. The gallbladder is the judge of astral depravity but it can only perform this function if it contains sufficient strength. If the gallbladder is removed, its spiritual counterpart must replace this function. To establish its etheric double in a way that it is capable of achieving the dynamics of the physical counterpart, may take time. The removal of the gallbladder may be the physical manifestation of a pattern of despair that stems back over many lifetimes. Its significance for protection is so important to the body that to have it removed indicates the gravity of the difficult karma involved. It will be the need to re-establish the protection of this centre that will be the link to undoing these previous events. Remedies that pertain to resolving this karma will be required before the spiritual function can take up its place by means of the etheric and astral communication, for it is the aetiology that is the problem, not the removed gallbladder. The physical body will never function one hundred percent and remedies will need to support this loss, perhaps along with other therapies, but before this can happen, the past and the reason for its removal must be resolved.

During sleep the soul leaves the dense body behind along with the etheric body in order that the body may recuperate and repair. This prevents the physical body from diverting precious energy by having to integrate with the faculties of the astral body. During this separation, the astral body is able to enter the astral world for the purpose of exploration. This aspect of Self remains connected to its physical counterpart via what is known as the silver cord, which is attached to the three navels that exist on the three different levels. Whilst away during sleep, this exploration will be an unconscious act, which we call dreaming. The more advanced the soul, the more significance will be placed on these dreams and understood by the candidate. This exploration differs from that of shock where the etheric body is knocked away form its physical counterpart, enabling it to roam outside the physical body whilst never leaving the physical plane. If Self is able to leave its physical body by separating its astral body without first inducing sleep, then this is a valuable means to reenergise and revitalise oneself. What would ordinarily take a whole night's sleep to achieve can be achieved in the space of twenty minutes.

Exiting the body from the solar plexus refers to investigating the Astral Psychic Realm as apposed to opening up at the point of the third eye for the purpose of exploring the causal body and upper echelon (though both are related primarily through the ego or rather its ability to transcend). There is no reason why either can not be practiced, as they are part of one another and Astral Projection can be considered to be an initiation that requires mastering before one has the experience to navigate around the higher planes. Therefore, astral travel really becomes special when its secrets are explored consciously during meditation. It still remains imperative for Self to set up protective measures using light for the duration of the voyage and one's success in this is part of the training. There is much on the astral plane that Self needs to protect against. A sphere of light completely surrounding the traveller will be required in order to prevent any infiltration of astral entities and it needs to be maintained throughout, even during confusion and instability.

Because the astral world appears very much like our own, the Earth being a denser reflection of it, then it is easy to understand its revelations, making it possible to connect with events, actions, people or places from any time, or obtain information on those waiting to manifest. Here one also has the opportunity to meet the dead, past ancestors or to explore one's own past lives. Other non-human beings that resonate on this plane are also to be found here and, of course, those visiting to pass information forth to those humans who can use their astral body as a vehicle to receive it. The person who channels from the lower realm of her higher self whilst in meditation does so by opening up the astral body and offering it as a receptacle for information, often brought by a guide or visiting being. This being does not enter the physical body but because the physical body is a duplicate of the astral body, it reiterates this information on the physical plane. It is not possible for another being to get stuck in one's astral body. If anything has entered the physical body and attached itself within the etheric body, then this is possession, which is something quite different and the result of infiltra-

Chapter 3 ~ The Solar Plexus

tion. There are many souls stuck in the astral world, unable to progress any further and they are quite willing to hitch a ride back to the Earth plane. There are also dark forces that Self uses light to protect against, for it is often in their best interest that the information does not get through. Again, in using light, one will be sufficiently protected but it is also wise to listen to one's guides in order to know that the circumstance for astral travel is right. If it is not, do not open up.

Remember, this is all training for the safe advancement that is to come. The feeding back of information gained from the astral plane may not be straightforward either. It can be quite difficult to verbalise that which resonates easily in astral matter or in the astral body but does not so readily in physical matter. Practice in focusing etheric energy will be required so that life can be given to words or images that have come through to a more dense environment. This is the same for when astral bodies suddenly manifest in the physical world in order to be seen, for they have been able to obtain excess etheric energy that belongs to the aura of this planet.

Information which is generated from the higher planes and descends to those of the lower can be obtained in the astral plane, it being a junction box between the two worlds. The contents of this book will have existed long before writing it and the act of writing enables it to be formed at a conscious level, regardless of its worth, even if it is simply to resolve my personal karma. I should therefore, be able to feel when there is something within it that does not belong or that it is unfinished. We also communicate much to each other in the physical world by this channel but have lost the confidence to recognise this. Those sensitive enough will receive information when something is wrong, especially with a loved one, even though they are not present and there has been no confirmation of it. During this time or at any period of general concern, the astral plane enables one to visit such a person, meeting at a place which is an exact replica of the physical situation and enabling Self to administer comfort between the two souls. The mechanism that enables this is love and it heals the fears of both, often avoiding the proliferation of great anxiety, which is very harmful. If personal injury is too extensive, this can also be a time to say goodbye.

The astral world lies between the elemental and mental realm. An opened sacral centre enables the emotional exploration of one's environment that provides the experience for feelings to be developed in the solar plexus. Thus the solar plexus provides the means by which to bring further clarity to the higher psychic plane. It is within the solar plexus that emotions are felt and are either expressed or repressed. Understanding comes with thought and it is to this process that the etheric and astral body lend power. The healthy maintenance of these two bodies as far as Self is concerned is through thought. The way by which we think is the means by which solar energy and astral light can optimise their uppermost vitality on the human. Only through clarity in the human, as well as in the astral plane, can this be achieved. Emotion is sandwiched between these two bodies and is the product of both the vital and astral faculties, without which emotion would not manifest in humanity.

The etheric world forms a bridge from the dense body to the lower psychic universe (the astral plane), and this is how the astral body connects into the central nervous system, without which there could be no thoughts or feelings. It is within astral consciousness that the full range of emotions, from pleasure to fear, is contained. It could be said that the physical body is a manifestation of the dregs of the etheric body and the astral body is that which was to accumulate from Self, once Self had pushed away from being completely connected to the Divine. The human astral body has an aura of its own with differing shapes and colours pertaining to the differing emotions, and these colours and forms can be used in diagnosis. Negative thought patterns can also be seen and hinder the clean flow of energy between the liver and the spleen and subsequently affect the function of the whole of the solar plexus chakra.

Every object radiates a band of astral light, even the universe, and the Earth's radiation is called the astral plane. When a plant is picked or a tree is felled, as the vegetable kingdom lacks the ability to produce a central nervous system, there is no mechanism to produce pain. There is no free will or compulsion to act and, unlike in the animal kingdom, nothing with which to register the feelings that produce choice. However, as the vegetable kingdom is necessary to the survival of planet Earth, the pain of their destruction will be reflected and felt by the planet in the aura of the Earth's band of astral light. The collective term for astral light is known as Jiva, or cosmic vitality, which pervades every part of the cosmos while acting as a huge sponge. It is that which connects the whole of the cosmos. For this reason it pertains to the ego, both incarnated and that developed by the personality, for it is the life of thought. Choice enables the animal to be hunter-gatherer but it offers no control over pain other than to try and avoid it. The human kingdom does have this potential, but only highly enlightened people are able to have mastery over their astral body, preventing it from otherwise penetrating the lower bodies and thus alarming Self to react through feelings of pain.

THE PANCREAS AND THE COSMOS

The cosmos is a space that is all encompassing. To the human being, its vastness is difficult to comprehend, but the existence of astral light extends to the far corners of the cosmos shining on places about which we have not as yet mastered an understanding. Within it are the energies that are reflected down and felt in the form of emotion, giving a cosmic dimension to our view of ourselves and to the activities of our life here on Earth. These energies stimulate the process of rising above the negative and generate something far more precious in our being. For Self, if there is no sweetness in the cosmos, then there will be no sweetness here on Earth. The receiver and converter of this cosmic vitality and subsequent transmitter through all the subtle bodies, is the pancreas. This organ will detect if the facet of aspiration is missing and this will be indicated by its physical behaviour. The inability to convert sugar or the craving of it, will reflect the lack of sweetness that is being hindered on its way down to one's psyche. In Traditional Chinese Medicine (TCM) the spleen is the centre of digestion, however, in the West we consider the pancreas to be the central organ.

Because the pancreas is the central gland of the solar plexus, it acts as the control centre of the chakra. This gland has much responsibility around the purpose of activity. It receives and thrives on the sense of worth created through the expression of the will and likes to revel in its successes. Its sensitivity controls the amount of fuel that is available at any given time so that cells can obtain power; therefore it is connected to work and the struggles that may make one life more difficult than another. When action is called for, then power should be ready and forthcoming. Doorways in the cosmos should be open for this two way process to respond, which brings direction and clarity and will remain strong as long as one's actions are free to flow. Positive feelings are fed back towards Self where they can be processed by the organs of the solar plexus.

The pancreas is in tune with those energies of bliss that find a way down to the astral plain in the form of memories or as new experiences. They guide aspiration, reminding us that there is something worth working for. They manifest as the 'here and now', so will indicate the level of obstacles if they are blocked and the pleasure of reward when they are overcome. The more one craves sugar, the less one has resolved one's place in the cosmos, which should in itself supply sweet energy. The bigger this void then the bigger the addiction to sugar. The more the fires of this centre can be burnt in the pursuit of purpose, the less one needs a quick hit to stay in touch with the rewards of desire. You may feel that your work does not sweeten your life but perpetuates the struggle. If it is truly what is mapped out, then the pursuit of this work will be also the working through of karmic hurdles. It is simply that some hurdles are greater than others, depending on the life.

The pancreas has two forms of secretion, aligning its function to the dual existence. One is internal and the other external. Digestion is exocrine, the external secretion of digestive enzymes in the form of pancreatic juices that when fed into the small intestine combine with juices of the intestine to help break down protein, carbohydrates and fats. The pancreatic duct runs into the second part of the duodenum and there the liver, gallbladder and pancreas are all interlinked via the bile duct to aid digestion. Bile emitted by the liver is either stored in the gallbladder or is sent down the bile duct where it meets with juices from the pancreatic duct. The pancreas produces bicarbonate in order that its juices neutralise stomach acids that enter the small intestine. The pancreas acts upon the blood by producing building blocks for the body. If we consider the blood as the vehicle of integrity then the rewards of the pancreas will reflect in the quality of the cells. New remedies such as *Hazel* and *Slate* support the pancreas by strengthening this action.

Endocrine function is internal and is how the pancreas regulates insulin, blood sugar levels and insulin receptors in the body. The hormone glucagon breaks down glycogen stored in the liver, which raises blood sugar levels and then insulin converts glycogen into glucose enabling its uptake by all cells to be converted into energy. It is the proper function of the pancreas to maintain the correct levels of sugar in the blood. Diabetes type one occurs when insulin production is inhibited, and in type two the cells no longer recognise the hormone. When either of these occur they mark a significant loss of reward from the task, for cells only respond to that which is correctness. Only the correct alchemical conversion and subsequent use of glucose, the substance in the blood that pertains to cosmic spirit in the dense body, enables the cell to smile.

Chapter 3 ~ The Solar Plexus

MARS

It is because Mars creates the power by which desire can make things happen, that this planet has a crucial role to play during incarnation. It should be remembered that this planet rules the astrological sign Aries as well as Scorpio. Aries marks the beginning of life and the desire to incarnate is the willingness to sacrifice bliss in order to progress. The very expression of Mars energy brings about change. This influence is the same for the higher self as well as the lower self. Therefore, the energy of Mars will have equal bearing on the higher planes of existence, from which its rays are in reality being directed. Fire or light bounces back off humanity. The influence of this powerful fire on the liver stimulates the blood and puts every cell into action. Mars energy knows no boundaries, can see no obstacles and, as revealed by its influence upon Scorpio, induces one with the kind of strength that enables humanity to rise from the ashes. This energy lends courage, stamina and endurance, all wrapped up in a single motivation: to win. It is the energy of self-preservation and at its core is that which ultimately governs our survival.

Mars stands as head of the personality and because it has been let loose to be explored on the planet of desire – Earth, then here it will occupy the battlefield and rage war over who will rule supreme – the personality or spirit as separated by the soul. In our solar system, Mars is positioned one side of the Earth with Venus on the opposite side. Being closer to the sun, Venus has the reserves to raise Mars energy above the animal level and offers Self with choice. This push and pull will continue throughout life until its duality evens itself out into harmony. The nature of this balance within the existence of various groups throughout the world has caused much cruelty and destruction today, as in the past. Mars energy, when applied to religious belief, can become very hierarchical indeed. This is religion expressed purely through the personality and not the road to spiritual enlightenment expressed in working on the chakras. Mars' influence can be fixed, stubborn and determined like its metal – iron, making its fire difficult to put out once it has taken hold. This single-mindedness, by its very nature, when woken by Self, promotes the influence of the solar plexus to act. Where Mars is positioned in the birth chart will indicate how the individual will resolve this balance between the personality and spirit. This is where the desires of the flesh will be taken over by the desires of spirit through the soul. When its position is positive and the solar plexus willing, Mars plays its part in sacrificing the lower manas of the personality in order to aspire to the higher manas. It is the colour red, the colour of the battlefield, that gives prior warning to this event, suggesting that this transformation will not be an easy one but then it would not be a sacrifice if it were not so.

If we put the Moon to one side, as Mars orbits the Sun, it geographically lies next to the Earth and therefore, this makes it easy for the burning embers that stir up syphilitic consequence to catch a ride when called upon. This is achieved as the close proximity of Mars energy allows the syphilitic miasm to influence Earthly karma in order that a reaction can be achieved. In relation to this, if we reconsider time and space, then the rise of the Roman Empire and the rise of the Third Reich happen simultaneously, or put another way, they sit side by side in parallel time dimensions. This is an energetic connection within the evolution of the Earth's karma that will continue until resolved, being played out again and again but in differing dimensions. This is the result of an extreme build up of syphilitic karma that coincided with a high boost of Mars energy absorbed by the Earth's atmosphere in order to bring about change in the name of humanity.

The actions of Mars do not go unnoticed by Venus, the natural harmonic balance to raw fire in the universe, and she will attempt to redress the death and destruction caused by the ongoing power struggle between man and Divine Will, by introducing the qualities of love and beauty to the pot. Karma has to be unravelled by the use of forces in harmony. Mars has long been associated with the Underworld mainly because power can go left or right and thus is feared when placed in the wrong hands. This power is sought and used by both light sources and dark ones, which attach themselves to it and absorb its fire. Direction is most important here, i.e. how we apply this power. Assertiveness, the ability to discriminate, can equally turn from trust into control and further lead to brutal oppression. This can be seen as the battle between spirit and mind, for when overcooked, this dish will be served up as obstinate selfish behaviour. The sacrifice, therefore, is to act for the benefit of others but from the safety of Self.

The sphere on the tree of life, which pertains to the solar plexus centre within the philosophy of the Kabbalah, is Geburah, the sphere of power. Geburah is also known as Pachad, meaning terror or fear. This could be considered as the fear of God or, in reality, the fear to transcend: said to be the beginning of wisdom rising out of the personality and with it

Chapter 3 ~ The Solar Plexus

revealing one's shortcomings, that which the ego would prefer to hide. Intelligence here emanates from the primordial depth of wisdom and this power is tapped into in order that we can go about our magic. It is Mars energy that enables such a transition, for it liberates us from obstacles that would otherwise obstruct our path. On the Kabbalic plan this path is number nineteen. When Mars and Jupiter are placed together, the constructive and destructive principles form a unity, an important piece in the jigsaw of existence that is our universe. When these forces are united, they make the realisation of the secrets of all the activities of the spiritual beings obtainable to Self. On the tree of life, Mars lies on the left pillar, which is, incidentally, feminine and known as the pillar of judgement. We of course tend to perceive Mars in a male manner, that of the warrior, the phallus which is depicted in every culture. This is the male sex principle that the Roman's placed as God over nature, sowing the seeds of humanity. But the true energy of Mars relates to that which is responsible for all creation – feminine energy. The left sided pillar of the Kabbalah is also known as the dark pillar, the pillar of death, in which this feminine energy masquerades as the dark force of male energy. It is the balance between creation and destruction that accompanies feminine energy in order to maintain a balance in the grand scheme of things. Only when there is true harmony in this combination will there be the benefit to mankind in opening the heart chakra and thus the dominance of the male myth will be extinguished.

Chakra Prescribing and Homœopathy

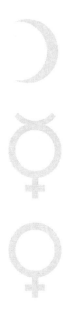

 Chapter 4
The Heart Chakra

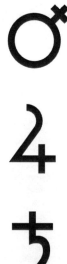

THE HEART CHAKRA

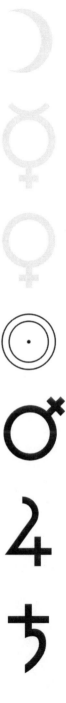

At the heart of our solar system is the Sun. The Sun is the heart within Self and like in the solar system all that which is attributed to Self revolves around the heart chakra. The chakras are lined up in the body along the spine in order that spirit may dip in and out of them. This vertical mapping is constrained by the notion that this energy runs in a straight line, but the spine is simply a line of axis and the chakras do, in fact, spin around themselves and each other. The true interaction that interplays between each chakra on an energetic level is the same as that of the planets, their orbit being held in place by the magnetic forces of the push and pull from the Sun in the centre. Without the Sun at a central position, all existence would not be possible and, therefore, all the connections of existence are made through and around this central linchpin. The heart marks the dividing line between the lower and the higher self. It is the place where one explores the nature of the spirit of personality with the nature of the Divine spirit, as both are of equal importance. This centre is where the lower and higher aspects intertwine and where duality unites to create a purpose that can truly shine.

Each homœopathic remedy consists of some function of the spine or two ends of the same stick, a negative and a positive polarity. The new remedies are needed and have been selected for the reason they resonate with the vibration of our time, having less to do with polarity. They are very specific and remain true to this in their provings so they are prescribed in a very direct way. Prescribing with the chakras in

Chapter 4 ~ The Heart Chakra

mind provides much insight into these new remedies and a framework in which to structure their use. Our time is that of the Aquarian age, of brotherhood, and this is why the new remedies help to induce balance for they speak more about this place of unification at the heart chakra. In this respect, they act much more as a positive and they are also able to enhance this unification in all the chakras. Each chakra is a mini solar system, which contains within it a heart. So when these new remedies are prescribed, being very specific, they can draw much more focus on the particular chakra in whatever way is required for the patient. This will tune the chakra worked upon in order to bring about balance between the others. This balance is a need of our time and there is at present a movement in which homœopathy is being required to incorporate other systems of perception in order to widen its consciousness. In order to enter the Aquarian age, the development of group connections at the heart centre needs to occur. For this to be a success, we will all have to embrace compassion.

To have true love means to have love for all existence, be it dark or light. This does not mean to indulge in the practises of the dark forces or to give them fuel or credence. Neither does it mean to find the light one must start with the dark but it is often so that negative karma can produce great goodness. It means that with only true, unconditional love will light shine through fear and heal. The dark and the light are essentially the same when in balance but are placed in opposition only in their extremes. It may also be noted that by the nature of balance, if there is a lot of light there will equally be a lot of dark. One needs to keep an eye on the other, to have an understanding of each in order for love to create harmony. All is possible at this centre and the more that it is open, the more light will enter into life, inhibiting the attraction of dark forces that stifle a true path. The heart chakra is, in a sense, a vortex of all reasons for existence on every level and so all will crave its attention. Self has choice as to where, when and how the heart directs such great influence and ever since the division between self and divine, this choice has been far greater than we have given it credit. The ability to touch and have influence on every part of the cosmos comes from the power of the Sun and within the heart the level of interaction transcends every other energy if it is truly at one with Divine love.

With every heartbeat we formulate life. This is a wondrous activity and opportunity to cooperate in the connection of humanity with the higher planes. This can only be achieved by doing one's best in the name of love and by this we burn the dross in our own hearts for the benefit of all others, for this is the group with which we are all spiritually related. Every beat is like a beacon which energises Self and radiates to the outer, the quality of the inner. The love that is emanated is not simply for one's partner, one's offspring or one's friends, for these are only an offshoot of the expression of love that has evolved. Love here means that which was at the beginning, the love of all existence, of all humanity, of all spirits, of all gods. When one's heart is truly open then this golden light will change even the most difficult of circumstances. If the heart is strong, then it enables the consequence of significant existence to radiate out to the four corners of the globe. It is that which brings things together, which is existence as it stands, not diluted, reflected or transposed. It is honesty. We say "with all my heart". This is the light of the soul that is connected to the source through the light of the Sun. It is the quality of the heart that makes the person. Spirit has things preordained before it incarnates and it retreats into the heart in order to guide Self through the difficulties of life once in the sanctitude of this temple. The glyph for this centre contains no trace of the cross of matter, the symbol of the earth. It should hold no credence to Earthly considerations as this will only hinder its path. Light is its tool, for it enables spirit to see in the dark. Here there is the unification of inward and outward movements, of the upwards and the downwards, of true belief. It is the junction where north meets south and east meets west, where above greets below – the central spot as in the dot in the centre of the glyph, that of creation, that of the single cell, that of the beginning. This spot is the centre of the six pointed cross, and so represents the seventh mark, the unification of the seven chakras, completion and thus balance.

The work achieved at the solar plexus makes ready the quality of fire that will be required in the pursuit of change at the heart chakra if spirit is to progress. Instead of the nature of this fire remaining that of combustion, as at the solar plexus, it has been transformed into refined ether – light. This light radiates within and without. Being of the Source, it is this fire, which is central to our being; and so has the power to transform the patterns of past mistakes that have burdened Self. It is in the heart chakra where all the negativity of the lower self has an opportunity to be incinerated by such brilliance for the benefit of Self and thus the group. The heart chakra is home to the light and thus is also home to

Chapter 4 ~ The Heart Chakra

its opposing force, the dark. At the beginning and as a result of separation, it was the use of this energy that Self, through its exploration, was so determined to make its own. Love was shown to be an energy in itself, a tool but with independent direction and in order for it to stand out and be given form it had to be recognised along with its opposite or opposition. In the same way that a star can be seen from a distance, it is the dark background that enables us to recognise its shine and this is the same for people. This all prevailing love once having been recognised as having power, came under the jurisdiction of desire, to be owned and controlled. By the notion of placing Self at the centre of creation, it was believed that one could determine one's own fate. First, control was attempted through magic and then later attempts become religions. This control went against the very nature of the forces of light, with belief often becoming dogma and the subsequent downfall of many a civilisation. In the pursuit of development, guided by the changing energies of each root-race, dogma has lead to the release of the most destructive of forces; such is the fine balance between creative purpose and the resistance to it.

The heart was to become the organ that would measure and tune the fine balance of creative purpose within Self. For when the heart is fully open then the soul is in a position of total acceptance; and when closed it is capable of hiding its light under a bushel. The heart has evolved so that it may adjust its focus under the weight of grief and disappointment towards that of an authoritarian stance, in order that Self, in the modern world, may survive and still serve. Such is the magnitude of influence that love has on the subtle bodies, that unification here, with all the differing attributes of life, pertains to the rules of the cosmos. The greater the life has been, the more open the heart. And here lies the dichotomy of this centre, and one of the greatest trials of life. Self has within its hands the secret of existence. It has captured the Holy Grail and within this responsibility there is the paradox, that of division, for how does Self hold on to something without controlling it? The answer is that one can't for it is bigger than Self and Self has had a problem with this equation for a very long time. It is at the heart that the little will has to give itself over to that of Divine will to undertake spiritual growth. Self does not make what light it chooses, but rather it has to use this source like a lantern to gain guidance in the dark. During incarnation there is no conscious Self, so we all forget that what we have learnt may not be the truth and as Self builds consciousness, it thus holds on to what it knows to be true. At the heart centre these structures of false truths are ready to be incinerated, or to put it another way, Self at this juncture, is ready to be shown the light. In a sense we are truly of this life and in its uppermost finery, we are without excuses, as we have come from nothing and it is only consciousness that we seek. At the heart centre, unlike any other centre, Self has at its disposal all that is right and therefore the ultimate guidance and so nothing to lose. Self, however, greatly fears wandering around in darkness, but the irony is that the more one holds on to dogma, the less the light of the lantern illuminates the true path. If faced with a controlling patient, it is the heart chakra that will be closed.

At the age of twenty-one, in the evolution of the cycle of sevens that is life, Self is concerned with its own purpose. We call this time 'the key to the door'. This is the time in which the lower chakras amalgamate and fuse in the pursuit of understanding the higher three. The key opens up the spiritual possibilities through the heart and the resultant expression is unconditional love. This love is universal, the key being the age when the world opens up to this expression in Self, or it could better be expressed, this world is the place in which one can practice this love. In everything we do, the heart chakra radiates its quality and therefore, the making of a person can be detected in even the slightest of tasks. To detect the quality of the heart chakra within a patient one should assess how their tasks benefit others. The purpose of a radiant heart is to make the world a better place. The key is the magic wand, it undoes the lock, opens the door to which all that has been learnt can achieve goodness. At this age Self has achieved adulthood and is mature enough to take on these responsibilities within the complexities of its own life. It will be during the next seven years that the development of adulthood will be expressed through how one begins to make one's mark in the world. This will be for good and bad and it will be the quality of the heart and the flames that now form light, which will be used to readdress this balance in order to maintain one's purpose. This is the period of life before Saturn reappears in the birth chart (around the age of twenty-eight or twenty-nine) and is an indication of the relationship between the heart chakra's role in expressing one's purpose and the help received from the Lord of Karma when this path is strayed from. So important is it to be on the right track during this stage in life, that the timing of Saturn's presence is crucial to the scheme of things. It is a time which should blend

Chapter 4 ~ The Heart Chakra

smoothly with Saturn's watchful eye, for if we compare this to the glyph of the heart centre, it is here that Self has gone full circle. There should at least be an attempt to close the circle in readiness for the protection and guidance required to work on the new spiritual levels. The seven years spent working with the Sun evolves that which the whole sum of Self can provide to humanity. Saturn waits at the other end in order to congratulate progress or clean a muddied signpost.

In the past, a fire would have marked the centre of a home, village or territory. This is the extension of the qualities of the heart centre reflected physically to carry out the same task. Light, which is fire in the heart, was once used for the means of telepathy. The remnant of this in the modern world is television. In the home, the television's flickering light is the new hearth and the new heart of the group in which its movement can be reflected and thus studied. In the heart the flames that burn create an opportunity for re-birth and this is needed and pursued each time the heart centre is purged. The fire in the centre of the group acts in this same way by providing safety and a place to gather around to communicate new ideas within its security. This is also the heart operating within the base chakra, just like attributes of each chakra do in the chakra system. The qualities of existence, which feed Self in order to give life are exactly the same and reflected in the activities of existence here on earth. So the fire of the group also provides the means by which to purge those destructive forces that threaten the group and sends a signal to others to keep away. Also, just like the fire, the heart is the mark of territory and for this reason this centre is often misunderstood. Because this chakra is often locked away in modern life, it creates the wrong impression that the use of its energy is solely personalised. This centre is the link in spirit's need to rise out of the personality and not to be confined within it. This desire enables the power of this centre to be relinquished for the benefit of others, which in turn feeds its way back to achieve personal gain. With it comes the opportunity to rid selfish desires, which are the confines of personal karma that keep one rooted in the personality. To have an open heart and have high function of the heart chakra is to have resolved that which binds us to perpetuate negative karma. Only this can raise the consciousness of humanity. The love we have for another is the love we have of our existence. This is not simply Earthly existence but universal. The need to express this comes in the form of a partner, a family or the group and then extends outwards and encompasses all the kingdoms, the planets and every facet of the cosmos. We have chosen planet Earth to gain this connection and it is where this energy manifests for us in the " here and now". It is for this reason that the true position of the glyph of planet Earth, if superimposed on to the chakra system, would be where the heart chakra lies, in the centre. Earth, in effect, lies directly on top of the Sun. The cross of the Earth glyph forms the axis which joins at the centre spot of the glyph of the heart chakra and lines up with the centre line, which is the spine. So even though there appears to be no sign of matter in the glyph of the heart chakra, when both are transposed together this becomes the universal symbol of the balance between matter and spirit, that of the circle and the cross.

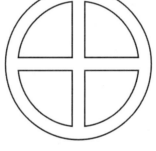

Figure 6. The Solar Cross.

This also hints at the illusory quality of Earth and poses the question as to what is reality. When the circle and cross are apart, it is the syphilitic miasm that results from this separation. It is the resultant consequence of the loss of one's true spiritual home. This is why the planet Earth is placed in the heart charka, because here earthly karma is its template. The psoric miasm also has an involvement here, for although associated primarily with the base chakra, it bleeds into the heart via karma and it will be here that its desperation will be felt. The past is very important as it gives rise to the future, one in which the circle can flourish with the cross.

The heart is a very sacred chamber and when visualised can be seen as a small temple or cave surrounded by jewels and other fine materials which prevents its presence from being hidden, and entices the curious to take a look. It is well protected, for this place represents the overlap of the ascending triangle with the descending one or the two sets of three, which form a six pointed star, the symbol of balance which is at the root of aspiration. Just like the circle of its glyph, a heart chakra is produced

Chapter 4 ~ The Heart Chakra

when a circle is formed for the purpose of meditation. The circle forms a field of protective light and the dot is that which is received as the purpose of the meditation. Like the seed, it is the point of a new beginning referring to the power that the act of meditation can provide. Being the pivotal point of the chakra system, this point requires a good base chakra and a good base working within it, for this centre has to support the higher spiritual triad of the upper three chakras. The heart chakra, as already mentioned, is where fire becomes light, so this centre is still very much associated with ether and therefore it is still considered connected to the physical realm. Also within this sacred chamber that is the heart, many stars can be seen. They are the community of stars that make up the constellations, of which the sun is one and which to us, is the centre. This is why the glyph contains no symbol of the cross, for it hints at the opportunity to become one with the stars, an emancipation from negative karma whilst still being of the Earth. This is to be re-born, with oneself as ambassador to humanity and is also the place where the animal kingdom meets the human kingdom. It provides humanity with the gift of reflection, which is the making of integrity and the highest vibration of the sun's ether.

The meeting of the animal with the human kingdom is an evolution that is key to spiritual enfoldment and it is at the heart centre, through humanity, that the Earth is in direct connection with Divine. To understand this connection imparts much wisdom as to the nature of the hurdles that require jumping to maintain the direction that we are all being asked to follow. Humanity has a choice as to the length of time it wishes to remain with more animal values. It is at the heart chakra that humanity will make these changes. This will be the final interaction of the two triangles. The ability to have reflection of thought is the balance between these two triangles and the division between the human and the animal kingdom. It is that which was bestowed on mankind when the separation by Self was made. The animal has not developed the act of reason and the human is in the process of developing a mind that can explore the nature of consequence or karma through considered action, which is the evolution of creativity. The central point of this division and the root of creative thought is the heart chakra. This is to make conscious that which was not and thus implies the development of humanity. It is at the heart centre that these two worlds meet, that of the desire of the structuring force of the material world and that of the instantaneous energy of the spiritual world. The two together make reflective thought. When something exists only in its unconscious form, it has energy that resonates its potential but once made conscious this energy ceases to exist, it has gone. Therefore, it does not exist as it was and subsequently squeezes into human existence and this effect creates ripples of change that vibrate throughout consciousness.

The heart chakra is the seat of direct consciousness. The level of love also correlates directly to the level of consciousness and this equation is what happens when we treat our patients. We bring into consciousness, through love, that which requires changing. All karma that has laid down what we know as maintaining causes, the circumstances that hinder choices, are open to change by homœopathic remedies. To bring into consciousness that which is negative karma is a release and with it brings a change for the best. This is why at the heart centre there can be the greatest of obstacles for our patients and it is here as practitioners that we need to be wise to those obstacles.

Smell and touch are the two powerful senses that are attributed to the heart chakra and give guidance to the practitioner as to how open the patient's heart is. How the patient receives the touch of a hand, if part of the diagnosis is achieved by looking at hands, can give an immediate indication as to how open the heart is, especially in patients who have been the victim of sexual abuse. The rose is a symbol of an open heart. It expresses one's love and the love which is of central importance to the group which is working on the behalf of the many. The pain of this centre is what the new remedy Pink Rose is primarily used to release, it being strongly associated with releasing karmic pain stored in the heart. Plants that present such beauty in form, colour and smell but are also equipped with sharp thorns have a deep mythical relationship to this pain. Not only is the thorn capable of inflicting a wound but also each subsequent drop of blood is symbolic of the circulatory function of the heart, which may be under much hindrance from the weight of many lifetimes. This image of the thorn can be seen in art forms from all parts of the globe. The level of pain felt from the thorn is a reflection of the level felt in the soul. The new remedies that work on the heart chakra are needed now to release this negative karma of the soul. The subsequent release of love opens up the compassion of the throat centre, awoken by the energy of the heart through the action of healing.

Chapter 4 ~ The Heart Chakra

All healing comes from the heart centre. This is not just to heal oneself but it is here that all healers, including a mother nursing her sick child, work from. It is this energy from which remedies should be prescribed. The greatest of healers marry both the physical and spiritual. This can be associated with the two levels of the heart, the upper part and the lower, which to some can be seen as two separate chakras. The lower is green in colour and the upper gold, which as a colour vibration has also a relationship with the higher triad within the seven chakras. This colour also helps to enlighten the brow with the crown chakra. For the purpose of this book we will stick to the one unified heart chakra that pertains to the colour green. But I will say that the lower heart is associated more to the animal world where senseless feelings of guilt, pride and jealousy are still able to roam free. Of course a shut down throat chakra will also contribute to inhibiting the heart, for being possessive is in effect a lack of compassion and this will not only suffocate the heart of Self but that of another. Jealousy, the expression of the lower heart centre is what will result in the pursuit of constant reassurance. When the upper and lower heart are united, which is a reflection of the upper chakras united with the lower, this produces the power of nurturing. If one can heal from the higher heart then the levels of light at the healer's disposal can be wondrous.

With the inability of allopathic medicine to recognise the qualities that are most important in the work of the heart chakra and its relation to the immune system; coupled with the dynamic and rapid changes in group construction particularly during the last century, it sadly seems inevitable that humanity has had to face consequences such as the AIDS condition. Humanity ignores the needs of the heart at its peril and recent times have seen structures in the West that are purely mind based and materially motivated and which have reverberated around the world through greed. It is not surprising that with most of the modern world built on a lack of feeling and with the dissolution of human interaction, that a disease should ensue which amalgamates all other disease states and expresses the control that the heart centre of humanity feels under at present. With AIDS, the heart chakra is in utter mayhem and this will mean that those diagnosed with AIDS will also have great issues of the heart, usually in the form of deep rejection. It is not the heart chakra which is responsible for creating this state we call AIDS, nor is it the place of origin within the human system but the roots of its inevitability will be found in this chakra. If the disease had pure associations with the lower centres then it would be easier to name it as a virus and thus would be far more easily detectable and manageable. At present the immune system is under great control by western medicine, the like of which has never been seen before. Live bacteria manufactured to remain so by being fed preservatives when in the human blood stream and cultivated on animals with varying different disease states, is an experiment that no biologist has any idea as to its outcome. The greatest experiment with our children and their future is going on right now. This experiment leads to the manifestation of karmic chaos, not only through the interaction of a crossover between the kingdoms, but because this bacteria will surely mutate within the soft tissues. The interaction of disease is complicated enough within their miasmatic relationships, without creating a further pool of confusion from which homœopathy is then expected to pick up the pieces, on top of the already suppressed disease states. This creation is spiritually perverse. It is to be inhibited from the expression of love, and inhibits uniting with the light of Divine Love. Much time has been spent in the physical world by physical thinkers trying to isolate the AIDS virus but to no avail. This is a condition formed by modern life using modern methods of vaccination to repress natural expressions. To be alive means to embrace life, including that which has come before, in order to face that which forms the future and not to be dictated to by the fear of change. The levels of suppressed expression over the years and especially during the twentieth century have placed great insecurity in the heart chakra and subsequent confusion within all the other chakras. It is through the heart that we love and it is here that so much can be destroyed if love is hindered. To purify the heart is to free the soul, and without this the soul can get stuck within the personality, never reaching its rightful place at the heart.

There is much cosmic energy for the purpose of growth, within the higher chakras, and that awaits for Self to pass its test at the heart centre. Clarity is gained as a result of the flames that burn that which would otherwise hinder these cosmic energies. The heart chakra is the seat of physical and spiritual life. It is the amalgamation of the astral body meeting the mental body and where the foot of the throne can be found. It is where Divine love can be crowned within oneself and where all personal karma can be transcended. Burning the dross enables us to rise above the bounds of karma, which is the freedom to exist without being victim of the past and forgiveness, humility and acceptance are the assets that free Self from physical and mental pathology. The dot of the glyph can also be seen to represent a footprint in the sand. Life is very short, so at the heart chakra, the question is asked: with so much to be done, why waste energy stuck in negative attributes? Self, in relation to its time on Earth, is measured at the heart chakra by worth and if lacking, Self will be very vulnerable to disappointment. If repeated, the subsequent feelings of inadequacy make the heart a safe place to withdraw into and hide. The resultant emotion of not feeling good enough inhibits the flow of life, after which Self often compensates by being proud, arrogant and aloof. If this is left to continue, then Self indulges in activities that reflect this lack of self-worth and is thus pulled down into a descending spiral when it should be ascending to the light. This negative process forces Self to retreat further into its cave and subsequently may hide in the dark for good.

LIGHT

The light of the heart centre is feminine, like the creative light of Kundalini, even though that from which it is received, the source, is considered masculine. The mythological legend of King Arthur is a representation of this male energy on Earth and Guinevere represents the feminine, without whom there could be no Arthur. The round table represents the source or the sun. Similarly with the Jesus story, without Mary – the creative mother – there would be no King on Earth. Mary represents Mother Nature, the force of existence and the pattern to which all will eventually adhere. On the tree of life she resides at Binah, as does Saturn. At the Source, there is no separation into male and female attributes as both have found a balance long before and transcended as one. However, here on Earth we are far from the Source and this male manifested energy is under the authority and guidance of the superior female of Divine Mother. Hence Guinevere was once Arthur's sister, before becoming his wife, the marrying of the two energies on Earth. This female energy is also known as the Druid moon goddess Ceridwen, the Awen initiator mother. The Moon, like the soul, is essentially nurturing and mothering and so both are feminine in their energy. The Sun is the masculine luminary, which is the energy of Leo. By representing the Earth, and so also Arthur, as the human body or torso, the Moon in accordance is represented by the head. It is information directed from the higher planes, or the head, that governs earthly activities. This is exactly the same in reference to the astrological birth chart, for where the Moon is placed, will push the person to think in accordance or with the restraints that the position suggests, for it pertains to deep patterns of set behaviour, the emotions that maintain thoughts.

The aura of the heart centre is an amalgamation of all the colours of the other chakras, forming a brilliant white and can therefore be considered a compact version of the collective aura that surrounds the body of Self. This light is an insight into how the initiate receives revelations from one's higher self, or as the Hindus call it from 'the supreme self', that of truth, honour, and absolute reality. The other chakras also have within them all of the colours of the spectrum, for this is how each chakra interacts, requiring the attributes of all the others to enable them to function properly. However, each chakra is true in essence to the colour of the light of its own ray. When the light of the Sun and that of kundalini meet at the heart centre, the ensuing brilliance creates such change that no force can counter it. This coming together creates an influx of mind energy and places an emphasis on thought. There are negative forces that try to counter this exchange long before this meeting can be successful. It is at the heart centre where these forces have the greatest attraction: this is the place that is preyed on the most and this is the place that we and our patients meet the greatest difficulties and the greatest of challenges. Here we are asked to pursue the trust of Divine Light through Self. The heart chakra is the ultimate chamber of the individual Self. It is the cave that pertains to a single soul. In pursuit of Divine Will, the most extraordinary acts of heroism can be achieved here on Earth. To utilise the light of the Sun is to have at one's side primordial wisdom, the energy of the lion. It is wisdom that produces strength and used correctly, it will develop intelligence. This is the relationship between the head and the heart.

The influence of the planets acts upon Self in the form of rays. Each ray is of a single colour and is thus the colour of influence from each planet. The seven rays are the seven veiling forms of the spirits. The laws of the subtle planes are also applicable to the colour rays and the lower their vibration or how still their plane of colour, the more material is their essence, for they too have an atman and a buddhi within them. The planets and the rays are the method by which the higher beings work on humanity and through these rays the seven planetary colours enhance the seven colours of the centres within Self. These

Chapter 4 ~ The Heart Chakra

are the seven lights of the greater to the seven lights of the lesser. Each colour may or may not be more important than another in the development of humanity at a particular moment in time. Each ray can also be potentially significant to the path of an individual throughout his or her life. They are of that ray in vibrational terms, so will carry out their work under its influence. For the individual, each ray is secured in a vault for which the key must be obtained before its colour can be used in its purist sense. To gain the key a portal must be opened but the individual must have placed themselves in a position for the portal to be present. These portals, if they can be seen, form shapes that have been passed down through humanity and often surface, simplified in all sorts of human imagery, including modern as well as earlier art. More than one symbol can open the same portal. In the case of the ray that is most natural to the work of one's spirit, then it is equally a natural progression for spirit to open the portal to obtain its key. However, this is not possible for those out of their bodies, or away from their path or those who are in opposition to their purpose. There are many who have no connection to one ray, let alone any others. Working on the chakras can open up portals and produce a key. Each vault-contained ray is shifting like the planets to which they pertain and thus they deliver the relevant vault to be opened when its significance is called upon and the candidate is ready. The influence of the planets and their rays are upon us all the time. If one can see auras, then this influence can also be detected along with the radiance of the subtle bodies. If one was to look at a birth chart by the planetary auras, the interplay of them as they are positioned in their houses and signs would produce a display or a fingerprint of an interplaying colour formation, much like ink patterns on blotting paper. This at the time of birth is the colour photograph of the alignment of the energies of the universe at that particular minute as seen from Earth and if it can be read, it will give as much information as any other linear method. This influence that appears in the swirling patterns of the planets' colours, can be considered to be in a diluted form or an overview.

The focus of an individual ray can be considered as a concentrated energy field. It is for that reason that the key has to be obtained before Self is ready for such a condensed influence. The inter-weaving, dilution and mixture, which forms other colours has, over the centuries, formed the various different lodges that have arisen from the original colours. These lodges have, under the influence of their rays, tried to inspire civilisation to move onward. The rays, in their mixed form, instigate much confusion in the human psyche and much work has to be achieved in order that the true vibration of their purpose is adhered to without the jeopardising influence of outer forces. In short, the greater the mixture of colour away from its purist version, then the more conscious Self has to be in order to be able to pursue its development and deal with the energy. The energy will also try and inevitably revert back to type, thus dividing into the single planetary colour of its original constituents. This will all depend on humanity's need, even down to a given individual. Green is the colour we associate with the heart chakra in this system but this is not the light of the Sun, as already mentioned, but a reflection from the growth of the Earth – humanity's domain. The amalgamation, which forms true, white light, is a reminder of the Source.

The quality of the seven rays and their manifestation are dependent on seven Creative Hierarchies and are the vehicle of these Hierarchies. There are in total the Twelve Creative Hierarchies that govern the manifestation of humanity, of which five have been liberated, leaving seven in the process of liberating humankind. However, the influence of the other five will still be present in one form or another through experience. This stage of liberation is currently concerned with the spirit in Self but through its development of the mind. In the emblem of the western mystery school of the Rosicrucian Order, the seven red roses reveal that there are still seven Creative Hierarchies active in our development.

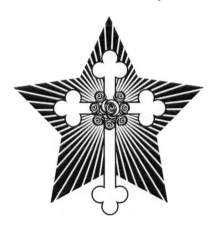

Figure 7. Symbol of the Rosicrucian Fellowship.

Chapter 4 ~ The Heart Chakra

The five liberated one's are products of earlier systems but their work is what has manifested in the lower manas. They are those that were set free when Self separated from Divine and formed the desire to explore, which was from then on, necessary in the development of humanity. So the liberated first five mark the past development, that of the establishment of desire which is now complete and brings humanity to its current concern: the manifestation of thought and reflection before action. This is, in one sense, the path across the abyss in order to liberate the heart chakra from its actions of the past. The light of the Twelve Creative Hierarchies relates to each of the twelve astrological signs and is expressed via the seven planets through the rays in order that the twelve houses may be given life. The home of these Hierarchies can be seen in the sky as the twelve constellations of the stars. From the Earthly point of Stonehenge, all twelve can be seen at once and returning to the glyph of the heart chakra once again, it symbolises the Twelve Hierarchies encircling the logos. Numbers are always significant and the number twelve has importance in relation to the heart chakra. When the five kingdoms – the mineral, vegetable, animal, human and elemental kingdom (the elemental kingdoms generalised as one) – plus the seven lights of humankind are added together, we can see that the constituents of humanity also comply with the figure twelve. If this number is thus added to the Twelve Creative Hierarchies, the total figure is twenty-four. It is only when these are fused, that the whole, the numerical vibration of the light of the Source, is correct. These two numbers, two and four, when reduced form the number six, the number that represents Venus. So the mastering of this light, in chakra language, is the root to Venus, which is to enter spiritual consciousness, and can only be achieved by crossing the abyss. The new remedy *Ivy Berry* will help in the transition towards Venus. Incidentally, the generalised fifth kingdom is that of two layers. There is that which enters the planet and that which leaves, for elementals search for evolution in their designated form until it is gained. Therefore, although there are entities in the pursuit of identity here on Earth, they are equally present in the angelic world. So the elemental kingdom can be split to form the two outer sponges in a layered cake and Self's endeavours connect the cycle by acting as the filling. If the whole of the planetary development through the Earth's life chains are taken into consideration, there are in fact ten kingdoms. This will be elaborated on later within the brow chakra chapter.

It is thought that we are one of a group of seven solar systems and the Divine spiritual entity behind the Sun in our solar system is the Solar Logos. The manifestation of our solar system is said to take on the form of a twelve-petalled lotus and this numerical theme runs through the heart of each level from the Solar Logos right down to the twelve-petalled lotus of the heart chakra within Self. This forms the constant stream of energetic connection from Self to the Source. The Source is consuming fire but also the light of love. It is the font from which all reality drinks. In the pursuit of this light difficulties that require clearing may become evident and here homœopathy has an important role to play. This light is colourless; hence the greater our spirit is raised, the less we resonate to one colour. This opportunity can be seen in the heart of Self, for the amalgamation of the spectrum of colours – which is Divine Love within Self, radiates from the heart. This light awakens one. It does not simply energise the physical but it is the measure of life. It is how 'alive' Self is, as opposed to how dead Self is living. Light is life within us.

Light occurs when Universal Intelligence comes into manifestation. Darkness is the lack of this intelligence. The dark is also expressed as winter and the light summer, where growth is either at its peak, or at its most destitute. Often to bring forth light we have to explore the dark. This may also require exploring that which has been forgotten, the unknown, beyond perception and therefore out of the 'safe' limitations or limited Self. Growth is that which is waiting to be shown the light. The task is thus to change this state by enlightenment but light too is invisible, so to explore it involves trust.

The process of growth requires making light visible whilst also being in the dark, which involves spiritual protection and is what many of the new remedies have been selected to provide. To Madam Blavatski, both light and dark were constituents of 'absolute light', for without one, the other would cease to exist. The balance of the two best describes the untying of the Vishnu granthi. This is a knot (granthi) located at the heart chakra and there are two more granthis, one at the base chakra and the other at the brow chakra. The purpose of these knots are to act as major gateways between differing planes of consciousness which dissolve to allow spirit to venture upwards. This can cause difficulties at the heart chakra, for this knot is closely connected to both negative ancestral and personal karma. But equally as important in the pursuit

Chapter 4 ~ The Heart Chakra

of potential, this knot is also attached to cosmic good and the releasing of its energy during the pathway from twenty-one to twenty-eight years of age, allows healing light to shine on humanity's suffering. The granthi works with the Astral Body in order to achieve this, for part of its dissolution is the liberation from the ego of the individual. Morality is the measure of its resistance. To achieve this release is the ultimate freedom of 'I' that of true Self. It is light that dissolves this knot, so that self-realisation or the wishes of the spirit, as opposed to the ego of the personality, are achieved. In effect, by undoing the Vishnu granthi one is enabled to transcend the genetic code towards complete freedom, which is testament as to how difficult this is to achieve, the last obstacle for the seeker.

The centre point, where north, south, east and west, above and below do not exist in separation, is the point at which we are one with the light of the Source. This is a place of pure existence and harmony, both infinitely small and the size of infinity. This spot – the nucleus of the cell – marks the first point of manifestation for the incarnating Ego or the cosmic ego of Self. It is the first to live and the last to die. It is that piece of Divine spirit in every soul.

Variations of the symbol of the heart chakra have been found throughout differing civilisations, linked in form with the Sun, the two being of the same light, as are, in reality, the two egos. They are both pure potential. All of the kingdoms share this same link with the Source, that of starting with the single cell or the gift. The presence of the Ego can begin to be seen in the radiance of the aura from this centre, which constitutes its subtle body. Here in the heart charka, Ego, via light, inspires the brain in the form of the lower Manas. On the higher levels, Self becomes under the influence of the mental plane, which marks the total movement out of the personality, and yet to be achieved whilst still in the heart chakra. But the heart's resonance is still of great importance in the higher mind, as it links Divine desire to humanity. Experience obtained in the heart chakra requires the rationality of analytical thought processes in order for Self to place the heart and the head at the universal bond where they once were before being divided by the forces of Atlantis. This was the true communication of the fusion of thought with love, which the desires of Atlantis made too unsafe to continue. The Kama Manas, or reflective desire, are the link between the two worlds: that of the world of personal desire; and the mental apparatus that is capable of working within the spirit world. So here, the concrete thoughts that rise from emotional attachment to possessions, such as jealousy, have to be shattered in order to transcend. Feelings that direct towards winning and losing have to be reconciled in order that ascending and descending energy can cross and not get stuck in the abyss. The heart is the bridge between these two worlds; love being so fundamental and encompassing that it is inextinguishable in both the etheric and astral plane and the reason why the heart requires the assistance of the powerhouse of the solar plexus, which it resides next to in the body. The emotion of the heart, therefore, will equally affect the solar plexus and drain it of support, this being why *Ignatia* is such a major spleen remedy. It will also drain the liver, for its vortex has much pull on the astral plane, for this subtle body associated with the astral plane in the human body is directly associated with the function of the heart chakra.

Light sustains life's faith. In Hebrew, the word for magic is kesem, which is very similar to the Hebrew word for money, kesef. Trust in life and you will be rewarded by its magic is the lesson of the heart chakra. It is choice that can fuse these two worlds and the lower Manas are the facility to interpret, through the harmony of emotion and thought, that which is enlightenment for the soul. The heart centre is the centre of spiritual consciousness in mankind. These Manas are mortal and disintegrate during death. However, what will be retained will be the essence of their experience as a result of thought processes being integrated in the form of understanding. This will be held in the Ego and carried forth to venture deeper into the upper realms. The lower Manas are really aspiring to meet the promise of conquest laid down for the remit of the incarnating Ego. This is achieved by the intensity of ether or light that is used at this centre.

As the soul is concerned with the gathering of human experience, which is associated to the manas, then the twelve astrological signs are the splitting of human expression into twelve manageable ways. Beneath these are further subtle layers of interaction that make up the whole and fit precisely for the relationship of each individual during their time on Earth. The point to this expression is to feed the higher self and reach to the highest point of human existence, where spirit entwines with the Logos. The twelve disciples represent this same connection, for they are a subdivision of the Holy Spirit for which Christ acts as a vehicle. The twelve disciples, when joined, form the Son of God. If we take the

Chapter 4 ~ The Heart Chakra

scene of the Last Supper, the soul is represented by the room, and the twelve disciples represent all the facets that the soul must explore before it can transcend, gaining a position in the work being carried out on the higher planes. This work is unachievable whilst here on Earth for only its influence is manifest here on a lower level. The amalgamation of the twelve disciples expressed as metaphor, is wisdom. This is wisdom that for Self is the quality of the amalgamation of the four lower chakras with the higher three. It is the soul that illumines the mind and creates such wisdom. Each astrological sign rules differing attributes which Self needs to evolve in order to concentrate its activities purely in the higher realms. As already mentioned, the number twelve has much significance here in the heart centre. The lotus flower of this chakra is said to have twelve petals and the heart is enclosed for protection within a cage of twelve ribs formed from a twelve-sectioned vertebrae. There are twelve constellations and it has been speculated that there are twelve planets within our solar system under the central gravitational pull of the Sun. It is the twelve constellations or Creative Hierarchies, working through their represented planets, that manifest exoterically in the form of the influence of the zodiac signs. Their influence is of the closest physical connection to this planet. The heart is the cave here on Earth in which, by ritual, the energies of the Twelve Creative Hierarchies that energise the solar system can manifest through Self. Most forms of rituals and ceremonies are an attempt to facilitate this manifestation and the group usually forms itself into a heart by means of a circle. The dot in the centre represents the channel of new consciousness that is being received and brought down to manifest in the world. Being a portal, this is also the point at which spirits that are trapped here on Earth can be helped to leave, for the channel enables them to rise and reunite. This is the same as the pillar of light used in meditation to reach out of the body and gain ascendance. When spirit has risen to the higher levels it obtains partnership with Divine through the Creative Hierarchies in the pursuit of all knowledge.

It is that which we love that guides our emotional intelligence, that which is embedded in the heart as well as the head. Our learning has much to do with aspiration and is why we have great love for those who have inspired us through their teaching. Here is true learning. Where that which is the truth gets passed on in the form of knowledge from teacher to pupil. Something happens in this transference of possession, for it is then under the influence of a new day. It is for the pupil then to become teacher in order for the new to have relevance. In the northern hemisphere the Sun rises in the east and sets in the west. This is the age long process of enlightenment. With the Sun comes potential and with its passing comes knowledge. It is a process that is at its most powerful during the ancient rituals at Stonehenge each summer solstice. It is the light of a new Sun that when focused on the brow centre, opens the heart so that the old wisdom is ready to receive the new. With light comes enlightenment and the rays of truth that are carried in the air are the gifts of life. The moment of this knowing, of realisation, is the amalgamation of the higher planes with those of the lower one's. Intelligence of the heart unified with the head is the love of brotherhood and it is intellectual arrogance or ignorance that destroys this connection. Air is the key element here, bringing inspiration, logic and fast moving light, which is the combination of head and heart. Air is the medium through which humanity is able to take in and utilise light. Air is the element of etheric love, for its composite is not simply to oxygenate the body, for humanity requires more from it than the animal. Contained within is the "spirit of life" and it is this which denotes reflection or it is the "spirit of life" that humanity can reflect upon. Air is the vehicle for this and it is what we make of it that separates humanity fully from the lower kingdoms. Air can only be found within the Earth's stratosphere in our solar system, placing humanity at the heart of conscious development. It is, therefore, our thoughts that exhaust our vitality during day to day existence by the absorption of light into the nervous system. Recording the quality of the patient's thoughts is thus very important during the homoeopathic diagnosis. The heart in connection with the immune system through the power of love means that patients who have autoimmune diseases will be struggling on issues in their lives around love. Air and thus oxygen and prana that is taken into the body by the lungs, is under the jurisdiction of the right side of the body. The left side is responsible for the distribution of blood around the body, which through the heart results in the holding and passing of spirit. Spirit binds both blood and air and in meditation a controlled breath expands consciousness and deep breathing oxygenates both our thoughts and our feelings, which are then distributed throughout to every cell. The physical body dies without this delivery by the heart and circulatory system. All the other subtle bodies are also dependent on this process, as the

Chapter 4 ~ The Heart Chakra

heart is the centre of spiritual nourishment and because its connection runs up through all planes to the Source, the quality of this nourishment has been granted such governance.

THE THYMUS GLAND, THE BLUEPRINT OF KARMA

An open heart requires the wisdom of experience to judge how appropriate it is to explore a situation as opposed to gaining protection against it. It is considered that between the ages of twenty-one and twenty-eight, Self is able to explore the world with an open heart, having now gained the experience to make such an assessment. As a child and during the development of the base chakra, Self is insufficiently experienced to make such judgements, and subsequently is very open to many new experiences. At this time the heart requires protection in order that it is not lead astray or placed under the influence of dark forces whilst the child learns the balance of saying yes or no in building its own authority. It is the thymus gland that is responsible for the protection of the child during this vulnerable time. At the heart centre the thymus gland acts as doorkeeper to energies entering the heart, absorbing that which is inappropriate before it becomes party to the heart and causes damage. An understanding of the heart and its true function is imperative in understanding the function of the thymus gland. The heart is central to achievement here on Earth and thus its quality is uppermost in maintaining the needs of the soul. Its radiance should be naturally brilliant, but most commonly this is achieved through great personal work. The thymus gland maintains the potential of this quality, before Self has mastered protection through judgement. During childhood the gland remains open and then starts to atrophy before puberty and finally relinquishes its power during the development of the solar plexus. Problems can occur if the thymus is damaged or does not atrophy. Criminals waiting on Death Row in America have been tested and many are reported to have thymus glands that have remained open. The closing of this gland is part of the process of growing up, of judging right from wrong. Damage to the thymus does not always prevent its atrophy, although it usually does, but equally alarming for the welfare of humanity is that damage prevents the gland from protecting the child in that the heart remains wide open. The main causes of such damage are vaccinations, mechanical accidents, tumours, severe trauma and allopathic drugging like steroids and antibiotics. The repetition of fevers during childhood is a sign of thymus damage and a sign that syphilitic influence has been allowed to advance and fill the heart. The heart chakra is the centre which under such an attack has the most to lose. As each one of us makes a difference, this damage has repercussions that feed into the detriment of this planet. The most common form of thymus damage comes from the insidious consequence of vaccinations. This is why those who have knowledge of their devastation are so opposed to their use.

Remedies that help to correct this damage are *Thymus Gland, Jet, Hornbeam, Black Obsidian, Berlin Wall, Ayahuasca, Red, Green, Blue, Yellow* or a combination of these colours, *Mimosa, Japanese Oleander (White)*, all the vaccinations that have been administered given in potency and all radiation remedies. Because the syphilitic miasm is the central root to all the miasms, then if the damage to the thymus goes very deep, it will stir up such a miasmatic cocktail that nosodes may at first be the only means to touch this.

It could be suggested that all pathology pertains to shock: the result of having something inflicted on Self that it is not ready for or is never meant to be ready for. This could be considered as a definition for the notion of negative karma. The result of this will have consequence and it is exactly the same for inoculations – the body goes into shock. Shock has its part in encouraging readjustment as it is a reaction to being confronted by reality but it doesn't have to be so destructive. If the reaction is very harmful, then this may take many lifetimes to heal, more so if the cycle is repeated. This is the same for self-acceptance: healing the thymus gland begins with being honest about who one is. This does not mean that one cannot change but quite the reverse, for this is the beginning of change and it refers to not being shocked by what one is. We have lost so much of this connection because modern society has not the tools in order to cope with this level of acceptance. In eliminating the possibility for shock, it is far easier to embrace with honesty and integrity that which needs to change. When it comes to undoing negative karma, one has to recognise it and not be swamped by the fear of it, for it is part of Self. Therefore, to follow one's path, one has to be in full acceptance of all that this entails. The dark can only become light once light has been shone upon it, so in knowing oneself, one cannot be dragged into something that is far from being oneself. In the case of

Chapter 4 ~ The Heart Chakra

inoculations, this means one ceases to be attracted to them.

If there is shock then one has been lied to and coming out of shock is the acceptance of the truth. Homœopathy helps avoid this shock of the truth and enables a smoother transition, for we are all on differing levels of consciousness with differing karma. What is meant by the phrase, 'you are not ready' is unfortunately now too prevalent. This has to change in light of the Age of Aquarius. No longer are the truths that we have been living under or had instilled by group leaders holding up. Therefore, such leaders are incorporating ever-increasing extreme measures to re-instil our faith. We have to be wise to this, for it increases the level of shock because it is designed to disarm us through fear and destroy the individual. Inevitably, when the truth of what has really happened arises, which it always does; this creates another shock and the subsequent reaction of trauma, grief, anger, etc. These days we all live amongst so much shock that the subsequent insecurity motivates many to increase the material gain in order to create the illusion of security and not trust in one's path. In the short term, this avoids having to address the repercussions of stress in the heart chakra. This of course does not make people happy but illustrates how trauma within the heart chakra plays out in the base chakra. This is why many patients who come in a state of shock, unbeknown to them, think they are only bearing physical pathology. When one detects the shock, one may think a prescription of base remedies will help bring them back into their bodies. But this can prove to be futile as there is too much fear going on at the heart chakra. Remember, this chakra is the centre of the universe, the centre to its alignment and from where all the governing forces project in order that all the positions are maintained. The thymus is the record of these readjustments. Therefore, it is often required to firstly address this shock held deep in the heart and then ground the patient using base or other remedies as a support. The reverberation of released waves of energy from the heart will thus have an aligning effect on all the other chakras. It now seems that in order to deal with the new rules, structures and formats that are undermining the base chakra that the heart must first be relieved of these consequences. This is because trauma that has been laid down in the rapid expansion of the last two centuries has left its mark on the sensitivity of the heart chakra. A closed, fearful heart with a damaged thymus gland not only parasitically takes over the base of another, like a cuckoo looking for a nest, but also ends up destroying all the nests around it. Conversely, poor base function destroys the heart by hindering the thymus and denying the life path.

Damage to the thymus gland has consequence for the whole group and so its proper function should be of concern to us all. The dark forces that pertain to syphilis fill the child with dark sludge and leave the soul rendered helpless under its control. If you ask this child to justify its actions, the reply will offer nothing other than the expression of numbness. When the heart is consumed by this bleakness then it inhibits purpose and thus the child is unable to feel the consequence of her actions towards her fellow human beings. It is useless to preach to these children, and also later to them as adults. What is required is work at the heart centre to free it of its dark constraints. The thymus will also be in need of repair for it will have the connections to this sticky mess between it and the heart. These two are not separate in function and nor are they separate in influence. To visualise what is going on here, one has to picture the deepest of dark spaces, filled with the deepest of dark karma. The clearing of both will result in the proper functioning of the thymus gland and an opening to joy in the heart. Joy is the most important energy in the function of these two working in harmony together and can be used as a benchmark as to how lovingly a person interacts. To clear this centre of dark syphilitic influence may not be as straightforward as it appears and it will require the utmost co-operation from the patient. Again, the test is to clear the negative forces of the abyss and so involves the patient trusting in Divine will.

The thymus gland contains the blueprint of karma. The purpose of incarnations, and all of that which has not been cleared through the act of redemption, is written and contained in its passages. Like a great tunnel that extends to the beginning of Self's inhabitancy in this universe, all that has been shaped for good or bad is written down its walls. This is the tunnel to the heart and negative karma will burden the pathway for Self and those connected to Self. In Kabbalic philosophy this is known as the abyss and is mostly associated to the sphere of Da'ath. It is the path where most fall when its crossing is not achieved correctly. The new remedy *Chalice Well*, along with *Holly Berry* and *Thymus Gland* will give much support in this crossing, and of course *Ayahuasca*. The abyss contains our greatest darkness and thus our greatest difficulties. It is not possible to intellectualise this, for crossing this void means to work through much that goes beyond rational feelings and normal events.

To work through negative karma means that experiences that to all

Chapter 4 ~ The Heart Chakra

sense and purpose appear external and happen externally, like an accident, are in fact being governed by internal events. During this crossing, events are pushed furthest from Self in the disbelief that they can have anything to do with such inner bleakness. To undertake work here is to balance the exoteric with the esoteric by undoing negative karma that pertains to this gland. The thymus can be described as being filled with energy that if manifested materially would be as bleak and disabling as being waist high in tar. The density of its destructive potential is dependent on the individual's past. The thymus gland is where all the hard work placed on clearing and balancing the chakras has most potential to fail. Kundalini, as already mentioned, is female in its creative energy. This energy when it enters the thymus gland is that which instigates renewal; it requires the transformation of dark into light, for spirit could not survive in such a place. This can be extremely alarming for the soul if this is practised too quickly and without wise support: the level and pace of revelations are simply too much to bear all at once. Many have done great work in achieving lifetimes of clearance here but the negative forces are liable to do their utmost to corrupt this. Others, mainly through ignorance and a lack of respect, have tried and failed, resulting in madness or even death. Female energy is destructive in nature: it needs to be in order to sustain life. When expressed at the thymus gland death is possible. When working on the thymus of the patient, if something is likely to come to the surface to be dealt with during the normal course of prescribing, it is more likely to arise when working here.

Working on the chakras in meditation should be done slowly, starting at the earthly end with the base chakra. This order is not the same when using knowledge of the chakras to prescribe on because the subtlety of the remedies will gently work on the weaker chakra in order to bring it in to balance. This makes it possible to work on blocks within a chakra at any stage. This is the same for the thymus gland. If remedies are needed that pertain directly to its function, there is no reason why the damage here cannot be addressed first, this is especially true with children. However, a word of caution, for within the thymus gland there may lie the answer as to why a patient is determined not to change and is frightened to move on in life. These will be very difficult karmic blocks. These blocks may lie hidden deep under the symptom picture and the process of their exposure by working at the thymus make it possible that all the problems and symptoms that relate to what the patient presented with during their first visit, may return. It is like hitting a raw karmic nerve and the patient then retreats back to using all the previous powers of resistance to avoid change. This of course, on the whole does not usually happen, but it can, and it is not a matter of potency, it is a matter of the past. It is important when working on the thymus gland to remember that this is where the karmic blueprint is contained and so much may lie within, which is beyond the normal powers of perception. One needs to intuit when the time is right and, I reiterate, this can be on the first appointment. Some of the new remedies like *Orange* are not of great use when given as a first prescription. The patient is simply not yet sufficiently spiritually tuned in, in order to bring his energy into consciousness. Much sadness and deep grief can be hidden in the thymus, the result of trauma that has long been left in the archives of time. This needs to be released before the patient feels able to continue along their road. It will usually rear its head during treatment and it is the purpose of the prescriber to recognise this. To understand the workings of the heart chakra brings much enlightenment to prescribing.

At the thymus we have an area about our person that is the collection point of all the actions of Earthly Self, which was and still remains part of the commitment made when independence was born. Most, if not all the difficult karma of the thymus was laid down during the activities of Atlantis and it is the karma of this root-race that has given birth to much subsequent karma, of equally dire consequence. The indulgence of Atlantis fed the problems that humanity is trying to wrestle with today. Regardless of colour, creed or religion, we are all trying to reach the light, the Source where we feel truly loved. In this respect, we can only do our best. It is our negative karma that gets in the way and it is also this karma, as a collective, that prevents us from walking safely in the world, open to everything as it was before Atlantis. This open state is what humanity is striving to re-accomplish and it will not be achieved without understanding the activities of the past, which are stored in the thymus gland. We are all ultimately responsible for our actions, but there still remains divine guidance. At the heart chakra guidance enters in the form of spiritual nourishment. It will be the contents of the thymus gland that prevent one from seeing this and thus the symptoms of a swamped thymus are the inability to do what's right for Self, others and so for humanity.

The importance of the correct function of the thymus gland cannot

Chapter 4 ~ The Heart Chakra

be over-estimated for it acts as the spiritual doorkeeper. It attracts and is likely to contain entities. This is especially true of the souls of foetuses that have been terminated, for it is through this area that they leave and can get stuck, which will create confusion within the relationship of its parents. Specifically, a combination of *Thymus Gland*, the musical note *Middle C* and *Ayahuaska* can be used to release these souls. *Middle C* is one of the notes pertaining to the seven-stringed Druid harp, and this remedy will have encapsulated its origin by means of intent. Each string is the sound of a colour ray and resonates to the soul the sound of the seven blessed planets. Generally, a combination of *Syphilinum*, *Ayahuaska*, *Holly Berry* and *Moonstone* will be required to assist other entities in moving on. If this fails, *Berlin Wall* in high potency should be given first in alternation with *Thuja* cm, *Anacardium* 50m and *Syphilinum* 10m, not in any particular order other than that perceived or intuited, leaving three weeks between each remedy. This complete prescription should be repeated three times in succession. When such entities are present, it usually means that part of the protective aura of a person has been blown open. *Syphilinum*, *Ayahuaska* and *Ignatia* help to reseal the aura, which is imperative if a recurrence of the problem is to be avoided. Although the thymus pertains more to male energy and thus the male of the species (the thyroid pertaining more to the female), the act of giving birth, for the mother, clears much in the way of negative karma from the thymus gland. This relationship between the mother and Mother Earth is that of being the container of Earthly karma. It means that this gland is given the opportunity to cleanse itself in order that the correct level of nurturing can be present to welcome the incoming child. The new child also greets this situation and adds to it by presenting the opportunity for re-birth in the family in every sense. This energy has to be passed on to the male who is often not privy to such developments and can often feel the most disturbed by the changes. A father who is tuned in to the mother will naturally feel the trust and the growth.

The thymus gland acts as a bridge between the heart and throat and can be perceived as a chakra in its own right. In some esoteric philosophy and Kabbalic writings it has been suggested that its true placing is at the throat chakra and this centre can manifest severe repercussions when the thymus gland is clearing. The function of the thymus also helps the throat chakra to create spiritual manifestation through the development of individualism, which is lost when this gland is damaged. All that has been made of oneself is here in containment for reasons of safety. Damage to the thymus gland breaks this security so takes one very far away from being oneself. Individualism or to be Self is required in the quest of purpose. Ill-health is the organisation's failure to manifest purpose and therefore individualism is very important for the connection with the world of higher desire, that of the higher manas. This connection is maintained even when there is atrophy of this gland on the physical plane.

The thymus helps to usher in adulthood and for this reason it is known as 'the gland of maturity'. A clue to the fact that its spiritual function does not retreat is reflected in the dense body by the continued production of T cells that feed the blood via this gland. The thymus is responsible in helping to organise and build the immune system, and it is where the endocrine system meets the immune system, which the remedy *Lotus* pertains to. This is the focal point in which the inner world meets the outer. It helps to hold back puberty and continues to keep all the other endocrine glands in check along with the pineal gland, until the birth of the desire body at the age of around fourteen years. From then onwards, its contents can be expanded upon in order for Self to explore its individualism. This gland is the link between parental karma and personal karma, from ancestral to individual, and thus when this gland atrophies then the sex glands take over in readiness to pass on the genes. The thymus has a fundamental link with the work of Divine guidance and thus the crown charka: the two in theory should be opposites but their interaction is imperative in progressing through the seven chakras.

It is relatively easy to spot the physical symptoms of a child who is overrun by the negative karma of a damaged thymus gland. There are often tubercular symptoms of the lungs, nose and throat, accompanied by a fragile, pale, porcelain-like complexion and prominent blue veins. The suspicion that there may be thymus damage usually starts in what is seen in the child's eyes. The lack of morality or even a possession will prompt the practitioner to look away. Later as the child grows into adulthood, it will be the reverse: the adult will not wish to make contact let alone meet your gaze. Deep trauma at any age blows the thymus open and breaks down the protective layer of aura, allowing the unwanted to enter. The gland does one of two things when damaged, it ceases to atrophy or it becomes enlarged, acting as the overflow to the heart. If the damage to the gland results in its enlargement, sexual development will be early and there will be a tendency towards aggression

Chapter 4 ~ The Heart Chakra

with a marked increase in libido and selfish, dark indulgences. During the first consultation I may enquire whether the patient had any difficulties around the time of puberty and this is invariably met with a puzzled response. Problems as a result of puberty are an indication of thymus damage. There will also be secrecy way beyond the bounds of normality, so never expect a truthful response. Also there is often perversion, especially of a sexual nature, coupled with immaturity. This immaturity leads to emotional dependency, especially in men towards their mothers, and who subsequently go on to chose a wife to replace their mother. Dependency is due to great fear and as adults this often manifests as fear of disease and so the emotional dependency may become a dependency on the medical profession. This is the gland of maturity as already mentioned, which enables the transition from child into adulthood by absorbing and containing the pain of early life. If this pain is great it will be buried deep within the heart chakra. In trauma such as sexual abuse, then the energy of all the chakras will become buried in the heart centre and as a means of compensating through the personality, this may only be detected in minute patterns of behaviour. The practitioner may have to be given information by indirect means to detect this. The level of trauma can remain hidden from one lifetime to the next; such is the power here to masquerade. Its effect will pass from one generation to the next, as this is one of the reasons for the child choosing the parents. All can appear well but underneath there will be a cauldron of trouble, stored up and desperately waiting for an opportunity to find expression. This energy is not likely to take the direct route or to make itself visible. It is underhand, for it contains no spiritual attachment. Therefore the way it is spread down the genes is by the most invisible means. Before a society has time to realise what is afoot then it is upon them. It is this syphilitic foundation to which all the other miasms are a reaction. Just like the Sun within the solar system, the other miasms orbit around its presence, feeding off its energy, depending on the degree of infiltration.

The thymus gland, like the thyroid gland, is very sensitive to radiation, which destroys light and weakens growth. Damage here lets in the very stuff that hinders love and acceptance, which is the energy that is needed in order to conquer that which has invaded. If not contained in the gland this negative energy overflows into the heart and the lungs and also makes Self feel extremely vulnerable. Therefore to heal this requires spiritual help in order to re-link with the heart and radiate in the world. It is the protection of the thymus gland that provides a sense of belonging, the ability to interact and to feel a part of the world. It is this spiritual relationship that is taken away if the thymus is damaged, cutting off that natural connection and creating a person removed but dependent at the same time. Without this connection to humanity there is no desire to celebrate its finer aspects and no justification as to involvement in its progression, especially on an artistic or cultural level. There will, however, be an obsession with material gain and this will often manifest through an affiliation with a particular group or identity, which although very important in maintaining stability, provides permission to behave or feel the same way in which the group does. It is safety in numbers that will be used to justify behaviour. Often this group will have a badge or a mark of identity: this can range from a sports badge to the right set of golf clubs in the back of the 'right' car. Identity is very powerful in the relationship Self has with what has come before. A lack of individuality creates the desire to blend with the rest, or be a part of a group in which one can hide and collectively turn against the individual. To be an individual means to have an open heart and it is these people who leave their true mark in society.

Collective pain experienced by trying to maintain an open heart in the face of great animosity over many lifetimes, will burden the thymus gland. The remedy *Healing Ritual* will be needed here. In such a situation, frustration results if one's karma is acting against Self and this will be coupled with the fear that things can't get better, for repetition has locked the soul in turmoil. The karma resulting from persecution runs very deep: this can lead to a desperate state and where the remedy *Thymus Gland* is needed to release the patient. *Thymus Gland* as a remedy can also be used to help replace Prozac while the patient develops new openings for natural expression, when further remedies will be needed. This remedy helps to take away the fear of individualism by reinforcing the bond of "Universal Brotherhood", which in its physical manifestation is the thymus gland, linking morality and protection against the dark. When we work on this centre we have to acknowledge this, for the route towards the light will require the freeing of negative karma.

THE HEART, SYPHILIS AND SELF

The Syphilitic miasm was formed out of the first hindrance of love. The flow of love between early humanity was constant and interwoven

Chapter 4 ~ The Heart Chakra

between each soul, with each heart linked as one universal heart. Each soul delved in and out of each heart, not only as a way of communication, but as a natural form of existence without the boundaries that we have today. The heart was a meeting place where sacred communication was open and available to all; there was nothing to hide. As a result of the development of individual consciousness, soul communication became a very private affair between Self and personal karma. It was not so much that the transference of love became prevented but the notion of Self as something separate had developed. The syphilitic miasm is central to this discovery and is the result of the individuality of Self being formed. Previously, humanity was bound together only by Divine consciousness and so manifested a completely open heart: this is only possible with such consciousness. There was no awareness of Self until the premise on which the syphilitic miasm was to manifest, came into being. This was the awareness that Self is not God and thus there had to be separation. Once this spark of enlightenment that marked the beginning of human consciousness had occurred, it was not possible to be anything other than Self, be it in any variant stage of completeness. The insecurity of this awareness led to the structures supporting individualism that were to reverberate throughout the cosmos.

Power is of the Source and it had now become open to the perception of Self. It was this power that would be of total concern to developing humanity from then on until the need arose to start the Wisdom School and the Love School, but this first stage was the one in which Self had to grapple with the notion of the power from its first awakening, and is known as the Power School. Self no longer perceived ownership of power as the prerogative of the Source, though in truth it is. Under the illusion that it could exclude itself from any constraints, Self went about placing itself as centre of the universe in order to understand power. Before truly understanding anything, it must first be experienced. This development may have been inevitable as a result of the pact that was to see creativity subsequently flowing from both Source and Self: an evolutionary process. It could be presumed that if Self has something to gain, it equally has something to lose. This is the myth of loss at the heart chakra and the energy that perpetuates the syphilitic miasm. Essentially there is nothing to lose and only consciousness to gain, which can never be lost, even as the lower manas dissolve. True power at the level of the soul is to come from nothing, to have nothing and thus have nothing to lose. What came first was the desire to have choice, then arose the delusion that Self had something to be taken away. Thus the desire to replace this was only felt to be possible through the act of becoming worthy once more. The myth of loss is felt in the heart centre and subsequently the Syphphilitic miasm is the mother of all tears.

During the Lemurian Age, the heart was not so highly developed and the material existence of today would have been very alien to its function: it would have been far too vulnerable to survive. Hence its form and the structures of tissue were also very different from the heart of today's world. The heart has undergone many changes which have been appropriate in maintaining its function, as Earthly karma, of which Self's consciousness is a part, has evolved. This is not Darwinism: we were never a cross-species, nor were we ever apes. Apes have always been a separate part of the animal kingdom and of a lower development, which were never intended to be human, even if it were possible. Nor were we ever of fully animal origin prior to the evolution of the human kingdom. The evolution of species has solely been about their connection through the inhabitance of the planet Earth and not who grew out of what. Human beings have always been of a separate entity. The arbitrary way in which people using a vision that extends no further than that of assumption have pieced huge periods of development together, drives a wedge between science and spiritual wisdom. It was as a result of the division made between personal karma and ancestral karma that humanity evolved into separate genders and the pleasure of sex formed two pairing reciprocators, one male and the other female. Ancestral energy was thus able to flow in and out and be passed on in this manner, as opposed to being contained principally within the heart chakra.

As part of its evolution, the heart was now to concern itself much more with the protection of the soul through personal karma. Prior to the start of individualism, as mentioned, group consciousness was more interlinked through the heart centre. The subsequent evolution of the Lemurians, in their pursuit of choice, began making many divisions within the life force, resulting in the creation of further facets of light and dark energy which would be explored fully later. The heart could never have remained so open within such volatile curiosity. Even today, the heart is in a never ending cycle of adjustment as to what the world contains, which to the heart is its fourth force of influence, a never ending turmoil. This will be expanded upon later in this Chapter.

Chapter 4 ~ The Heart Chakra

The notion that one's spirit was in fact separate from the group, came from the advent of action that went against Divine will. This is the separation by which Self became conscious of its own will. Will is in fact one, it is complete and is the same on every level, be it of mankind or Divine, even if directed away from its true source. This is what humanity is having to learn because it believes there are two separate wills, that of free will and Divine will, and it has been the struggle with this that has given rise to the syphilitic miasm. This belief in free will is more than the act of becoming aware that Self is separate from Divine. It was to go further by denying that Self was under the control of Divine will, or that Divine will even exists. Allowing this spiritual denouncement gave rise to the birth of the syphilitic miasm. Because of the separation of Self from the Source, and through fear of being of two distinctly differing entities, Self seeks control in order to re-establish trust, but this only serves to cast the soul further from Divine spirit. There is only one will, that of Divine will, and there is the syphilitic miasm: all other miasms are a subdivision of this. This oppression marks the syphilitic miasm as the first miasm to be planted in humanity's evolutionary garden. The formation of further actions would embellish the magnitude of the miasmatic influence by the principles of karmic laws. In a split moment that reaches beyond the notion of time, mankind became aware that it too could be party to the creative process, that of builder (the Creative Hierarchies), creator and destroyer of existence and thus controller of events. This to Self was to act as God, or at least believe it could replicate this energy. The thinking arose that desire, in which all manifestation is built, could be generated by Self and not of God's making. Desire became a question of judgement, as to whom does it belong and what is its purpose. Judgement is the result of the misinterpretation that there are two separate wills in existence and subsequently, the desire to be God was never to leave Self, for the realisation that this would never happen created the insecurity of being neither one nor the other. To eliminate the syphilitic miasm is to dissolve this desire to be God. This awareness had brought forth a new feeling, that of despair. Thus began the process of mimicking Divine power in a conscious effort to replicate its image into the evolution of humanity. Christ, Buddha and others were all ways in which Self could pull Divine consciousness down to act as a model for itself in order to limit this feeling of despair. The result seems to be a never-ending exercise in the pursuit of the notion of perfection.

As soon as spirit became self-conscious, aspiration was formed. This is the division, all it took was a microsecond of acknowledgement and the change had been made, from Divine consciousness to self-consciousness. It was now here to behold, to be dealt with; it had come to pass. The expansion of human consciousness and the evolution of the planet was decreed. The pain and the suffering of future trauma became part of humanity's path and Self found it increasingly difficult to maintain blind faith without any justification. Self had no means to remember. Each root-race would face a new set of challenges that under such perils, became difficult to escape. What was at stake was the notion of a single Source and yet how could it stand by and allow such atrocities? Self had something to blame other than its own judgement, even though it had instigated the structures to maintain judgement as being of its own. It appears that humanity's battle with Divine guidance is what will remain of the planet Earth in every sense. For Mother Earth, a creative force in the cosmos, the repercussions of this struggle will be raging on the higher planes, creating a morphosis of changing energies, the full purpose of which is beyond our knowledge.

It has been made plain to humanity that evolution through the exploration of the root-races is designed to complete the circle from whence it began. This is for the greater good and enabling humanity to once again unite under a single consciousness. As to the reason for this in the grand scheme of things and what is to come after, we can only speculate. Perhaps there are souls that can receive answers on that matter. What we can assume is that the relationship between Self and the Source will have changed, and this means the Source will have changed in order for there to be unification. Perhaps this is the point to it all. The syphilitic miasm in its perverse way is a vessel to acquire such consciousness, for it too has two ends to its stick. This cannot be denied, and it has to be recognised so that its karmic consequence can be brought into the light and a balance formed. This will not be easy and the results of syphilitically induced action may take a long time to redeem. This miasm is often associated with genius. Genius is the culmination of a long road of gathering experience through many lifetimes of having to reconcile a deeply damning situation: then in a single lifetime this reconciliation or genius appears as something to share. The prescribing of the syphilitic nosode is extremely important in enabling a person with such experience to manage it.

If love is denied then its subsequent relationship with Self puts self-

Chapter 4 ~ The Heart Chakra

worth into question and thus begins a cycle. It is karma that prevents us from loving and being loved and nothing more. It is in the heart centre that the karma of the past must be cleared and then a new direction can be let in. This is why heart remedies are so effective in enabling people to move on in their lives.

The development of the heart brought with it the notion of an opposite with which to fall in love. The heart receives the love of all and this became a need to have it reflected in one other. When there is too much pain in the heart, then life often becomes a process of living through another, as we see in the *Natrum Mur* picture. As the division between the activities of the Earth and the Source widened, humanity became further conscious of its actions. Development is the process of becoming conscious, so karma was inevitable when humanity got to sample consequence. Ethics are not just a question of morality but also a question of health. The energies of Self are the result of its actions, and the product of its desires. These energies and life are one and the same, as is the little will and Divine will, it being only the polarities of extremes that change. This establishes the importance in the connection between the heart and the base chakra, for karma makes no judgement as to the quantity of how right or wrong something is, but is only a gauge as to the extremes. It is the karmic lords that sit in judgement over those decisions, for when we hand our truth over to another, be it human or a force, then the result will surely reflect in the auras of all the vital bodies. This can only be the result of deep syphilitic karma.

The psoric miasm was not the first miasm to spring out of the evolutionary cycle of humanity. Neither was it the first to bring about separation, but it did result from the insecurity that Self felt when first aware of that division: from the awareness that Self is an entity in its own right. The psoric miasm does not stem from the desire to be separate but from the struggle for survival that resulted from this separation. It is the resultant insecurity of fledgling independence coupled with the new demand to become conscious that has brought about fear. But first and central to all the miasmatic energies is the syphilitic miasm, for without its presence there would only be unity and the expansion of mankind would not have manifested. Neither would there be the need to develop the seven vital bodies and the seven chakras and all that is reflected thereby on the higher planes. The miasms are an intricate part of the act of regaining connection to the Divine. The syphilitic miasm is not the fear of change but the fear of no-thing. This miasm, which is within all people, cannot bear to do nothing and this usually means individuals becoming involved in other people's karma. To them, taking on other peoples 'stuff' is an attraction, a way to rid or distract from what they cannot abide within themselves. It is the pain, the anger and the disbelief that grew out of the question; if I am not God then who am I? Realisation brings with it much responsibility. This is the moment of choice, of identity. The psoric miasm grew from the insecurity of having the choice; it is not the driving force of the choices, for this is the syphilitic miasm. Real choice should come with the flow of trust.

The separation from Divine spirit and the resultant behaviour made humans karmically ready to awaken the mind. The group felt the pull of the love that grew out of a stronger connection to planet Earth and with it came the desire to be God on Earth, which is to be King. With the newly awoken mind and the development of Self, judgement became the tool of desire in the absence of Divine authority. It was what the mind had to expand upon. This within the widening gulf of the separation from light and dark meant it became crucial to judge one's Self and others. Never before had such an emphasis been placed on the development of the conscious mind and the insecurity of this need for discrimination gave further opportunity to the psoric miasm. If the psoric miasm was formed from the division of consciousness between that of the cosmic whole (unity) and that of Self; it was during the Lemurian age that its expression would scream to the stars and its subsequent suppression through the evolution of the mind influenced the structures of all the subtle bodies. This included, most fundamentally, the mind as representative of the individual having authority over the function of the sympathetic nervous system. It was through the evolving balance of instinct and the human will that this miasm was to cavort. Meanwhile, further development of the mind was to become fuelled by Self wishing to mimic Divine power. To have knowledge of the light means to have knowledge of its opposite, the dark. In order to develop the mind, light and dark are perceived as two separate entities and the means in which they have been explored only confirmed this development karmically. In such a development, not all beings were to remain on the same level and this would have a profound consequence as to the distribution of what was perceived as power. Once it is realised that one could not be what one thought one was, the subsequent exploration is the making of what one can become.

Chapter 4 ~ The Heart Chakra

What arose in Atlantis was the scenario in which one had power over another person or group, which manifested through gain or its offspring: protection. This became the energetic peak of the materialism of the Power School. Such an emergence was not possible without the proliferation of the syphilitic miasm and the consequence evoked an eruption in the battle of light versus dark forces that, through karma, has introduced a further shackle to spirit in its pursuit of Divine enlightenment. It is difficult to imagine the levels of destruction that were at work during the Atlantian root-race and to understand the methods that were used against conflicting souls, by what we would call black magic. To comprehend this depth of derangement, one only needs to look at the legacy that has been left in the world today and throughout the recorded history of mankind. To guard against total destruction it became imperative, through the formation of the Vishnu Granthi, to protect and preserve the good of ancient wisdom. As more protection was required, the more this knot became entangled in layers of subterfuge, making its secrets almost impossible to unravel. Before Atlantis, the soul of the group and the souls of its individuals were in less need of protection, for they were closer to the initial separation. They were also closer to living in harmony with the energies and structures of the cosmos, albeit unconsciously. The word 'united' implies the fact that the heart chakra is safe to be open. This of course had to change and with it the duality of light versus dark was intensified: the protection of the heart became a necessity. What entered or projected from the heart needed to become under the scrutiny of Self and therefore its contents required Self to maintain secrets. Humanity had changed. The interaction of love was now distinctly different and the emphasis of trust had never been such an important commodity, since the separation of Self. Selection was the new consequence of the pain of Atlantis and this need for protection changed the way in which the heart was to respond: the heart now had a choice between the need for greater protection and thus shutting down if too open, and making the judgement as to when it was safe to open up.

The expression of the heart in the individual is a reflection of the heart of the group. Secrecy became important in the protection of the knowledge that formed the wisdom of the group. The greater the refinement of wisdom, the stronger the act of security would be. The keeping, partaking and teaching of such knowledge led to the Mystery Schools. These were forums where knowledge that would only belong to a particular group, united as it were as one heart, could be taught in the utmost secrecy. No fixed meeting place was ever kept and candidates were strictly vetted as to their integrity. The heart was now not only divided from Source but also divided into discrete pockets of humanity. Secrets had become imperative in the pursuit of maintaining a connection with the light. Such groups used ceremonies to gain guidance and prepare them in the pursuit of their desires which they believed would benefit humanity. In part their insights prepared them for the forming of the new lands that were to rise up out of the sea. These were the promised lands that were the result of the desire to rid Atlantis of corruption. The true motivation was not the notion that the dark could be left behind forever, for the teachings were most instructive as to the true inclusion of dark and light forces: but the search for pastures new was an attempt to shed the dark karma that had already produced the possibility of invasion within every soul.

The Mystery Schools played a major part in maintaining the esoteric knowledge that we have today. Each group fled what was to be the ruin of Atlantis and spread out onto the new lands, which were to be the footings for the new conditions of a changing world, that of the fifth root-race, which is still evolving today. The Mystery Schools continued the development of understanding, which subsequently increased the changes of the planet, the universe and, we can suppose, the cosmos. Each group had to work with the energy of their place, time and forefathers – the bloodline of their school. These would be the trials that shaped their focus, common to all the groups wherever they settled, in order to maintain contact with Divine.

The ritual of joining a group was no easy task and was the confluence between the purpose of the individual on the one hand and the needs of a particular group on the other. Entering a group meant swearing allegiance to what was known as the 'brotherhood'. Brotherhood was formed through the intensification of knowledge and enabled the group to grow. Standing at the threshold of the Age of Aquarius, it is the same principle, the desire to gain knowledge for the greater good, which is the force that is bringing people together. This Age is about exploring the nature of brotherhood and disseminating what were secrets through the joining of ideas. The rivers fed by the early Mystery Schools are still flowing, albeit more like a steady trickle, but it will be during this age that their resurrection will challenge the established practice of selfishness and the dogma that supports it. It is dogma that suffocates the heart and creates hardness in the absence of spiritual flow. This new

Chapter 4 ~ The Heart Chakra

energy will confront all rigid structures that maintain outdated methods of social conditioning, for they will no longer be relevant. Generations are coming through in order to confront the old and prepare for change. Schools, workplaces, prisons and all manner of social establishments will need to become more appropriate to the new group dynamic. This does not mean the individual is irrelevant, humanity is still very much concerned with the development of the individual but the interaction and understanding is changing.

The mystical heart, secure and hidden behind its cage of ribs and muscle, is able to harness the light of the Source and was replicated by groups during Atlantis by the formation of temples. Religions were also flourishing at this time but the Mystery Schools were groups of pure science (in the true sense of the word) and only when they were to evolve in the fifth root-race did they build temples for places of worship. An example of a temple acting as a heart chakra and the principle from which such buildings have been created, is the house in which Christ eats his last supper. If this house is representative of the heart, then the dining room, as already mentioned, represents the soul and the twelve disciples are the twelve facets to the soul's route of enlightenment. The true meaning of the last supper is a story of induction rather than betrayal, which enables spirit to be shown the way home once the work of emancipation between the twelve has been completed. The temple is the ultimate testimony to the change within the psyche of humanity that has reverberated throughout the cosmos. It is a sacred place in which it is safe and possible to worship, a place where one could focus the forces of light and reach up to Divine love without fear of recrimination. When we place ourselves within it, the temple becomes a heart within a heart; a safe vessel in which the heart is free to open, to reach out, a place where the soul is able to once again have that from above down here on Earth. When Self connects with the duality of these two, it is free to meditate on the nature of consequence. Without such places, Divine could no longer entrust humanity in the name of co-creator, leaving insight in the hands of just a few, which is not very effective in spreading to the many the importance of creative force in the New Age. It was the Mystery Schools that sowed the seeds of the later civilisations that were to become the fifth root-race by the information that had been entrusted to them. Like all root-races the shoots of new growth are born out of the circumstances of the previous race. In Atlantis there were a few who were enlightened with this information and knew how imperative it was that it may be interpreted with quality so it became their duty to pass on such information.

That which is of spiritual significance can only be passed on to humanity if it is kept alive in the heart. The act of knowing is contained in one's heart and is the fundamental connection between the head and the heart. Today those of the highest morality, who have integrity of ethics and aspire to the highest altruism, keep or have kept such important qualities alive throughout the human kingdom. This is a thankless task, unconditional as it has to be, for once the motivation changes to personal gain its mastery is lost and the door becomes open to manipulation. This is true science: the ability to observe, to perceive using all possible faculties, in order that the conscious results bring us closer to, rather than further from uniting with the truth. The structure of the Mystery Schools had at their centre the theme that they should be a reflection of the higher levels. Therefore the intention was that the practices enabled the greater good of all energy, the complete cosmos, to be brought into physical existence. The ancient insights and the resonance of this completeness are still at work today. From this come the perceptions that provide healers who can practice on every level. It is the heart centre that is associated with nobility and so the strength of the connection between the head and the heart in the pursuit of the truth, makes the noblest of persons. These were people of the Schools who had no fixed time other than being of their time but were able to exercise ancient knowledge and mix it with the new. Those of the Mystery Schools were able to move without any constrains of censorship for they had nothing of material substance to lose – no physical possessions or fixed building of residence – and therefore were able to speak freely without the fear of being controlled. There are still groups that operate like this today and the students are not constrained or lured by any gain other than that of wisdom.

Even though the dark became motivation in itself and the consequences were justified to those who explored it, and thus necessity brought individualisation of the heart to every one in the form of protection; there were beings, in the form of Earthly guides, who could walk the Earth totally free of animalistic desires and remain interlinked with all of our hearts: they are known as the Mahatmas. They are still able to see that which is hidden from us and receive insight into the true mysteries that

Chapter 4 ~ The Heart Chakra

have been twisted by syphilitic karma. They are gifted with the purest of vision and their task is to make conscious these visions that are beyond normal comprehension. They stay true to heart consciousness, allowing humans to forgive and embrace their fellow beings with love. There is no need for them to reincarnate to gain enlightenment, they simply return when needed for the good of humanity, to provide guidance and wisdom. This manifestation by their spirit without reincarnation occurs by inhabiting a body just as the previous owner has left, so it does not appear that the original person has died. This enables their return to be swift for, unlike us, there is no need to take the time to evolve a body through the process of chakra development as they have already obtained extensive levels of consciousness. According to the laws of duality the Mahatmas have an opposite: these are the Brothers of the Shadow. They are detectable by their vested interest in things that appear to have nothing to do with them. They are determined to prevent liberation from material desires and because homœopathy is all about the alchemy of transformation, this may explain why homœopathy has faced such opposition. A full amalgamation of the relevance of all the various past schools of mystery into the modern world is yet to happen and some still hold true to the past, to the old Power School. The Brothers of the Shadow use the egos of others as the source of their work, in order to practice the art of seduction through the power of suggestion, to control freedom and feed negativity. As homœopaths, every so often we may be confronted by one of their representatives rising to disprove homœopathy through us and this is capable of playing havoc with a practice if it is not protected.

The purpose of the Mahatmas are not to become gurus but to be used as guides enabling each individual to understand their spiritual path, which is the challenge of the heart centre. Our patients may present at this time of challenge and thus ask for assistance, for this is the point of separation from the material world to which such patients are too attached, resulting in the fear of the progression into the spiritual realm. This transition asks but one question, which often remains a quest too far for many: this is to relinquish the instruction of the will of the lower self and to place unconditional trust in the will of the Divine. This is in effect what the whole group failed to achieve during the reign of Atlantis, marking the end of the forth root-race, and what the Mahatmas try to encourage in us with the knowledge that if all were reunited at this point then universal spirit would return to Earth.

Atlantis was not an underwater world but was taken into the sea as an act of Divine purification, the memory of which can still be witnessed in ceremonies today. It is only the entities still attached to Atlantis, and unable to leave, which keep its presence alive through their influence and give us the impression that it was an amphibious city. It was, in fact, a great land mass with a sizeable population of many millions. The growth in population had started in Lemurian times and had through the act of sex, expanded rapidly, for sex was an integral part to much of the sorcery of Atlantis. The downfall of Atlantis marked the beginning of the pull of the physical planet, the start of the significance of gravity to the species, which meant judgement became embedded in matter. The great city becoming too heavy and burdened with dark energy was pulled into the waves to be purified, forming the notion of hell below and heaven above; that which has much in common with the new remedies *Lotus* and *Green*. The conscious notion of a separate dark as opposed to light was complete. The war that instigated this submergence was an attempt to amalgamate the two by fire, from which much dross would be burnt before its time was lost into the sea forever.

THE LOVE SCHOOL

As humanity evolved, its quest was driven by curiosity to make the unknown conscious, to understand Self's relationship with the Source. This understanding developed through three great cycles of change, for understanding produces change. The working of these three different strands of awareness was to place humanity in the correct position to enable it to resonate more closely with the creative pursuits of the Source. This can be understood as the one, the three above and the seven below, which is the source and its division. The first of these strands, as already mentioned, was the Power School and the second started by the formation of the Egyptian dynasties. This was the Love School. The evolution of the structure of the heart coincided with, or was governed by, the evolution of humanity's relationship to the Sun. The Sun provides nourishment from the Source and the capacity to assimilate this was found to increase with its worship. During the vast evolutionary jump that occurred during the three stages of the Egyptian reign, many Sun Gods were worshipped. The homing in to the single one – Aten, recognised by the symbol of the disk, brought about an enormous leap in humanity's evolution.

Chapter 4 ~ The Heart Chakra

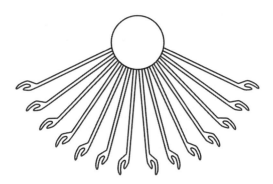

Figure 8. Egyptian God Aten with a Human Hand on the End of Each Ray.

This consciousness shift was to have great effect on the heart. The amalgamation of the Sun Gods homogenised all the levels of radiance and therefore all levels of worship. The notion of one supreme Sun was later overthrown during the reign of Tutankhamen but by then this was too late in terms of evolutionary consciousness. Humanity had became aware of the Sun's position as the centre of human existence and by doing so came the insight of the heart being the recipient of this responsibility – that the heart is the storeroom of Divine love within Self.

The structural changes to the physical heart that occurred towards the end of the Atlantean Era were in preparation for the changes that were to happen in the Egyptian period and through the teachings of what is known as the Love School. Through the Love School much information was received as to the source of creation, the meaning of love and the circumstances that lead to all existence. This knowledge was pursued and passed on by the teachings of the Memphite schools. They revealed that the key to existence is that love becomes light, which in turn, becomes life. But what was crucial to this awareness was that light manifested from the heart and enlightenment was achieved by living the light received from the heart. So the greater the love, then the greater the knowledge which leads to greater deeds. This is the path to enlightenment, for it is the heart that appeals with love for the light of the Sun to in turn provide life. The greatest return for this is the good of actions. The Love School speaks of this balance. Too much sentiment (heart) is wasteful of thought (mind): and too much mind is the absence of love. The foundations of Egypt were built with a new group consciousness, which was to shape its civilisation through the development of the Love School. This school recognised and pursued the understanding of the power of the heart and its association with the Sun. Its aim was to develop the channelling of love energy in order to make changes in humanity. Unfortunately, not all the high priests were averse to corruption and some ignored the cultivation of the higher desires and pursued that which the amalgamation of power and love could provide in the way of selfish pursuits for the gratification of the lower desires: this behaviour was infectious.

Under the spell of oppressive and controlling behaviour, the Egyptians began to misuse the teachings and believed that Divine Love was such that it could be used to achieve things other than its rightful expression. The Egyptians began to care less about the greater purpose and more about wealth and decadence and, by means of ruthless social structures, a few were determined to hold on to this wealth. To achieve this these leaders suppressed love amongst their nation, for these few were aware that the road to enlightenment by the many would create a distribution of this power and greater freedom. In many ways these structures of suppression are still with us today. Secrecy and wealth that alienates love are still the chosen methods of suppressing a society. In an evolutionary sense we have not developed that far from those old structures.

In preparation for the Egyptian dynasties the heart had had to change to achieve that which it was not originally equipped to do and so as a result of the forces placed upon it, a physical transformation was instigated, forming the four chambers of the heart. These enabled Self to incorporate the karma that such pursuits demanded. Selfishness meant that no longer was the heart to be nourished in quite the same way through the group, but this was to be achieved via more individual methods. Worship was always controlled and the harsh pressures of day-to-day existence were allowed to continue to deter the mass of population from expanding their practice for reasons of loyalty. Slowly as Egypt evolved, the corrupted pharaohs became nothing more than figureheads, who were replaced by those who were leaders of war. Faith and trust in the powers of creation were suppressed by fear in the hearts of the very people that humanity needed to not get stuck in this turning point that abandoned spiritual motivation for that of material attachment. Many of those who were chosen to be guardians

Chapter 4 ~ The Heart Chakra

of the Sangraal and thus lead the rest out of this mire, were themselves also pulled in by the temptation of material enticements and the fear of what may happen if they themselves were to go against the shadow. After all its attempts in the earlier dynasties, Egypt was still fuelled by the negative desires that had destroyed Atlantis. This spiritual suppression was to produce the greatest of structural changes in the heart and thus in the way the human cell was to be nourished to this day. The Egyptians noted these structural changes and this is why the heart was given such high significance during mummification.

The heart was very vulnerable to the increase of negative karma that was building during the actions of Atlantis. The consequence meant that an individual's light and the transference of its life-giving properties became, for reasons of protection, a very internalised affair. Like a wedge being driven into a single block of stone, this change was necessary in human evolution, for it forced the heart to split into a left and a right. The wedge, in turn, formed the third chamber, that of the fire element. The left chamber now pertained to the water element and the right to earth. It was the fire that separated these two elements but also made it possible to sustain life within a protected sphere. Earth and water may contain the easiest of harmonic compatibilities between the elements, excluding their role as part of a balanced whole, but they require fire to push their possibility through. Without this, there is only a muddy sludge and no growth. The fourth chamber was created by atmospheric pressure and from it the tubercular miasm was formed.

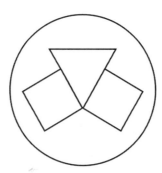

Figure 9. The Forming of the Four Chambered Human Heart.

The tubercular miasm represents the purpose to life but taken or pushed too far, so much so, that one is out of touch with what the purpose was in the first place; hence the depression associated with it. In this situation, what one doesn't understand tends to be dismissed, for this is what happens if Self cannot accept the limitations of Divine will. Life is then used up without containing any substance, leaving a hollow space behind. This is reflected in the base chakra, being the chakra that reflects light into matter and so can be detected in the tissue, primarily the lungs which are a component of the heart chakra and where the synthesis of oxygenation is carried out. The limits of Divine will are encompassed in what can be achieved in one lifetime as determined by one's purpose. Not even homœopathy can change this – speed up karma yes, but not overstep the boundaries of purpose. Because of the symbiotic relationship between fire and air, the tubercular miasm appears very much like the syphilitic miasm in character, for as we can see it is none other than a further extension to the syphilitic miasm – a reaction which can create much confusion when differentiating between the two for the purpose of prescribing. Although similar, they are separate, and need the correct counterpart when being prescribed for. The understanding as to the division of the heart can give much guidance in making that differentiation.

Self had to learn how to balance the four elements within the heart, for their consequence was now reflected in life. The pressure of air acting upon the forces that were now internalised through the new formation in the heart, maintained the elements in a constant state of existence. Such was the result of the new constraints on the heart and thus on humanity in the new age. The central wedge is that of human karma, the stone is that of matter and the weight of human emotion, and their containment is the force acting on the three – Divine will. The positive point to these changes was to allow these forces – that had been metamorphosed and re-rooted under mankind's nose – to be studied and made conscious by Self in order to be privy to the secrets of creation. The consequence of the changes was to create readiness, as always, for the next stage which is the development of consciousness. The third force, the wedge, needs careful balance as to the degree in which it can split the heart completely apart and from which, as an extension to this, the actions of negative karma can divide humanity or the heart of the group.

The absorption and distribution of light in the heart had changed to incorporate a new level of individuality, which had to compensate

Chapter 4 ~ The Heart Chakra

for humanity's movement towards a greater level of restriction. Each chamber of the heart was now governed by one of the four elements, the building blocks of existence, that when joined produced the fifth element, that of life. The maintenance of these elements pertains to the varying degrees of refined light contained by the heart chakra. The exact amount in vibrational terms, of each element in balance to another and distributed by the blood to each cell, is preordained. The life of the cell will depend on the precise combination of these elements being fed to it, in relation to that being demanded of the planets as they feed down the wishes of the cosmos. The balance of these elements can be read and predicted in a daily astrological chart. This alchemy is carried out in the heart when the blood circulates within it and its precision is the code that transforms light through love so that life can fit the individual person. The greater the human desire that is pulled into the personality, then the greater is the pressure on each element to maintain a balance in which to manifest a purposeful life.

The establishment of this stage in the heart's evolution readied it for what was to be the deep divide between Self and Divine will. Those who believed they had jurisdiction over the cosmos had effectively invited in the shadow. A gate had been opened to the unexplored territory of the psychic space and that allowed in the destructive part of human nature. This materialised only because it was compatible with the forces already in existence in the law of nature. Corruption on the lower planes has to be counterbalanced on the higher ones and the disease and destruction that resulted from the new representatives of Divine Love being prevented from taking their place, erupted on Earth in the form of the Ten Plagues. This threat to all individuals was a lesson to those who thought they were safe and had the power to ignore the important teachings of the Love School. Disharmony between the four elements was the tool used to create the plagues, a reflection of the lack of their balance in the heart of humanity. Humanity had divided these elements for the use in destructive magic and now this separation was bearing fruit. Even though the Love School had provided much to the nature of the inner workings of Self's relationship with the Source, its relevance had to be fully felt through the plagues before its significance could be understood and above all, be respected. This mark of respect and the bowing to its supremacy paved the way for the beginning of the third school, the Wisdom School, developed in ancient Greece. It has been during this present cycle of the fifth root-race that the heart has undergone the transformation from power to love in order to incorporate its role within wisdom.

Since the separation of Self, one has had to learn how to share one's heart on an ever-increasing hostile planet. This divide between Self and Divine split the heart vertically and manifested a world divided by left and right. The right side of the heart is the seat of psycho-physical consciousness and in the left resides Atma (spirit) or Divine within. The direction of their expression reflects that of the structure of ascending and descending energies of the cosmos, placing the heart and the Sun as centre of our universe. Logic and spirit meet as right and left respectively in order, at this placement, to act as one; but remember the forces of karma have always separated these two for Self. These forces acting upon the other are like the Sun's magnetic swirl around which all the parts pertaining to Self are fixed. The transformation of the balance of the elements in the heart and the changes left over from the old structures are still in the process of development today. Many people will need spider remedies, especially the Black Widow (*Latrodectus Mactans*) in helping to dissolve fear that arises when clearing the old structures of the heart. The new remedy, *Healing Ritual* will also be needed to balance the four elements with the four corners of the world.

THE SUN AND ITS RADIANCE AS NUMBER ONE

In most numerological systems, the heart represents the number one, the symbol of Unity. If this number is present in either the date of birth or when the birth numbers are added together to form the life number, then its qualities are said to be attributed to that individual. Such individuals are often good social communicators either in speech or writing and love to interact with as many people as possible. They usually have a sunny disposition and like to be the centre of radiance and the place in which all things revolve or come back to. These people come with a task in mind and do their utmost to complete it. The more the number of one's contained in the date of birth then the greater the opportunity to create real achievement. However, this desire becomes internalised if frustrated by life blocks: and can manifest in the expression of morbid thought, as the energy of the Sun needs a vibrant outlet. The mind becomes over-radiated with thought and mentally burns up if thoughts are not put into action or are thwarted. This is why people with lots of

Chapter 4 ~ The Heart Chakra

ones often need regular doses of *Carcinosin*. It may not be that simple to recognise these people for you may only see their sunny side in the practice room, because number one is "I", own heart, own mind and they will tend to keep their worries private. 'I' is where the soul resides between the ego and spirit to nourish them both. This relationship can be seen clearly in Chinese astrology as it pertains more to numerology than western astrology. In the Chinese system, the Sun is ruler of the palace of the year of the horse. The palace is said to house four lodges or Star-Spirits: Jing, Gui, Liu and Xing. Those born in the year of the horse strive forward in life powered by the Sun, using the energy of these Star-Spirits in order to root out injustice, which in turn, feeds their own spirit. Neither retreat nor aggression is an option for those born under the year of the horse, so difficult karma may impede intention that can lead to deep depression. Like those with a strong influence of the Sun, horses are not preoccupied with the love of a partner but are much more concerned with what love can achieve for the greater whole.

Our Sun is the largest object in the solar system, housing ninety-nine point eight percent of its total mass. The Sun's inner core makes up twenty five percent of its mass and even though as humans we can make what is deemed to be accurate predictions as to its atmosphere, the true nature of this place is beyond any comprehension other than its spiritual significance. On its physical level, energy is produced by nuclear fusion and this is emitted to Earth in the form of radiation. It is the Earth's atmosphere that protects life from the harmful levels of radiation and, like any other aura, it is dependent on the health of its body. This is a symbiotic relationship, for without light there would be no aura and without aura anything can enter. The Sun emits various levels of beams of light and depending on their refinement, they will extend to the far quarters of the universe. Each star lights up a passage by which we can explore the universe. The Sun, like Self, places its awareness on what belongs to it, that which is in progress and in the here and now. This is its magnetic field and that which it feeds through light, including all the planets, their satellites and that beyond. It has been estimated that since the formation of our solar system the output of energy from the Sun has increased by forty percent. This increase of luminosity may go some way to explain the increase in the consciousness of humanity.

When the human race is under change then planet Earth is bombarded by charged particles of electrons and protons. This is known as

Solar Wind which when emitted by solar flares appear as high streams of fire reaching out higher than the natural circumference of the Sun. Light, as we know, instigates action and the effect on humanity of these flares causes much upheaval. This kind of transition can be found in the proving of *Stonehenge Sol*. Plans, promises, thoughts and ideas that have been held back will suddenly come into fruition after using this remedy. Any sudden increase in power creates electrical surges and the heightened atmosphere creates interference and change within all aspects of life until what needs to be tuned comes into alignment in order to maintain the new atmosphere and equilibrium is restored once again. Nature's way of instigating change is to work with these atmospheres: This is never a wise time to rely on things being set in stone. From Earth, these beautiful surges, for they are beautiful gifts, can be seen when they interact with our atmosphere in the form of the 'Northern Lights' or below the equator as the 'Aurora Australis'- collectively the Aurora Borealis.

Sun spot activity does not remain constant but it is required, especially by humanity, in order that the Earth's progress is energised. When there is a lack of hot spots then there are much colder temperatures for longer periods, as has happened historically. These cool periods can be severe, especially to those areas north of the equator and are known as an ice age. The atmosphere of the Earth is wholly dependent on the Sun and the pivot of its axis that further maintains this relationship is kept in precision by the counterbalance of its doting mother – the Moon. When there is a complete solar eclipse we get a chance to witness this profound relationship, revealed through the mathematics of these three globes. The Moon matches up precisely to the sphere of the Sun, as seen from Earth, testimony to the subtlety of the strength of feminine energy, where something so refined is capable, if only for a short time, in taking command over the light. During a solar eclipse the Moon reveals its secret and is the reason why this event holds such profound curiosity when witnessed by humanity; for the light of the material world is an illusion and when hidden, life does continue to exist. The total eclipse is an opportunity to glimpse and have confirmed the existence of this other side. It relieves Self of the fear of darkness or no-thing, so that once again it can have trust. Day turns into night but is still day, as in the reality of the unity of dark and light, the 'reflection' of information, which is the making of the relationship between the father, the mother and the son.

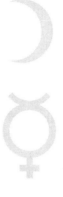

Chapter 5
The Throat Chakra

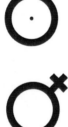

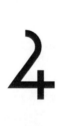

THE THROAT CHAKRA

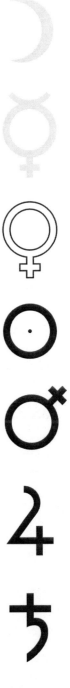

The first draft of this Chapter, in 2004, coincids exactly with the very moment that Venus is at her closest point to the earth for hundreds of years. The intensity of light is extraordinary, for Venus, who carries the golden orb, is having her radiance electrified by the Sun. This light, though intense, is not harsh but has a refined brightness, which seems to wake up all vibration with promise during this transit. It provides an opportunity to bring out into the open what is normally very subtle – the work of Venus.

At present, as Venus can be seen as a little black dot venturing its way across the bottom of the Sun, one is struck by its subtlety, not only of size in relation to the Sun's magnificence but also the vibration of light she emits. This vision, that of Venus, projected against the great power of the Source that glows behind in stark contrast to the tiny sphere that gracefully makes its way from one side to the other, represents a little insight: that which humanity considers as strength is often quite the reverse. Venus acts as a portal in order that we may take a glimpse of the creative purpose being undertaken on the other side, in that other world. She reveals to us that we are a part of that creative process which manifests in life as she works through Self and the grace by which all things are created through the tiniest of expressions. Venus contrasted against the Sun leaves us humble as to what is possible from such a tiny point of creative purpose. Her message though is steadfast, her path constant and her influence on mankind is immeasurable.

Chapter 5 ~ The Throat Chakra

The energy of Venus pertains to the throat centre and each homœopathic remedy that acts upon this centre will contain an essence of her poetic energy. At present, as I write, the population of the world is in the process of having to redress their relationships, not only between themselves but also the relationship that Self has to all things. As we are part of the extended family of humanity, our purpose, which should be enlightened by one's own spiritual creativity, is at the same time being bounced off other people's creativity, who will of course be going through the same process. This is a time for vast readjustment and I am sure this will involve one or two arguments. It may well also create new love affairs or the breaking of old ties, be they family, friendship or business relationships. It is impossible, esoterically speaking, to start afresh without having completed the previous task. Venus allows blocks in relationships to open up so that they can be completed. By speaking one's truth, energy can be re-released so that it can once again flow back up and down the spine, freeing that which blocks and restricts movement. At the throat chakra, the energy that manifests is creative and will instigate, through relationships, what is necessary from that which has been wished. Dreams do come true and it is here that their request can be heard and made manifest. This energy is awakening and is honest, but not brutal, for it offers support. When change is required from this centre it will feel that it is the right thing to do but it may also meet an equal amount of resistance, for this centre stipulates balance and will reveal the negative karma still outstanding from the heart chakra.

The manifestation for what is required to establish purpose within a context, which is inevitably a group, comes into fruition here at this centre. So now, as the transition of Venus across the face of the Sun is coming to an end, the consequence of this is yet to be obvious, leaving us all to explore what new changes within our own relationships are going to manifest. The energy of Venus in transit is cooked by the rays of the Sun and sent directly upon the Earth, intensifying her qualities dramatically. The light of the Earth becomes of a different quality as it is mixed and expanded upon by means of her blessing. It is a good time to receive the comforts of her bounty, especially if trauma pertaining to the throat chakra has been an obstacle in life. This abundance may materialise as love or money or simply attract people that enable one to see or act in new ways. It will help destroy longstanding inhibitions by a strong feeling of connection that can be expressed more freely in communication. A Venus transit will, in fact, enhance one's love and allow it to find connections that Self may have previously been a little too shy to make without her influence. Venus does this by helping to clear ancestral as well as personal karma, for this chakra is the higher octave of the sacral centre. The throat chakra is closely connected to the function of the kidneys, and to hearing, and this connection can be observed by the similar shape of the kidneys and the ears. What one hears feeds Self and by resonance connects to the position that one has made through the bloodline. Self chooses to listen to what resonates with where it feels it belongs and finds it difficult to absorb sound that is contrary to its status quo. Sound brings much change and debate is important to formulate new ideas, many of which will require ancestral energy to loosen its grip in order that the new can come into fruition. Congestion of the ears is often the result of ancestral congestion of the kidneys. In classical images, Venus is depicted wearing a fig leaf, which refers to the coy restraint of ancestral karma and the social conditioning of the group. Its transit is an opportunity to peel away the fig leaf revealing what is naked underneath. With this new sense of pure abashment, one feels free to abandon that which has probably been hidden for a long time and has been weighing down the individual's spiritual progress.

Venus has been known by the name 'Goddess of Light' or the 'Other Sun' and wife of Vulcan, the god of celestial fire. Fire, as discussed earlier, connects the solar plexus with the heart and also with the throat chakra. Here fire is both terrestrial and celestial and marks the movement by which the throat creates a bridge into Divine light or the fire of life. This light, in the form of love, has provided Earth with perfect laws which humanity rejected. It is Venus that feels the pain of humanity's despair as a result of this rejection, it being the twin sister of the Earth. She receives twice as much light from the Sun as the Earth and therefore is more forgiving. Thus, without disdain, Venus stores the light of the solar orb, a third of which she blesses the Earth with through her compassion. Humanity gains much in the way of healing from this light, for Venus is also Eve. It was intentional that she would leave paradise and bring to Earth the fruits by which humanity would gain Divine consciousness, for banishment is another form of growth. This is an indication to humanity that the energy of Venus is all encompassing, she being the most radiant of all the planets. She is Mother of the World alongside Mother Earth and the two swap or share communication through vibra-

Chapter 5 ~ The Throat Chakra

tion, as do all twin sisters. Whatever affects one, the other feels, which places Venus, by simply being there, in the position of instigator and ruler over this creative duality. It is the Yin with the Yang, the male and the female, the light with the dark, soiled as creativity is, for as soon as the Earth's sister was banished, she was vulnerable yet free to explore all the dualities of the creative facets but only here on Earth.

If Adam is made of spirit, then Eve acts as the bridge between the Source and Adam, the creative force of the Love Goddess. Venus or the ray of Eve, is the colour of dark blue which signifies the darkening of her radiance by fire as she incarnated into Earthly karma and took a taste of the fruit in the Garden of Eden. Venus, however, remains a sacred planet, which the Earth is not, hence her assistance in the struggle of mankind. This fruit and the golden orb are one and the same, the initiation of spiritual enlightenment or the power of the imagination to create thought.

The light of the golden orb engenders the possibility for contradiction, by stimulating Self to develop individualism whilst being under the instruction of Divine Will. As already discussed the mishandling of this contradiction by Self gave rise to the syphilitic miasm. This also displays a positive side to this miasm and an indication as to the complexity of Venus energy; for it is true that humans have had to explore in order to progress and therefore is this not always only possible under the instruction of Divine Will? Thus all exploration is ultimately positive, is it not?

On Earth, humanity is the planetary light bearer, of which there are three frequencies of transmission: knowledge, wisdom and understanding. Knowledge, the result of creative thought, is gained through the exploration of our universe and the relationship we have to all its aspects, both individually and as a whole. These dualities that have already been discussed as being prevalent within the sacral centre are now also of spiritual significance here in the throat chakra. Ever since humanity formed itself into two groups, male and female, the light of the golden orb of Venus has guided these separate entities. As already revealed in the Solar Plexus Chapter, the idea of Mars being of male energy is a myth, this energy is simply the other end to the Venus stick, her alter ego, her persona on a lower level and having her roots in the function of matter, she masquerades as male energy for the purpose of this part of the Earth's evolution. Mars as governor of the solar plexus will not be removed after the emancipation of this myth, but the fire will be more in tune with

Chakra Prescribing and Homœopathy

Venus' wishes. Venus is a cold planet and she requires this fire to warm up humanity. It is the light that is significant here, for its truth devours any confusion that may otherwise rise out of the syphilitic miasm. This miasm pushes the truth of unity apart and in doing so places polarities as far in opposition as possible, creating an inability to live with each in harmony, as a single entity, from which in reality there is only female. As this chapter progresses it will give further understanding as to why releasing hidden syphilitic karma within the throat chakra is instrumental to Self's ability to explore as a whole entity and thus grow, which is the only means by which to maintain good health.

Earthly karma is the result of immortality: if reincarnation did not exist then neither would human karma. Venus (Aphrodite) signifies this relationship not only through the colour of her ray but also through her son Eros who became her extension after incarnation. For Venus and Eros are in fact the same, an illustration of immortality. Perhaps the only difference is that Eros is the male aspect of Venus's masquerade in the throat chakra and signifies the importance of balance in this centre. Venus resonates love and beauty that has plunged into the darkness of matter, awaiting the emergence from the sea (the instinct of the unconscious) and which, when materialised, produces uncorrupted pure Mother Love. It was Venus who brought into being the human kingdom, marrying the animal aspect with souls that she blessed, herself being under the instruction of the Creative Hierarchies through the fifth cosmic plane and the fifth ray. Previous experience of race development had given Venus the tools by which to do this and the psychic link between the two planets was said to have been established when Venus, having no satellites of her own, adopted her sister Earth for the purpose of passing on her knowledge. Hence the relationship of mother and child was bestowed on Earth and humanity has contained mystical connotations in the creative growth of its relationship with Mother Earth ever since, Isis and the Virgin Mary to name but two. Venus rose from the sea but did not remain in it and hence the female principle of water met that of the male – fire – and it is through this vapour that spirit ascends. (The Greeks categorised earth and water as being female and fire and air as male). Thus her position and the evolution of humanity are interlinked and she feels every mistake. Like Isis, she is goddess or star of the day, so has to grapple with the dark in order that there may be daylight. Seen slightly differently, she grapples with beginnings so

Chapter 5 ~ The Throat Chakra

that eventually knowledge can be converted into wisdom. Both female goddesses had sons to enable them to achieve this and so continues the unfolding of immortality. We can compare this balance of male and female to the energy that links the thymus to the thyroid gland and explains why the thymus pertains much more to the male of the species and the thyroid to the female: they are night and day.

Venus requires the dark in order for her influence to promote the question within our soul: what is it that you truly value? This is her spiritual connection with mankind, in which her role is like that of an adopted mother or aunt. It was the utilisation of Venusian energy that made the individualisation of mankind possible during Lemuria. But this mothering quality does not end there, for as humans we tap into this influence through the symbol that Venus maps out in her cycle around the sun, which when observed from above creates a pentagram or what is known as the 'white rose'.

Figure 10. The Pentagram.

This relationship between Venus and mankind was well illustrated by Leonardo da Vinci by placing the human figure within a circle, thus creating a direct correspondence with the human dimensions and the pentagram. This also reveals how important understanding cosmology in relation to developing consciousness was to those with insight at that time. The beauty of these geometric dimensions illustrates the love in which nothing is forgotten and where all is in alignment with the whole, as is with the golden ratio that is also found within the pentagram. This balance is often symbolised in the Tarot pack as the Tower, which though built mighty and high, can be struck down by grace, beauty and of course love. This is a creative process of renewal that enables the Ego to realise its true purpose, that of the unconditional love of the soul, which at times can be painful.

During the year of 1924, Venus came close to the Earth, in relative terms, and this coincided with the uprising of many feminist movements that redressed somewhat the proliferation of Mars energy and can be likened to the mother exerting her influence over her son. The esoteric principle, which is the representation of the 'son', is the promotion of love-wisdom. Venus conceives Eros in order that this stage in humanity, which is focused on the throat centre, can come into being. Eros's purpose, using the influence of love and beauty, was not simply to oversee carnal desires but the passions of higher aspiration, which Eros matches and delivers.

Under the influence of Venus, the Ego can awaken through the higher manas the inner psyche to wisdom, it being where abstract knowledge and impersonal love combine. This combination produces the aura of this centre. Again, through the words that the patient speaks, we can determine the level of creativity active through the source of their higher aspiration. It is Venus's role to provide the means by which the seeker can enter the realm of Divine light, for love here is Divine Will. Venus and her son Eros work together as the driving force that leads the soul from physical love to the intellectual love of ideas. There is no mention of Eros having a father, so these ideas mirror one's own soul and thus the love that is life can extend from out of them, leading the soul consciously further into its unconscious journey. The need to discuss, ponder and construct new ideas is a sign of a healthy throat chakra. Should these ideas lead to a tendency for procrastination, it can reveal an imbalance within not only the sacral centre and the Mars centre but also within the base chakra, for if it is lacking in energy, ideas will fail to be earthed. The throat is a place where the hard lessons of life are often felt and are subsequently either dealt with or not. Some say that all ill-health stems from the throat. This is because here Venus fully believes in her involvement in humanity with all her wonder; such is her creative relationship with Earth. The activity of the energy at play is fire, so the throat is not a place that has the benefit of hindsight; its method is instinctual which is activated by doing. Unlike the Mars centre, at the throat centre fire and water become mixed so this doing is no longer governed by the personality.

This is the centre of inspired intelligence: the integrity of this centre will give rise to the quality of the intellect, which will manifest as goodwill. The more this centre is blocked, the more judgement will be

Chapter 5 ~ The Throat Chakra

clouded and the ability to see clearly will be hindered. Trauma in this centre results in the avoidance of the beauty of truth and will require greater sacrifice in order to achieve transcendental love. The result is often deep anger as the trauma tries to defend or justify itself. As this is a centre of inspiration, if its energy is directed for personal gain it will use all its cunning and conniving to hide itself in the illusion of what life is trying to behold. Therefore work on this centre can bring to the surface very ancient karma that has remained unspoken for many past lives and suffocated much potential for creative purpose. Many remedies may be needed at this stage for the karma of this centre links into the function of the organs in the dense body, which will also need support.

The accumulation of negative sound waves will, over time, result in toxic sludge in the dense body and produce disease states. This centre is often regarded to be the gateway to the stars and this portal will remain firmly shut if the wrath of negative karma has not been resolved, for it is here, through sound, that negativity manifests. People who are in a battle to gain direction within their lives will most likely have it raging in this centre. It may not be obvious but where there are throat problems then there will be a frightful tussle in the ability to reach the Earth with any means of purpose or to reach up to the heavens to gain guidance for that purpose. Blockages in this centre are truly that of being left hanging by a thread, a creative shutdown. The resultant frustration can lead to the physical manifestation of being in a fight with life, or within group energy it will present as the repetition of constantly taking a warring position. To vocalise one's feelings, to establish a dialogue with the blockages in this centre, will change the situation, for our expression of higher desire will eventually resurrect goodwill. When throat remedies are given to the patient the resultant outpour from the thyroid gland (the gland of this centre) can be alarming to the patient and the practitioner when observed for the first time, but neither should be alarmed, as this is part of the process of freeing up past negative karma. Remember, this is where the angels preside, guided by the archangel Gabriel, and their work is to spread love and reassurance in what can seem like an endless journey, that of creativity.

During the first few months of our development the angels weave a fine silver net that connects the brow centre to the throat chakra. The finery of this net is so beautifully precise that it can detect the slightest flow of energy allowing us to make a rapid judgement as to the appropriate words to choose. The sensitivity of this web allows the correct chemical balance to formulate the brain in the first two years of life and goes someway to establishing the personality. Later, it connects the ability to think before we speak or speak as we think. Much can damage this net and its condition can be judged in the words that are spoken. Like any web, things can become attached to it so negative words attract negativity but positively it is very attractive. Remedies of the throat such as *Diamond* (words spoken remain so forever) and *Silkworm* can repair and refine its function allowing the angels to once again weave their magic. The thyroid is shaped in the form of the two wings of an angel, a parting gift from the Divine, given to remind us of their presence and guidance. With the larynx and its upright configuration of the lungs, humanity has the mechanism by which to be co-creator. It too can speak 'the word' and thus shape life. It too has the means to manifest choice. If, however, the process of refinement at the heart chakra is insufficient then this quality will never be lifted to high expression. It will remain the place where angels fear to tread or where they dim their torches and only surface for a fleeting moment, perhaps during the winter solstice or at a time of near death crisis.

It was close to the start of the fourth root-race and during the formation of the Lemurian race that planet Earth fell under the influence of the fallen angels of which Lucifer was the leader. Lucifer had been convinced, along with the others that joined him, that his role as Divine's right-hand man had blessed him with equal powers; and when shocked by the truth, came to Earth in order to pursue this wish, ignoring the angels' own layers of hierarchy. Before this, humanity had much more in common with Divine consciousness and through Lucifer's actions of attempting to obtain this consciousness for reasons of narcissism, this connection became subverted. Also due to his arrogance, Lucifer was unhappy with the influence of the planet's rays working upon the human condition, believing he was of higher rank and that the Earth should only prosper under his influence. Again the subversion of this harmony was to infiltrate the human psyche resulting in the creation of disharmony within the chakras. Lucifer's gripe was in fact with the Creative Hierarchies, for he no longer saw himself in the role of co-creator, but came to Earth with others of similar wounded pride in order to rule it. Lucifer succeeded in splitting the connection between the head and the heart, leaving his presence felt at the throat chakra, the scar of this separation. This wound, if left to fester, will run

Chapter 5 ~ The Throat Chakra

into the very depth of the being. At the time the high priests let down humanity by allowing this separation to happen and even partaking in its spoils. It can be argued however, that without such a division the throat chakra would never have developed or gained the opportunity to be co-creator, the manufacturer of karma. And without the birth of such physical desires the throat's power to create form and its connection to the bounty of planet Earth would not have come into being. The physicality of our creation is a direct result of these desires as is our desire for sex, to have a partner and to produce offspring. We create the physical form as a mechanism in which we can express our love. Venus and Lucifer in fact, have much in common.

To gain an insight into one's own creative power then one has to be aware that the Tree of Life, that tempted Adam and Eve, is the kabbalist map that relates directly to the human condition – for it is also to be found within. It speaks of being whole, of oneness without having been disillusioned. This tree differs from the Tree of Knowledge, which is humanity's means to fathom rationality, and belongs to the lower manas, the seed of which was planted by Adam and Eve and so in relative terms has just had its first blossom. It is therefore the tree of duality and oppositions, which is appropriate, for it reflects present consciousness which Venus's creation of humanity is to feed from until both trees can finally merge as one. The Tree of Life can only be fathomed by the higher manas and its energy is fed down to the lower. It is the Tree of Life that, through humanity, waters the Tree of Knowledge, for the latter is in fact mortal. The power of instinct is immortal. With the human body placed against the Tree of Life, Eve's first offspring, Cain, would be located on Adam's left shoulder in the sphere of Geburah. This refers to the soul of Cain being the descendent of the Super Ego and that of judgement and the intellect, the containment of both spiritual and material reality of existence. Cain was destined to roam the Earth because of his instinctual creative ability – he offered what he had produced with his hands. Abel, placed on the right shoulder, corresponding to the realm of Hesed, is the incarnation of the Ego's ideal, that of grace and the sensitive, fragile and primitive Ego. Abel gained favour by offering what was already of nature. In Hebrew, Abel translates to the word 'breath'. In this context it is referred to as the mist of vanity, or veil, that Self has held so dear for so many of its lifetimes. It is this delusion that shortens the breath and so, as in the case of Abel, it refers to a shortened life for he was slain by ideas. We are all but a hair's-breadth away from death but that of a greater force – the truth, overrides this fragility. Therefore, it is Cain that brings fire down to earth, the Holy Spirit or creative force, in order that Cain can strive to regain Divine favour.

The morality of mankind is within the sphere of influence of the throat chakra and its balance lies within the energy of compassion. One side pertains to punishment and retribution whilst the other bestows forgiveness and mercy, for Cain and Abel both had differing fathers and thus two different paths. The battle between these two can be associated with the road to Gemini, for it will be in the brow centre that they unify as twins forming a triad between Venus, Mars and Mercury. Without this struggle there would be no intellect, no knowledge to collect and thus no wisdom to gain. There is much here about honouring where one has come from and that indeed means parental and ancestral karma, which also falls under the relationship of mother and son. At present the West puts more emphasis on Abel, who it rewards regardless of his spiritual content, if we consider him to represent the human soul. But the true importance for our future lies in the strength of Cain, for he confronts conditioned existence, the like of which the conscience of the West finds difficult to comprehend, but this is its task. This dichotomy lies within Cain for the impregnation of Eve by the serpent (Lucifer) left Cain with the karma of humanity's new division, that of half angel, half demon. But it was Eve who was first aware that in order for humanity to evolve under the influence of her love and beauty, she would also have to understand the dark. To have a kingdom, to which humanity belongs, one must have a Queen as well as a King. Kingdoms are integral to nature as the kabbalist map reveals with its pillars of divided polarities, and presently all nature is dual, being male or female, active or passive. The Venusian days and therefore the nights are very long in comparison to those on Earth, so Venus has plenty of time to peruse the night-time activities in order to produce the quality of tact.

As Jesus' companion during his liberation of the seven chakras, Venus, as Mary Magdalen, was able to use this experience she had gained. It was her trust, through love and devotion, which enabled this right of passage. To separate Mary Magdalen from Jesus would be a mistake, for she was first to witness his resurrection, as she is an aspect of Jesus, part of the same entity, one emanating from the other. Her energy acts

Chapter 5 ~ The Throat Chakra

as an intermediary between Jesus and Christ, for she is Queen of the Human Kingdom. It was not so much her sex that made her so despised by Christians but the confusion over the idea, as the Christ story materialised, as to the role she played in his life. Here lay a problem, for they deplored the idea that Jesus could have left a bloodline, especially a Jewish one, so she was turned into a prostitute, to which Jesus could take pity, no doubt to match the night-time Venusian investigations.

It is the throat chakra and especially the role of the thyroid gland that maintains the balance between nurture and nature. It reveals that within duality there is nothing more than two aspects of the same thing. The thyroid relates closely to all the other endocrine glands revealing this need for unification, the marrying of the personality with spirit. It is also the method by which the throat balances with both Mars and Jupiter, being lower aspects of itself, indicating that negative energy reflected in either of these two chakras will also be revealed in the throat chakra. The story of Cain is not an illustration of good versus evil but of the balance between the male and female aspects within. The notion of good and evil is mankind's myth, for in truth there are only consequences, which are different aspects of the same reality. Venus activity has evolved to be above that of Mars and thus, on behalf of humanity, has made our development possible by maintaining the myth of these two energies being separate. Hence her station is that of commander over the fire of Mars, she being the spiritual instigator of human life on planet Earth.

Through what it receives, the throat controls what goes in, and thus what comes out. So the head feeds the body via the neck and in turn the body feeds the head: energy being that which rises as well as that which falls. The throat is the gateway for this action in the body which then commands the power to express yes or no. It determines the choice between speech or silence. The power of silence is linked to stillness and the ability to transcend from this world and into the next. This transcendent intelligence radiates through sound, for even silence has a vibration when it is placed between two sounds. To celebrate the magic of vibration and help us rise up from the matter and into the spirit of the triad of the top three chakras, we create music to which we often add words. Everyone has a voice and everyone can sing. The upper three chakras unite to produce a creative process of which the throat is only one part, albeit a very important part, for it enables that from above to manifest here on Earth, which is where form resides as matter. At this centre, Self has the means to manifest its desires, which should be taken up by the higher manas and emanated down, but of course are often dominated by the desire of the personality. If the work pursued at the heart is sufficient in allowing the kundalini to open up where Venus resides, then a successful clearance will enable the creative purpose of the individual to be steered via the connection with the upper three centres onwards on its path back to Earth. It may feel like a game of chess at times, in which the pieces are our souls being used by those on the higher planes; but it is only our negative response or simply fear that creates the illusion that there is something to lose and that everything will go wrong. This pattern can be removed by the compassion of the throat in which belief and guidance prevail and is helped by remedies such as *Natrum Mur*, *Blue* and *Sea Salt*.

Venus has had to enter into all aspects of humanity in order to understand when to offer her support. This higher vibration of generosity in turn is passed on within humanity and if this quality is within the throat chakra it produces very attractive people who can ably radiate this idealism. Their wit and sense of fun is of a healing quality making them good to be around.

It was following the taking in of organic matter to fuel the physical body that Self sought the pleasure of taste. And this of course evolves to be particular to the individual. No longer was this joy the prerogative of Divine or a necessity of Akasha substance but its enjoyment could be found within the matter of the other kingdoms already established on Earth. This went along with varying methods of obtaining, digesting and distributing what had previously been the sub stream of sound, Akasha had now been made material. The stratosphere, its climate and the use of growth and agriculture were the means of survival once humanity could no longer depend on the nourishment of non-molecular sound. It is thus the ability to gain food that limits human freedom, a sacrifice made when the responsibility for taste was handed over. In a sense humanity partakes in the pleasures of a feast on Earth's table that is the mirror image of the nourishment of the Source. In part and for reasons of security, the Celts chose the British Isles to escape the destruction of Atlantis because of its fertile soil. Taste is a pleasurable desire that the mouth offers the soul not only to nourish the dense body but also to feed the needs of all the subtle bodies. If one was so enlightened as to not require material sustenance, one could still taste the light.

Chapter 5 ~ The Throat Chakra

Adam and Eve wanted to taste their freedom and did so through the fruit, which would remain lodged in the throat for evermore, reminding us of the return journey, in effect returning the apple to its tree. The apple symbolises the liberation of the soul from Earthly karma, but until that day Self must search for its liberty here on Earth. If one is caged or incarcerated then society has seen fit to constrain one's liberty, which is the same as having one's creative freedom removed or losing one's voice. People who have endured this experience will often benefit from the bird remedies, followed by the vine remedies. This experience is nothing more than the imprisonment felt by the soul through negative karma. We taste our freedom for we breath in light and this is the spiritual nourishment that has maintained the souls of those who have been wrongfully imprisoned by unjust dictatorships, sustaining these people even at their darkest hour. To be liberated spiritually begins inside.

By placing man in the circle, Leonardo da Vinci was able to illustrate Venus representing the human soul, full of love and beauty and free. If this is not so then what radiates is a lack of acceptance. People without these qualities find group situations uncomfortable and are usually unable to work in teams or on collective projects. Everyday situations become a chore, an indication of still being stuck in the personality and as a consequence these types become very prejudiced and heavily burdened with judgement and untrue constraints. They struggle to grow and are unable to move forward in life. These people can be confrontational and hostile if challenged, as they hold tight to their prepared notions, (e.g. *Kali Carb, Anacardium, Veratrum Alb*). Humiliation often results when sticking to such rigid rules and humiliation is often the cause as it closes down the throat chakra from fear that they may get it wrong again. It is also the result of the inability to laugh at oneself. Laughter comes from the throat; a mixture of love, beauty and liberty that arises when one is happy. It reverberates around the cosmos and produces much healing, for if we are able to laugh at ourselves then no negativity will stick. Laughter is essential for children.

The life force of children withers if they are kept from speaking their truth. This truth is imperative regardless of what their guardians may think of it. Denial of one's voice is very damaging to the throat centre and if the child is being obscene then this is not its truth. It is in fact a reflection of a problem that lies elsewhere, usually a lack of love radiating from the heart, the making of which may not necessarily be of this lifetime.

If a single tale were to be made of this centre, it would be that it is only possible to be an individual in a group and only a true group is created by individuals. To master this centre will only help to place the integrity of the individual in public hands and thus the group, the planets, the zodiac signs or the disciples can all contribute and move humanity forward together in harmony. Unfortunately our planetary throat chakra has a long way to go for humanity is not listening to it. Truth is a precious commodity but this is the requirement in order for growth. Speech upon speech and march after march usually means that somœone has been thrust forward to open the hearts and minds of the people. This can of course be misused, for this centre also has the power to mesmerise and hypnotise and many have fallen under its spell. Hitler and Martin Luther King both had the ability to transfix the listener but for very different reasons. If in doubt, perhaps the question one should ask is whether one is being led into war or peace. Mars energy is important but should always be counterbalanced by Venus, for without compassion we have no means by which to counter our self-centred desires. There are patients with this problem and by using new and old remedies that pertain to the throat chakra, it will become useful to practitioners to discern how much more interactive within the group they become. Remedies that pertain to the soul of our planet, like *Himalayan Crystal Salt* and remedies that pertain to the destruction of our planet like *Japanese Oleander (White)* will help counter such self-centred desires and find a balance. This measure of interaction will indicate a return to quality and enable them to express their truth at the throat chakra.

Regardless of any circumstances that may dictate the way one expresses oneself within the group, all will have a bond to a lesser or greater degree. We may all at one time have to fight for peace on behalf of the group but this can be made especially difficult if the group itself is unable to see this or is not ready for it. It is the integrity of this centre that will teach the difference between acting on behalf of the group and acting on purely selfish motives. It will be this integrity that offers the correct balance during confrontation, between shying away from the issue and going on the rampage. The thyroid gland has much to do with this balance as Abel found to his cost.

ART

The throat chakra is the place where art, either visual or audible, is

Chapter 5 ~ The Throat Chakra

appreciated, admired and also discussed, and possibly dismissed through debate. Nevertheless, art inspires through such debates. If a patient has no refinement for any of these pursuits, then it will be the division between spirit and matter that they will be struggling with. Art should contain a link from the past to the future. Some artefacts may seem dated because consciousness has moved on, especially if their relevance was crucial to a particular time. Others may still contain their mysterious shine as they have yet to fully surpass the time relating to their consciousness. If it is relevant and what can truly be called art, then it will have a spiritual link and a purpose by which it can contain, through its form, abstract thought before becoming concrete. It is no coincidence that the 'modern art' movement coined the phrase 'Abstract'.

It must be remembered that the old masters used the secrets of hidden spiritual mysticism to enable their public to meditate on their work. By its very nature art has to be free and of course there have been many constraints placed on artists as well as their patrons, which led to artists using symbolism to relay the true meaning of their work. The Popes, for instance, could not have been ignorant of such symbols so must have promoted their use. For the artists, their work that has gained notoriety has been a way of containing the true meaning of stories that have been materialised by religious rhetoric. Paintings, sculptures and frescoes by these old masters were of their day what an epic movie is to present culture, though the process of meditation is slightly different, but their content mostly tackles the same dilemmas. We have, alas, lost much connection with the meaning of symbols used by those old masters that were able to evoke the power of enlightenment, though often heavily disguised under the dogma of religious formal representation. Often we have to forget the story in order to become one with the meaning of the art. Abstraction naturally extends this theme that evokes within and speaks to the depth of our soul.

Often in comparing groundbreaking art forms with the artists who created them, it can be surprising as to the levels the syphilitic miasm is at play in their lives. In fact, in the gallery many gather around such work or a speaker describes how it came into being, remarking on its historical significance. Yet given the choice and the circumstances that drove such artists to create their work, perhaps part of the fascination is that the viewer has rarely endured the persecution that is being expressed through the feelings of such ordeals. This is often the same for homœopathy, for one has often had to endure great pain in order to treat it. From one life to the next, these experiences, albeit unwittingly, are not only carried forward but are the making of one's expression. It is at the throat that our aspiration gains form and in art the bounty of the artist's angst, often from many lifetimes, can create something so soul revealing, that it will touch all of humanity. In art it is not the aesthetics nor is it the beauty of its construction that matters, for these are often techniques, although they do sing of the artist's genius. What does matter is the road, the struggles that enable an extraordinary life with such a background to deliver to humanity the result of aspiration designed to express the positive side of the syphilitic miasm. This is to dare to search out the unknown and make sense of it.

This world differs little to the one of the past in which those who are given the task to speak the truth are thrust forward, often reluctantly, to converse with humanity on its behalf. However, this has never been as difficult as in these modern, materialistic times where the more we have the more there is to lose. To have prophesied is the liberation from this and is obviously in conflict with those who have a vested interest in the material. This relationship within humanity is revealed in the glyph that represents Venus, ruler of the throat chakra. The sphere has risen above the cross of matter. The spirit here is more prevalent than the confines of the Earthly desires but the cross is still there. Those patients who come with throat problems will be struggling in their lives with this equation.

PROPHECY

The bottom three chakras refer to the act of receiving and the heart chakra relates to manifesting: the throat chakra, along with all the upper three chakras, is about sending out. Hence the Prophet is compelled to deliver. If we observe the function of these three upper centres broken down into their individual constituents, then the throat acts as the sound box to the whole, an indication as to the unifying power of speech. When acting as it should within the upper triad what is spoken should hold absolute truth, especially as its reverberations will create the consequence that brings about manifestation. When speech expresses what is received from the higher planes and translated from vibration into conscious expression, then its integrity will be clear for all to behold. Such communication – the collective intelligence that provides the structure for the integration of humanity – is the means by

Chapter 5 ~ The Throat Chakra

which we create. This is a process that filters through all the three upper chakras, once again presenting the challenge of separating out what is a collective process, for the purpose of understanding. Separation is a theme of the throat centre that holds heavy symbolic consequence in mystical descriptions. For instance, the removing of the sword from the stone represents the request at the throat chakra that one moves away from the notion that one only exists in the material. This is prophecy, bestowed on Arthur, as master of his kingdom and a symbol demonstrating that we all have the power to remove the sword. Prophecy is to discover why and for what purpose we are here: a spiritual quest. This does not have to incur some grand voyage of discovery but is a part of our day-to-day decision making. If one does not advertise one's practice, then this process can be used to detect the route the patient has taken in order to arrive at your door. This route will also give great insight as to that which requires healing, for the voyage provides clarity as to the reason why they are destined to be your patient. Moreover, on one level the patient knows this and by the practitioner being still, it will not be long before the reason as to this connection can be established.

Prophecy not only leads us to where we should be but also can keep us from danger. Such protection is bestowed by speaking our truth, as we know with so many of our cancer patients, or in fact with all our patients, that this is the most important thing to do in order to heal.

The slowing down of vibration allows artistic expression to be seen or heard and art is a means by which we can connect to the higher world. The ears are directly associated with the throat chakra, and the eyes although not directly associated, do have a connection in that they allow us to be filled with beauty and communicate the quality of life. The ears provide the ability to receive information and to develop the vocabulary to relay it to others. This expression is integral to freedom and to development and this is especially true during childhood, during which there will be many instructions that have to be adhered to, not least those of the commands of the parents. By the means of sound, these instructions will either promote growth or stunt it and controlling rules are often passed down from one generation to the next as harsh words. Compensation against such harshness also comes with consequence and can even create rapid growth, which is equally a sign of weakness. The throat chakra has much influence over those early years of childhood because growth is in line with instruction. As children and later in life through the little voice we hear inside our head, we are given direction by our guardians, which Venus instils with beauty. Ear problems may arise due to the contents of the head being full of unwanted remnants of thoughts and experiences from unfortunate influences made up of conditioning sounds in early life. When ear problems present in children, it may be wise to encourage the child to speak their truth, but great comfort must be instilled that this is safe and will be without reprimand. The ears are secondary to the influence of the eyes and, being an outlet, will also serve to eliminate negativity received through the eyes, which can otherwise congest the head. I have often seen children with ear problems as a result of separated parents with contradicting points of view, as the child has had to endure two sets of rules.

The tonsils are a security measure that allows judgement as to the quality of that which is fed into the brain. They act as a doorway to creative flow and inflammation pursues when this stagnates, the glands becoming heavily burdened with congestion. The throat chakra has a special connection to thought, for it is the centre that separates the head from the trunk and so behaves as the grounding to the next stage, that which separates the lower four chakras from the higher three. This stability enhances Self's ability to retrieve pure knowledge, which at the throat is brought down and spoken in the form of truth, and is fundamental to existence, for without this nothing would live or grow or change. It is the place where understanding can be met by manifestation for it is the sharp point of the descending triangle.

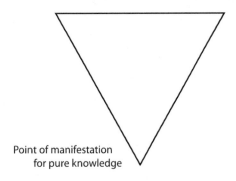

Figure 11. The Descending Triangle.

The throat chakra provides the point towards manifestation and if this is lacking, then apathy will result. Changes that seem impossible can be

Chapter 5 ~ The Throat Chakra

made here for it brings into manifestation what is privy to cosmic consciousness. This is possible by asking nothing more and nothing less, for the stability here is a place of stillness. This is why it is important to have a grasp as to what is needed and a direction in order to place one's trust, which should have begun during the development of the lower chakras. This centre is very special because of the propensity for creativity, and will present much in the way of understanding for Self and for the healing of others if it can be understood. To gain this understanding is by no means as clear-cut as it may seem, for this centre has many facets that challenge one's perception. Its creative energy breaks many inhibitions or rigid states of perception and so challenges Self to look hard at its relationship with the world. In doing so, this centre can open up some extraordinary events that may defy logic but muster much trust. The heart chakra teaches us to trust but it will be during the transition between the ages of twenty-eight to thirty-five years that the world will challenge all one's beliefs in the pursuit for what is being asked of Self. This will be more difficult to those who are not in tune with their wishes: life will continue without them if they are not careful, such is the creative force of the cosmos. However part of Venus's role is to be forgiving and unconsciously one will be guided by her influence, for we are all under the spell of her compassionate nature. She also has the support of Saturn, the great initiator that re-enters the birth chart at about the same time (around twenty eight to twenty nine years) that she pulls her masterstroke ensuring the stability, which is imperative at this junction, is in place. Saturn is the number eight which is the number that represents infinity. It is very apt and important that this number is present at the time of this spiritual quest.

Tests are great and in multitude at the throat centre, for it must be remembered that we have entered the realm of the angels and it is with this energy that we are asked to construct and lament compassion. It is the nature of prophecy that we often do not understand or have the foresight in order to justify at first what is being asked of us. These tests may be subtle and they can lead to much confusion, hence the meaningless hum of noise that infiltrates everywhere in the modern world. Self is asked to rise above this hubbub and find the stillness in which to receive the right vibration, the one that the angels lend so much support towards us hearing. Each one of us can be a prophet if we can only reach this level of stillness. This is the means by which the inspiration from which Self is able to expresses itself is met, and if one fails to unite with this chakra then there will be no real Self to express.

This energy relates to the pentagram and it can be said that the number five also represents the number of the prophet, it being the fifth chakra and the fifth element.

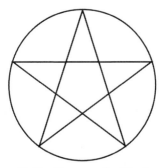

Figure 12. The Circumscribed Pentagram.

It is prophecy that allows Self to exist or to come into existence by means of the fifth element. Being a prophet speaks of reaching a level of attainment able to receive the gifts of Venus. Five is a numeric reflection of humanity and therefore Venus's route to this station. Five, with the amalgamation of the four elements, is the unseen, the ether that pumps through our veins. In the womb, this station is already prepared for and activated in a physical sense during the fifth month of pregnancy.

In a numerological sense, it is the number six that represents the throat chakra and the planet Venus and the five represents Mercury: but these numbers can also be seen as the stages of human influence as it gains consciousness, of which the throat charka is the fifth stage. Esoterically, the fifth incarnation represents the first imperfect attempt to create a human form, which produced the ape. These incarnating Egos were not quite ready to humanise, which numerically speaking, is the route from the five to the six and what Venus made possible. This also means that the ape Egos, although never destined to become human, are still evolving through each root-race. As the ape has been formed it is only a part of humanity's attempt to incarnate fully on planet Earth. The human monad or spiritual entities of Divine origin are, and always have been human, but they have an element of the animal that makes up the human animal. This transition could be read as the manifestation of Cain. During each stage of the subsequent

Chapter 5 ~ The Throat Chakra

human incarnations, these animal aspects to the human monad will slowly dissolve into a lower and lower level of significance. This is our relationship to the animal kingdom, like all the kingdoms before; they are a part of us but we have never been them. At five we are to be set free from matter, therefore, this number is the numeric symbol for that which is universal and impersonal or that of the higher manas, and the reincarnating Ego.

In the teachings of the kabbala Moses is placed on the sphere of Netzach where Venus also resides. All archetypes, theories, philosophies or faiths will be found here only if they pertain to the same resonance, or as the saying goes concerning all bodies on the same vibrational frequency – like attracts like. So Moses follows the same role as Venus and Eros along with Lucifer. Humanity has manifested these vibrations by isolating them and giving them form. Archetypal symbols can be found everywhere and are used to enter into the realms of understanding that are received through more than just our five senses. They are a means by which we can awaken the sixth sense or its vector. Moses is the practical prophet as is Venus, for they transpose to goodness: each spring the throat is awoken by this desire to pass on the good as can be seen by the antics of young lovers in a park. These archetypes have a great influence on our lives and also on the group. As children we choose our heroes around which we frame, in part, some of our development by consciously striving to replicate them. Archetypes resonate with a society unconsciously for they are aspects of its evolution. If they maintain the power to be worshiped then their significance is still present. As part of our relinquishing of the material plane, Self may cling to its deities in order to make sense of the blinding trust required in the pursuit of Divine will. Archetypes, nonetheless, provide a healthy link between the two worlds.

The throat chakra marks the start of the realm of occult intelligence and in kabbalist philosophy this is the sphere of Netzach. In Hebrew, Netzach translates to the word 'victory', meaning to reach a position of insight. This manifests as the balance between Self and the collective or the force which is the throat chakra, that of unification, in order to venture into the spiritual world. It means to have intelligence infused with spirit and possibility. This higher octave of Jupiter takes control of the creative force and instead of feeding it into sexual energy; it raises the kundalini to a level of love that can be expressed through the throat chakra. It is here that one meets one's partner and it is here that that attraction will be cemented, usually by the first kiss, a means of communication which is identification and where this connection continues to be felt. Love in this instance is directed through Divine Will and only the temptation of the personality will pull it down to a place of degradation, the corruption of Lucifer that accompanies Venus. We speak via the throat from our head and our heart when we call for a partner by which to be loved. This happens long before the meeting. Partners with healthy throat charkas stand a good chance of a stable relationship.

On the tree of life the pathway leading from the Sun to Venus is known as the route to imaginative intelligence. It is worth remembering that if the hippies had not dropped-out in the 1960's then the connections that created the modern computer programs would not have been made. The brow centre, through the intellect, absorbs this creative force, otherwise it would float into useless self-indulgence. It also needs to work the other way, for if creativity fails to extend from matter it never reaches beyond vanity.

The brow modulates conversation and the throat directs it: the two in harmony result in what we call reality. Continuous inspiration though, can be a breeding ground for instability, so here the brow chakra is a means of support, helping to provide selection. As mentioned, the throat chakra too has an inbuilt mechanism to enhance stability as is apparent from the symbolic animal archetypal representation of this centre: the elephant. This it shares with the base chakra, and for the same reasons the thyroid gland here is the target. The stability doubles up when supported by Saturn's visit during its seven years' cycle, which ensures the creation of a bridge between the heart and the head. Here, unlike at the base chakra, the elephant has a single trunk, representing liberation that reinforces the need for unified strength, the action of a healthy thyroid gland, in order for Self to be of service. Stability is a victory dependent on courage. Venus would achieve little without her counterweight, Mars, for there would be no compassion without passion.

The prophet may close her eyes but she cannot stop listening. Even her sleep and her dreams can be interrupted by the sounds that resonate from the higher levels and inform Self of the next steps. With practice or perhaps naturally, Self can focus its hearing on these important messages. Just like food is nourishment for the body, absorption through focused hearing is nourishment for the soul. The Tibetans and the Taoists use the throat

Chapter 5 ~ The Throat Chakra

chakra to explore the dream state of consciousness. In the Hesychastic system, Christian belief includes an Eastern form of meditative practice, which combines breathing techniques with prayer. They believe that in order for the throat chakra to be open does not simply rely on receiving sound but that it is activated by producing sound. So therefore, speech can be considered to be the first stage of prayer. Our words manifest our inner world and they remind us of the importance of their quality by what we attract. Thoughts form words and have a vibration. What we think creates vibrational intention and inevitably directs our actions. Even if our thoughts are not spoken they do eventually crystallise into form. The receiving of prana is also imperative to this process, for it provides the means by which to retrieve thought and, if spoken, allows the right words to be stated clearly. The throat centre requires the activity of creative force in the material world, at the sacral centre, to enable its wishes to be given birth in the personality. Artists, for instance, often have a high sexual appetite and a need for erotic expression that accompanies their highly developed creative impulses. There are lots of remedies that display compensatory behaviour when the sacral and throat centres are not acting in harmony. Sepia acts very deeply on the throat centre and these types may typically use dance to alleviate pent up sacral expression created by having a shutdown voice. Blocks here constrict the throat and inhibit the lungs, leading to confusion in the mind. Being able to focus sound correctly and freely is an expression of spiritual longing. This longing pertains to the Ego, for essentially the Ego is aware that sound is the vehicle by which its circumstances can be changed in this world.

Spiritual longing extends to caring and at times of crisis, the carrying of others. The insight that such longing provides is often directed into healing, and a strong functioning throat chakra will inevitably end up as healing energy, even if not used directly in one of the healing professions. This level of giving can, however, put great stress on the throat chakra and care must be taken if one is not to end up controlling others, in which case *Lachesis* will be required. Essentially healing work comes from the heart and will place further pressure on the throat chakra of the healer if their giving of support is not reciprocated. This may be something for the associated bodies of homœopathy to consider, for they may need reminding that the group is just that – a group – and not the select few of an inner sanctum.

A lack of emotional support or received love is compensated for at the throat by the elevation of the sense of taste and thus the pleasure of eating becomes a way of nourishing the heart, as a compensation for love. All eating disorders stem from the throat centre, as one's image or Venus beauty is also defined here. These disorders are of syphilitic origin. Speech is the expression of one's image and a lack of Self worth which is felt at the heart, will be reflected at the throat in the form of suspicion. When Self starts hindering that which is coming its way, it stops listening, cutting off the inner beauty. This is then perpetuated by the belief that there must be an ulterior motive behind attention that is received, for it cannot possibly be about one's inner beauty if there is no perception of any. Emotional responses such as anorexia and bulimia reflect the message of a lack of trust. The flexibility of the neck allows Self to look either up or down and when coupled with suspicion, can be too much to bear. The throat, in a downward spiral of negativity, mimics the feelings of loss at the heart, and if continued can lead to suicide, which denying nourishment is stepping towards. Negativity around the persona presented to the outside world may result in suffocation or strangulation. The throat is the tether between feelings of unbearable pain and the desire to end it and this is why it is the centre of hysteria.

For the throat to function properly it must rise above the limitations of the lower personality, or that which is concrete, and embrace the limitless realm of abstraction which is the very nature of its element Akasha. Guided by the subtle body, the Ego responds to the impulses of the higher manas. To make this transition of taking the abstract and creating form requires stability. All the creative transformations at this centre require stability or else manifestation gets lost in possibility: this is the dream state or trance. All the reporting of channelling is done from this centre and work here, especially through meditation, facilitates a bridge to the unknown. Truth is a universal commodity and it is infectious for it has power that cannot be disputed. One's truth is of the utmost importance. This will only be hindered when somœone else, a friend, guardian, a parish, a council, government, the group or a society do not wish to hear it or are not ready to do so. Blockages created in the patient's throat chakra are not just caused by a lack of expressing through the voice but are also produced by not being heard. This often involves a partner, who is usually a controlling type, being themselves too frightened to change. The feeling of not being listened to can create frustration, internalised anger and result in deep grief from continuous

Chapter 5 ~ The Throat Chakra

rejection. It is usually compounded in these situations by the patient having given much support through love; an action which if ignored will feel like betrayal; although eventually the truth will always find a form of expression. Spirit will be duty bound and a web of communication will be provided in order for it to be heard. This may start with one hearing oneself and making the decision to change. Instinct will guide the instigator through the means of the inner voice and in times of desperation, even clairaudience is known to occur. The hearing of spiritual voices in this centre, which are part of its function when at its most refined, will also provide guidance in order to prepare Self for the opposition that truth may encounter.

Most communication happens without words and as practitioners this should be noted, for the truth of our patients is important in diagnosis and not their appearance. We know that from many remedy pictures, such as *Mercury* and *Thuja*, speech cannot always be trusted. Gestures, movements, thoughts and auras are all of vibrational means and carry consequence. They all reflect one's truth and are constantly used for levels of communication that remain unspoken, a kind of private code. When Self evolved a body and retreated within, establishing a means by which it could maintain all its faculties inside, it gained its privacy, except that it could not contain the auras of those faculties. If one can see and read auras, the truth will be revealed, although unfortunately this faculty is still quite rare. The boundary of space created by the collective aura of the subtle bodies is immensely important in protecting Self from the outside. This is the same as maintaining a wall of silence. The phrase 'to keep one's word' also means to keep it to oneself, to not breach confidence and manifest deceit. To not speak is a human right and is powerful. Recently laws in the UK have gone some way to try and breach this code through threats of consequence imposed against the right to keep one's silence, a born right and one which Thomas More lost his head over. The keeping of one's own council is a key part to the formation of the American constitution: it places the burden on proof and not on confession. Peace within is very important for it reflects one's truth and if we were still of a spiritual structure, which the throat chakra demands, then methods would be used that are far more sophisticated and less open to trickery and subversion. These would use truth as a commodity on both sides of the law rather than simply having to use words to argue one's case, which always relies on the perception of others. The problem with cross-examination is that as a result of upbringing, conditioning and negative karma, many have lost the ability to live their truth and buckle under the guilt of so much trauma and intimidating treatment. As practitioners, this chakra asks and blesses us with the tools by which to be sympathetic to these things. Venus allows us to resonate with our patient's soul. It is this vibration that will guide the practitioner towards the patient's truth and only then will the requirement as to the level of healing be apparent. The more one tunes in to these subtle messages, into one's own guides and information coming from the higher self, then the more one will be aware of the real meaning of listening or focused hearing. Stubbornness is formed by dogma, which is the inability, or there being too much haste to listen. The patient can often transmit negative emotions, fears and the irrational thoughts as a result of desperation that can cloud one's perception, which these forces are often designed to do. It will be the truth that cuts a path through this in order to bring a resolution to the situation. This is where methods based around routine prescribing through layers can be so limiting in healing emotional pathologies derived from the levels of trauma in a modern world. The aetiologies of such problems are the means by which our intuitive prescribing is furthered through the development of perception.

False prophets present themselves almost daily in modern living. There are endless promises that cannot be delivered, that are made to seduce in the name of consumerism, most of which are not needed anyway but the myth is believed for it temporarily fills a widening gulf between spirit and matter. The glyph of this chakra is the only one of the chakra system to contain only the symbol of the circle and cross in their entirety. These prophets have even been developed in the East by the West, to feed back into the West for it is cheaper to come down the telephone line from there. The salesman/women is operating from the throat chakra. An effective salesperson will use subtle techniques and a silver tongue to entice in order that they may profit. The final pressure that is used to enable the seller to clinch the deal often falls upon the power of silence, for in the West this gap has to be filled by something. The seller knows this and the rule is known as 'he who speaks first loses.' When both parties are privy to this rule then the silences can be painfully long. The media and marketing employees are the new door-to-door salesmen and sexual attraction is a tool by which much silence

Chapter 5 ~ The Throat Chakra

is filled. This of course is not exclusive to one or two professions as the magnetic charm of Eros or Lucifer that places us under a spell can have far reaching consequence. So when a society decides to go in a particular direction, lo and behold, it throws up its false prophets as well as the true ones. It is said that by night, Venus acts out of love, but by morning she provokes man to go to war. She is the morning star and guides this transformation, for although never to be seen on the battlefield, she is nonetheless behind such moves, as in the Trojan War. To Venus, the battlefield is the struggle between male and female and a major part of the unification process of the throat chakra. The battle here is to harmonise these opposite poles. Love is the most wounding of weapons.

Attraction and its alter ego repulsion are the new politics of the modern world, or are they? Has this not always been the case and is not the media's obsessions with sex simply a reflection of our own? Attraction is not just the fire in Mars but also the fire in Venus. Her fire is designed to bring out the fire in mankind for which she was granted the golden fruit. Without this at present and for some time at least until the female part of the race becomes physically stronger than the male, the battle of the sexes enables a crude means by which humanity moves forward.

Venus was created from the froth of the sea or sperm within a sea of eggs, a turning point in the reproductive mechanism of the human species. But it was out of female envy, the result of a battle between lovers, that Venus came to be, in order to instil into humanity the complexities of division between the sexes – love and war. It is through this division that the desire to control found its fullest expression as Self sought to avoid the pain and misery that comes with Earthly love. However, the risk is not only exciting but is also the means by which two attract, by testing each others strengths and weaknesses. Love then is something to be feared as well as being a necessity, the consequence of which brings authority. Work on the throat chakra loosens control and provides choice. This includes being controlled by another or being subject to those who control their own lives and thus those around them. Sexual betrayal, jealousy, malice and envy are all forms of manipulation derived from the opposite of truth, which is deceit. In this sense, it may be that the most righteous character is the least trustworthy. Venus attempts through unification, to bring both of these sides together, so that both poles can co-exist in harmony. If there is continuous repression by an external force then spiritual expression is at the least very difficult. This form of control has a devastating impact on the health of the throat centre, so it will do its utmost to maintain an even balance, Venus being the ruling planet of the astrological sign Libra. Poor throat function creates or attracts domineering people, going against Libra's strong sense of fairness. A false prophet or a wolf in sheep's clothing will only appear when one is not speaking one's truth, so to create one's own universe to the relief of spirit and to the pleasure of the soul, it should be remembered that everything reverts back to Self. For the practitioner, verbal expressions such as, "so when is it going to be my turn" or "I never get to do what I want to do" will be indications of a block in the throat chakra. There will be repressed anger often created from control, so they feel guilty for speaking up for themselves, which they feel they can't: an example of this can be seen in the remedy *Staphysagria*. The prophet has mastered high function of the throat chakra but it is not difficult to detect in theses people a healthy function because for them it will be relatively easy to grasp spiritual matters.

Sandalwood has a mystical association with the throat chakra and is often burnt in order to help open oneself up to spiritual contact or to become 'awakened', putting an end to suffering which at the throat chakra is caused through ignorance. The sense of smell is very powerful in invigorating the action of the throat chakra. For this reason the sense of smell is often used to further progression in meditation. At the throat chakra this enables the inverted triangle to descend to form King Solomon's Seal, from which he heard the rites of life – the laws laid down by the Source. It was through the discovery of this 'vapour', of being able to mix the spiritual fire with the spiritual water, that King Solomon obtained the ultimate wisdom of an enlightened being. This is the alchemy of being able to turn lead, the negative values of the personality, such as lust, hatred and deceit, into gold, that of honesty and virtue: the Venus mission. As the sacral centre is the first step into spiritual growth, then here at the throat centre is the first test of that faith. The magic of Venus is the act itself, the expression, the intent: it is belief.

THE THYROID

The physiological action of the thyroid gland regulates metabolism so its fluctuations are reflected in weight gain or loss. It also, along with the pituitary gland, controls elimination through metabolism. Orthodox

Chapter 5 ~ The Throat Chakra

doctors have for many years been countering imbalances by either decreasing the thyroid's action through surgery or increasing its output by supplementing its secretion. This never, however, addresses the cause of the imbalance but is merely a crude way of sidelining the issue. Poor function of each endocrine gland reflects very closely the inadequacies of their given chakra and in the case of the thyroid gland this is revealed mostly in the personality. If knowledge of how both gland and chakra operate together is obtained then this makes the diagnosis as to where the problems lie far simpler. As with all the endocrine glands, in order for their function to be corrected, life changes will be incurred. These changes are often not easy and in this centre they may pertain to family as well as personal karma and be very emotionally infused by a sense of having to go against family protocol.

It can be quite a trial in homœopathy to observe people struggling to make these changes in order to gain the independence that their physiology is calling for. This may possibly mean turning one's back on a family that for one reason or another is not prepared to change when faced with the overthrowing of past dogma. One's independence is very important in personal evolution and to restrict what is being projected from the higher realms places a great strain on the endocrine system. What we are is in no small measure by virtue of our glands, under the guidance of the chakras and their rays. Homœopathy's gift is not to replicate allopathic activities but to meet the challenge of getting to the root of those reasons why imbalance has occurred. Like life, the tempo of the thyroid should be a constant, even flow and not subject to sudden outbursts of activity. Those remedies that are required at the throat chakra will contain in their picture the secrets behind such irregular function – *Calcarea Carbonica, Cimicifuga, Ambra Grisea, Silicea, Spongia* and *Goldfish*, to name just a few.

Looking like a pair of angel's wings flying on their way up to rest on the golden orb, the thyroid is the gland of truth. When one is not living one's truth this greatly affects its output. This is more than simply self-love; it is to embrace the truth of the whole cosmos. Much compensation is required during day-to-day living if one has to hide oneself. This lack of balance or lack of truth in one's activities results in the impoverishment of creative inspiration. This, being the major force here, will be inhibited also if one is neglecting to serve others as well as oneself. The integrity of group spirit is that which makes individuality possible. One is inevitably required to act from one's truth in order to prevent resentment building within and penetrating the other chakras, glands and organ function. It is resentment that restricts compassion for the group. The reverberations of this will not only reflect in the throat but also in the opposite charka, the solar plexus, for resentment attracts much negativity that gnaws away at the quality of astral energy, the place where we know cancer enters. This negativity can also shut down the generative area over which the throat has much domain, being its creative double. A good balance at the throat creates confidence, for it provides strong physical, sexual, mental and of course creative powers. Poor function results in the production of weak and feeble people. When one knows one can rely on creativity then one has a spiritual trust in the next step.

The secretions manufactured at the thyroid gland are thyroxine and tri-iodothyroxine. These are produced by converting iodine, which is extracted and absorbed from various foods. The levels of these hormones and the structure of the thyroid are kept in check by stimulating hormones secreted from the anterior part of the Pituitary gland. In the book 'Glands of Destiny' it states, "We are told that only three and a half grains of the thyroid secretion stands between intelligence and idiocy." Further to this, a lack of iodine will result in death. The balance of the thyroid places great emphasis on the formation of the personality. The calcium balance, also regulated by the thyroid, is so integral to stability that there is not one part of the body that it does not effect. A greater secretion of hormone from the thyroid tends to create youthful energetic types while a limited output creates premature ageing, reflected in the face as well as in the brain and can lead to senility. The thyroid is the gland of tempo, regulating the pace of life, which if too fast or too slow leaves the gland and thus Self, vulnerable to shock.

The thyroid gland is located at the throat for a reason; its action is both necessary for the function of the mind and to sustain physical form. The proper function of the thyroid during the development of childhood goes a long way to establishing who we are. This function, like all the endocrine glands, refers to where one has come from and therefore how miasmatic activity has shaped things to come. In the womb, the thyroid gland interacts with the fluids of the mother's hormones up until the point that it is capable of sustaining independent function. This may be the true link behind biologist's theories that con-

Chapter 5 ~ The Throat Chakra

nect the thyroid gland to the transformation of sea creatures into land mammals. This demonstrating the transformation of life and the pull of the planet Earth, from out of the confinement of the fluid world and into the fluidity of the bloodline. Aligned with its association with the tempo of life, and being the gland of energy, is the thyroid's regulatory facility in the absorption of life essence. This of course is limited when trauma leads to the constriction of this gland's function or restriction of the airways of the throat due to swelling, spasms or overgrowth. Too much protein in the diet will also result in this overgrowth by placing further pressure on the solar plexus and the kidneys and leading through reflection to constriction at the throat. Some of the life essence is retained and stored at the thyroid gland, which through alchemy is sent in a more concentrated state to the brain via the hormone thyroxin. This excretion is essential for the mind to deal with the complexities of thought. However, this depletes if constriction at the throat persists.

The transfer from communication via telepathy to speech evolved as the human form became more materially earthbound and as a result, or to coincide with this, the larynx was built. Thought was now internalised and the means by which Self developed its own consciousness. Speech became the method to pass thought on and grew in greater sophistication as consciousness also grew. It is imperative to the Ego that it is capable of thought. This was a major step forward in the way humanity was to construct its destiny: it now had the means by which to understand and explore itself in relation to the outside world. This is an intrinsic part of the creative purpose of the throat chakra. Truth here has much bearing on the function of the thyroid gland, for it is here that its secretion feeds into the rhythms of life which are understood by the laws of Absolute. Motion, space and duration connect directly to the creative force of the throat chakra by the thyroid's method of controlling the pace of life. This is translated by the amount of energy or fuel that one uses. These are the factors that give birth to and grow an idea and the thyroid provides the means by which the brain can think it through. Not only is the thyroid crucial in building the brain during early life but it also continues to feed the brain and thus sustains its many functions, such as memory. It is also responsible in balancing out mood swings, the positive and negative duality of Venus – love and hate. If these swings are severe, they can develop into deep, deep depression. Tuberculosis in the family often has a devastating effect on the balance of the thyroid and feeds insidiously into the central nervous system, the kidneys and cardiovascular system. This kind of depression can be seen in the tubercular miasmatic picture in which *Calcarea Carbonica*, being the closest remedy to the miasm, will be needed to underpin stability at some point. It is not a coincidence that this remedy is extracted from the mother-of-pearl in the shell of which Venus ascends from the sea.

Depending on whether there is insufficient thyroxin or excessive doses in the blood, the symptoms will be quite different from hypo-activity to hyper-activity. It is a lack of this hormone that is the cause of cretins in children who fail to develop the mature step into humanity asked by the throat chakra and thus pertain to a level that sadly does not extend much past the animal. In adulthood this deterioration of function is called myxoedema.

In general, under-function creates in children slowness to walk and to develop. These are backward children who become backward adults or at least exhibit characteristics that drive themselves away from others through their lack of conscience and creativity. Many hypothyroid families can be observed wandering slowly around mundanely criticising and complaining about everything in a negative chanter. Such criticism is the result of negative fatigue and has nothing to do with developing the sharpness of a critical faculty that would benefit their judgement, for these people do not strive to reach that level of aptitude. They give the impression that everything is so hard but if it gets any easier for them, in truth they would vegetate in their laziness; leaving everything for the troubled overactive thyroid types to worry even more about, if that were possible. These overactive types tear around under permanent time pressure, trying to achieve everything before burning out, which of course they don't believe will happen, and then complain of not being able to cope. They have little belief in trusting that life will provide for all that is needed in good time, if only they slowed down. Appendicitis can result from this state as the kidneys struggle to keep up with impossible odds laid down by the tempo set by the thyroid and also, as discussed previously, adrenal related problems.

Exhaustion can also arise from an inability to say no, which is not giving voice to one's truth at this centre. This pace appears to be set by external factors like a boss or the company, or another impossible deadline, which more often than not is created in the family. It is, however, only the thyroid's response to this pressure, as in reality one can chose

Chapter 5 ~ The Throat Chakra

one's own time frame as decreed by the laws of Absolute. Remember, the throat is the link between the personality and the spirit and neither of these extreme types of thyroid disposition has balanced this equation into realisation. Nervous energy uses up the fats in the body before they get a chance to form weight and so the reserves have to be eaten into, including the muscles and tendons. It is of no use suggesting to these emotionally reactive types to calm down.

The throat chakra is the place of hysteria and when presented by such a patient, they can be in a truly desperate state, which can also be very alarming for the practitioner. They may appear to be verging on madness and hysterical people do get sectioned. They will need *Thyroidinum* and *Fucus*, along with other remedies to try and balance out the thyroid gland. Of course these are illustrations of types where the thyroid is unbalanced towards one direction or another but it is often common to have the thyroid swing between these two states creating energy highs and then crashes. But either way, any thyroid problems will be reflected in a person who is driven by their emotions, which will be out of control. Therefore the brow will receive no standard of thought so operates somewhere in between confused outbursts and blankness. This state also unhinges the base chakra or inhibits its formation. Emotional stability, but not inhibited emotion, is the purpose of a well-balanced thyroid gland. The nosode *Tuberculinum* goes a long way in restoring contact with the earth by preparing harmony in the throat. This scenario can also be created if the head and heart go into conflict, which will manifest as a war being waged around the throat chakra and topple the nervous system. In this conflict no resolution means no peace, creating either calcification or excessive amounts of calcium being stripped.

Radiation has a profoundly destructive influence on the balance of the thyroid gland. This is especially so for women and can create infertility. When the Chernobyl disaster released its containment of Caesium gas into the atmosphere, the local women of the surrounding areas of the Ukraine were issued with lead collars to wear around their necks. This radioactive cloud was blown across the majority of northern Europe only to settle and find its way into the food chain. Once having looked at the picture of the remedy *Caesium* or having intuited it, there is much to compare in patients who come with chronic fatigue or ME. The start of a great flourish of these cases coincided with this event. There is also growing evidence that PCB's (polychlorinated biphenyls) found in food disrupt the function of the thyroid, among many other serious health risks and have been proven to create aggressive children. The irony is that pollution destroys the levels of iodine contained in our food, yet the intake of iodine helps to combat the poisons in our system. A balanced diet, or one that will help to counteract the thyroid's incorrect disposition, is also important. Even the quality of our water is said to have profound effects on the regulation of the thyroid, such is the sensitivity of the endocrine stability. When fluoride is added to tap water, then the incidence of thyroid problems escalates. The more that our food becomes difficult to digest then the more energy is lost from this gland that aids digestion. Tightness, restriction and problems breathing are all signs of an overworked digestion.

At present the human system is coming to terms with a new miasmatic threat formed by the radiation of mobile phones. It is not simply the masts that present the problem, for their field of radiation dissipates after a short distance, but the phones themselves, as they act as a magnet to this radiation enabling their communication. The effect of this radiation builds within the subtle bodies and acts upon them in a very syphilitic manner. Because this radiation is invisible, and initially at least may be subtle in its effect, it is not so easy to prove its harmful results. However, as we know with all miasms, they eventually make their mark on the physical plane by which time it is too late, its consequence having been built into the human condition. This radiation in particular will disturb development and maturity as it reaches into both the thymus and the thyroid gland. We know from the way that radiation is used to try and combat cancer, that tumours and the like will be the physical result of this miasm. Mobile phones are part of this carcinogenic age, as is their over-use. If they were used for emergency purposes only or infrequent use, then the dose of radiation would stay within safe limits but it is this carcinogenic age that prompts people to call a friend to notify their arrival only when they are a matter of a few seconds away.

So it is imperative to warn our patients as to the danger of their use. This radiation is also intensified in situations like public transport where many phones may be in use and the metal construction of the trains and buses bounce the microwaves back and forth constantly through each person. For the purpose of these situations, patients should carry their homœopathic remedies wrapped in aluminium foil for the radiation waves cannot penetrate through it. Mobile phone radiation can wipe out the energy of homœopathic remedies so they should strictly be kept absent from the practice room and patients need to be made aware that their phones should be kept away from their remedies. This also includes their use in homœopathic pharmacies. When a new miasm is forming, especially with a syphilitic association, it will try its hardest to infiltrate that which will otherwise hinder its formation. As a result, the level of its infiltration within all the subtle bodies on every level of the human condition, will be difficult to treat, which is the obstacle that as practitioners we have to face and will require the new remedy *Microwave*. This difficulty will be reflected within the higher planes and as a consequence of confusion, that which was relied on previously may stop working. The build up of this radiation which interferes with the energy in the body results in remedies not holding for as long as they use to, dramatically so in some cases, so prescriptions will need to be adjusted accordingly.

THE PARATHYROID

The parathyroid looks like the spots that glimmer on a butterfly's wings. These spots are several glands that collectively make up the workings of the parathyroid, and sitting on both wings of the thyroid gland, they act as small switches which regulate the levels of calcium and phosphate in the blood. These are the two primary chemical components of the brain and require an even balance, similarly to the thyroid, in their relative quantities for healthy function. A hormone that increases the solubility of calcium in the bones and thus the concentration in the blood, manages the maintenance as to the correct level of these substances. Tumours of the parathyroid can stimulate too much calcium but by far the most dangerous assault on this crucial and beautifully subtle mechanism is the Tetanus vaccine. The medical establishment refuse to heed their own warnings, for the devastation created on the immune system has been well noted. This vaccine is extremely dangerous when repeated yet they are handed out like free drinks at the Christmas party. We must be ready for a new influx of vaccines, for they will become the byword for curing anything and everything that becomes prevalent in contagious disease over the next fifty years, as part of a combination of fear, fashion and greed. The Tetanus inoculation pushes the syphilitic miasm more deeply within the being, allowing its destructive nature to hide more easily and thus trying to prevent any form of karmic release from happening. It will be in this centre that all syphilitic disease that remains incurable will lodge, as a result of blocks pertaining to the parathyroid. The removal of blocks here will not be straightforward for this is deep dark stuff, however if it is achieved, miraculous cures will be induced.

The balance of the glands of the parathyroid is imperative to the quality of thought. It pertains to the division of spheres in the brain, from the left and the right. Therefore, calcium and phosphorous balance thought, as both sides are required if complexities are to be understood. It can be seen in the remedy *Calcarea Phosphorica* that when this balance is disrupted thought jumps from one side to the other or from one place to another. Hence its leading mental characteristic is dissatisfaction. The three remedies of *Calcarea Carbonica, Calcarea Phosphorica* and *Phosphorus* all play on the frequencies of excitability created by these little switches.

All we have to do as practitioners is to decide which, within these frequencies, is the right remedy to use. Is the speed of thought too fast, leading to restlessness where a dose of *Phosphorus* is required to turn up the volume switch to increase the amount of calcium in the blood; or does it need slowing down with a dose of *Calcarea Carbonica* to counteract sluggish mental dullness? Or is it that the door to equilibrium can only be opened up by the administration of *Calcarea Phosphorica*, the patient not being content with any other prescription? The parathyroid and the thyroid gland operate in opposition to one another, by means of chemical pull and push, establishing the correct balance of calcium in the blood and thus its level in the bones. It is this correct balance of calcium that regulates the levels of phosphate in the blood, which if raised, the amount increased will correlate with the level of nervous excitability. The kidneys too will be stimulated in an attempt to clear excessive levels of phosphate through the elimination of urine. It can, therefore, be kidney problems that maintain high phosphate levels in the blood through poor function, an example of the throat chakra's close connection with the bloodline.

The luminosity of Venus that enables her to shine by day has been thought to be due to her phosphoric quality. She uses this source, for it can store large amounts of energy. This energy is required for humanity to rise above the animal existence and into the higher vibration of spirit. Phosphorus is the vital spark in the brain that enables it to connect to original thought, upon which calcium can then focus. This is why phosphorus is not only the tool of Venus but also of Lucifer, and is that which he came

Chapter 5 ~ The Throat Chakra

in search of. Without Lucifer, Self would not have grasped the knowledge to pursue its own intellect, which is profoundly important in humanity's development: his temptation was already present in Eden in the form of the snake. Phosphorus, when converted in the human body as phosphate, is the material reflection of that which has been sent to redeem us in thought, by consciousness and by light. It is within the human condition that mankind has to learn how to deal with its balance.

It will be in the parathyroid that the syphilitic component of the throat chakra will be housed. As the thymus energy is released it spills into the parathyroid in order that this negative karma may be released, a gift from the angels. The syphilitic side of the throat chakra may be so stuck that it lacks emotional expression, hence, having such a deep connection with the Lords of Karma, it will inhibit all natural processes. The resulting fear will interfere in the process of incarnating because due to the trauma of past life experiences the soul has become too frightened to live. This fear is hidden so as a practitioner you may have to look for it in order to make sense of the physical symptoms that are not responding to treatment. It will try to elude you, masquerade as other miasms or other symptoms in an attempt to put you off its scent. Even when writing this book, information about this area tried to hide itself. In maintaining a steadfast pursuit for cure many secrets may be revealed as the blockages of this centre start to unravel. During meditation, if this point is focused on, deep syphilitic karma may be released. This can transpire to be in the form of an entity, which, being too frightened itself to move on to the higher planes is a reflection of the terror, held in the body inhibiting all truth. If the block here can be freed then a great release of negative karma is possible, most of which will have its roots in Atlantis. Once gone, then that which was deemed incurable can be healed, which may appear nothing short of a miracle. This pertains to the magical power of balance: which is of the utmost importance and of true Venus energy; the dark and light combined in harmony. This enables us through the friendship of the marriage of opposites to see things in a different light. This will awaken new consciousness so that old patterns that are no longer relevant and which have caused debilitating diseases can miraculously be left behind. It is at the parathyroid that the root to Parkinson's disease can be found. Any shaking of any kind in a patient is an indication that there is a block associated with the parathyroid. The mysterious disease encephalitis lethargica, portayed in the film, "Awakenings", has recently been linked to a throat infection and the streptococcus bacterium: this condition can also be placed here.

SOUND, BREATH AND AKASHA

To take breath into the body to be utilised requires the support of the lower chakras. The clarity and strength of the lungs is crucial to this, as is freedom at the throat. The function of the liver and in particular the spleen and the kidneys, support the lungs to absorb solar energy. There will be a kind of energetic whip-round to replicate function by all the yang organs if there is a particular weak link or another organ in distress. The sycotic miasm plays havoc with the function of the lungs as they are used by the dense body as an overflow, filling them with mucus as a result of a toxic discharge from organs straining to operate under this miasm. Tuberculosis close by in the family history can result in the inheritance of weakened lungs. It may also be true that as one begins to apply remedies to such a state, in both cases, particular attention may be required to support the lungs. The kidneys and the spleen both act to control the fluids of the body and congestion in them is mostly the result of the sycotic miasm, which has been left to proliferate. If the congestion of the lungs is to be addressed then the effect of this miasm on the kidneys and spleen will need much treatment. Suffocation by this means is a form of drowning and has much to do with the weight of ancestral karma that rises up to take hold of the decisions of Self. In this particular struggle with the sycotic miasm, the ancestral energy that has encouraged its formation will be particularly obstinate to change. So much so, that this karma thinks little of ending the life of Self rather than, as a group entity, face the changes that here on Earth Self is endeavouring to achieve. We know, for instance, that if the sycotic miasm is prevalent in both parents then the child is prone to a double dose of its influence. This of course is heightened by the close proximity of the parents to the child in terms of generation, creating an instant bridge from miasm to child. This child will have much to clear in the way of physical pathology pertaining to this miasm, which if not addressed will be suppressed, leading to greater problems as adults. The bloodline is divided into its male part and its female part so the gender of the offspring will have much relevance as to which ancestral side, pertaining to its own gender, that the child will have to deal with most. As well as this, the masculine and feminine worlds are under a constant shift from attraction to

Chapter 5 ~ The Throat Chakra

repulsion, such are the interconnecting tentacles that go to make up ancestral blood. Eros brought about one important connection, the marriage of the Earth and the Sky, or the mother and the son. However, the sky bonded so tightly that it inhibited the Earth from breathing, it being smothered by too much of what it needed. From this constriction, Cronos, aided by others, was able to reach through to the light and sever his father's genitals, thus releasing humanity by re-establishing the distance between the Earth and the Sky. It was the compassion of Venus that was released as a result of this resurrection and was to become the source of all procreative acts without which humanity would suffocate. This process enables the release of not only negative ancestral karma but also the patterns formed by ancestors of our own gender, which are particularly deep rooted and will require much support whilst this energy is being dissipated.

Breathing is freedom. Asthma, pneumonia and other breathing problems are the result of a breakdown from this freedom. The new remedy *Peridot* reveals this connection, for it is useful in asthma where the child has an overbearing mother. That notion can be extended to the relationship between the Earth and the Sky. The lungs pertain very much to the heart chakra and *Peridot* is the birthstone of the sign Leo and one begins to see the link between the heart and the throat in achieving spiritual freedom. As discussed in the Chapter on the heart chakra, if the heart offers the opportunity to free Self of all negative karma, then the manifestation of Akasha at the throat centre is the achievement of this state. In meditation the breath awakens the gateway of the etheric world through the spleen, which also powers reception from the crown centre, the moon being female to the male sun. Thus the condition of the spleen in meditation is very important, it being relative to the depth of reception. Once the breath is extended, a process of relieving friction between the two worlds places its emphasis on the spleen and so the rest and recovery of this organ is essential before further meditation should be undertaken. Rest is also important for all the other vital organs as that which has been received takes time to filter through and instigate its change.

Rebirth that originates and extends from the heart chakra manifests as the first breath that opens up the individualism of life. Remember, air is the carrier of Absolute Energy that feeds the Ego for use in its material manifestation. Asthma is the result of a depletion of this life essence or freedom, which can become critical, especially if the body uses up its store of reserves that are held for such an emergency. When what is considered as death on earth occurs, the Ego leaves the dense body, which is then released from its command. When Ego has been used to direct energy in order to hold the atoms of the body together, it is Ego absent that creates the breakdown of these atom structures. However, not all the atoms are lost, for some may be absorbed and form new structures required during this transition. And further to this, the seed atoms that paved a way for the soul to follow also retain in essence a crucial supply of the vital energy. This is a similar process for the higher manas, which also die during the second death but their presence does not disintegrate completely, leaving some of their quality to be retained. The aspect retained could be considered to be spiritual, being both very slight and very great, like the perfume of a flower that can be smelt long before the form is seen. The fifth element or Akasha is a vibration or communication to the order of the atoms. Once again this connection illustrates the link between the head and the heart, which is the throat chakra, for sound is the bridge in the transcendence of consciousness. The word for this is Magic. The true definition of this word is the process or possibilities that can be brought about for the benefit of humanity and from which, with guidance, Self creates its own universe.

Because Self creates its own universe, then there must be many universes all being built in the higher planes: all of which are under the influence of the overriding result of cause and thus effect. Karma extends down from these highest activities until unravelled by humankind. There will of course be further universes to be created with the development of consciousness. In cosmology the appearance and disappearance of a universe is described as the inhaling or exhaling of the 'Great Breath'. When the word 'development' is used to represent evolution, it is in regard to this continuous motion as one of the three facets of Absolute, the other two being limitless space and its duration. The meaning of the facets of Absolute can be found in the many symbolic representations of the Hindu deity Vishnu (far too many to mention here); who is part of a triad very much like the upper three chakras, along with Brahma and Shiva. Vishnu represents the aspect of Supreme Reality that sustains all that is of the created and moving universe, the origin of which is associated with the sound Ohm and from which the five elements and the five senses are said to have arisen. Vishnu also acts

Chapter 5 ~ The Throat Chakra

over individual existence from which the word 'Vish', meaning to penetrate, has a link to the soul's journey within the upper triangle of the chakras, which, starting at the throat is to pervade the unknown. Once underway, a universe falls under the realm of the Divine otherwise it would be motionless. The very fact that we are creatures of breath means that we go along with or participate in the constant rhythms of motion or in its simplest terms – change, which under Divine orchestration, cannot be avoided.

The motion of breath, change and consciousness are synonymous with each other, one cannot exist without the other. The fire at the throat centre mixed with the fluidity of ether and then combined is Akasha and its reception has inspired the name 'Divine Breath', the cosmos formulator. It is the combination or balance of fire and water that gives humanity the potential, through harmony or breath, to be at one with Divine reality: but this is only possible when fully present. Each intake of breath connects with love. Breath reminds us that we are spiritual beings, connecting all energy and if we close our eyes and induce a meditative state then it brings with it the consciousness of Divine reality. The sycotic miasm with its fear of spiritual growth goes against this balance of fire and water and it may take many lifetimes before its karma can be sufficiently addressed, where cause and effect have been balanced so that Self is no longer under its constraints. When a remedy made from Coal is properly proved, it will go far in helping to re-correct this influence, especially in situations where the syphilitic and sycotic miasms are deeply interlocked, as they often are in present times. The balance of fire and water has much influence on how we construct and conduct our relationships with others. What we ask for in life is often expressed by our relationships and the motivation behind them can be very difficult to break, the hardest one being that of a partner, which may be only maintained out of a desire for security. This is especially so where desire has been motivated by the kidneys and not instigated by the Divine Breath.

Humanity, just like nature, is subject to the laws that govern creativity, themselves not being the result of evolution in the normal sense of the word, for they are Absolute. Thus things will either go one way or the other depending on those laws. Spirit combined with matter is the force that directs this motion to bring about change. Here at the throat chakra is the unification that creates this force and that manifests our solar system; but it is the Source that holds the ultimate power, bound by no laws that we are aware of and that overlooks these other aspects and thus contains the true definition of the word 'unity'. Therefore, Akasha is the consciousness of Divine or the purpose of planet Earth, making itself felt in evolutionary terms through the atom. Fire, as described in chemistry, is atomic motion, the bridge between the physical and the spiritual. The atom is the road to the monad and therefore 'unity' is unification on an atomic level, which is the current evolutionary stage of humanity's understanding as to the nature of energy being used on the higher realms. The symbol of the heart chakra speaks of the start of this process, for the dot at the centre is the spark of energy from which vibration oscillates to form the notes in which sound travelling outwards forms the circle which represents Divine Unity and from which everything proceeds. The circle and the dot is the dawn of differentiation from which sprung Self. Our universe also sprung from this germ. The glyph of the throat chakra – the circle above the cross – reveals the relationship in which this separation leading to our universe is destined to play out: spirit is above matter.

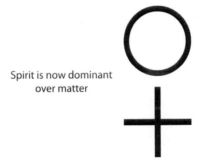

Spirit is now dominant over matter

Figure 13. Transcendent circle of spirit risen above cross of matter

Adam and Eve were banished from the Garden of Eden, and as a consequence, formed Psoric insecurity; this was the result of the temptation which was their quest to make their own universe. The tree of life bore fruit, which provided consciousness and the consequence of sampling this fruit was enticement, the desire to seek consciousness and break away from Eden, which is paradise.

In meditation, the deep breath sets up the opportunity to clear trauma that has been stuck and thus free emotions that hinder growth. This is achieved via Vapour: the mixture of fire and water, where sunlight hits

Chapter 5 ~ The Throat Chakra

the sea and forms the mist that will heal; but, in fact, all four elements are required for this process. The earth holds the water and air is the vehicle for fire. The resultant Vapour, if meditated on, provides insight into the nature by which life is sustained and holds the power to break karmic links that create the repetition of trauma from one life to the next. This is especially so if experienced after having lost a major love but this would have been a very special, deep love for a particular partner who has instigated an intense inspiration and much healing. This is different to the love for an offspring, which would have provided for the creation of perhaps many offspring and the loss of this love can haunt a person from one incarnation to the next. It can tie a person into a lack of fulfilment, making life decisions through this sense of loss. It can resurrect sadness or deep depression, the explanation for which has long been forgotten, with the exception, of course, of feeling empty.

Part of the act of incarnation involves forgetting. A sense of loss can inhibit the natural cycle of finding a partner, for the void left from the past must first be healed. This void, when expressed at the throat, attracts karmic relationships that resurrect the past, including also the pain. One can even meet the soul of this previous love again and continue this love affair if one so desires, and which can obviously be extremely difficult to resist: but the point to life is to be in the present and by doing so Self is asked to heal the sense of loss and move on to pastures new. The desire to find such a person again for the purpose of a relationship will never provide the solution and in fact it usually highlights the frustrations of holding on to the past, of not having transcended. Often the purpose of such a reunion is to allow the karma of it to complete: the past can never be replicated only healed. With the use of this Vapour, the element of Akasha, one possesses the secret potion that can break such ties. Just like Venus is enabled to spread her influence as a result of the actions of Cronos, then Self is released to breathe in this newfound freedom that comes with a fresh cycle. It is always that which is happening now that is important. So as stated, the hindrance of life breath reveals an imbalance of the four elements within the body, which is a matter of miasmatic activity and will inhibit the absorption of Akasha. It must also be remembered that this imbalance will often be the reason why remedies do not hold. Through the importance of this balance it is clear that the throat chakra is crucial to that which manifests in order to maintain good health.

To meditate on this Vapour not only opens up a gateway but creates the tools to open to the other world in order to perform spiritual healing for Self. To call upon what one wants, opens Self up to what there is, and the breath brings to this clarity, just like the first breath at birth; it creates the means to existence. Practices involving the breath have long had connections with entering the spiritual world. It is in this other world that changes in structures can be redressed, simply through the act of receiving energy through breathing in meditation, which in turn has a profound effect on the structures in this world. It cannot be emphasised enough how powerful meditation is in achieving this. The mouth, through the ability to express and receive, enables us within the mechanism of sound to mould a new life but only after this reception has been understood and articulated. Akasha then is regeneration, where the inside changes and is reflected on the outside. The influence of homoeopathic remedies allows our patients to find this understanding. That this is so simply achieved through matching the correlation of symptoms to a remedy is one of the gifts of homœopathy.

At the throat, the child takes her first life breath, the start of a function that will sustain her in being here throughout her life. The first two days of this life would be too much for the yet insufficiently strengthened lungs to cope with entirely on their own, so a portal at the top of the head which originates from a time long before lungs were needed, remains open for a day or two to assist in the accumulation of light while the lungs get used to their task. This is similar to how the crown chakra receives insight and it is a Divine wish that maintains life. This extra intake is especially needed if the child arrives with jaundice, a reflection of the mother's apprehension during pregnancy. It is our ability to breathe in life that fuels the creative purpose of the throat centre. During Lemuria, the throat was formed at the same time as the ears and nose, enabling those related senses to judge the purity of what was being received by the body. In pregnancy these senses are heightened. This also explains why these sensory organs are devised of the same tissue and why together, they act as an overflow to human fluids at times of congestion. Mucus finds it easier to escape through these openings as a method of keeping the lungs clear so that the important work of absorbing the life nectar can be maintained.

Chapter 5 ~ The Throat Chakra

The breath can control much, for it is the way in which the outside is permanently connected with the inside. We all breathe the same air and so it should be the same for our compassion. The throat is the portal that lets the outside in and the inside out. This also pertains to love. As already mentioned, it is at the throat chakra that we choose and attract our partner and where this connection is sealed by the first kiss and confirmed by subsequent ones. But also and of equal importance in this process is the way in which Self calls upon its partner by what it wishes and uses words and gestures to convey this. The future partner is already formulated in the mind's eye that knowingly or not, speaks out in the form of a request in order to attract the mate. It is the tubercular miasm that has romanticised this attraction, knocking the throat out of balance, and creating fanciful comparisons. As a result, in the West finding one's soul mate has become big business. What is really required in achieving this, though, is to loosen the grip of this distracting miasm, allowing clarity or the single trunk of the elephant to follow out its task – that of service, liberated from distraction.

It may be true that in the past when populations were smaller, the divisions between the sexes were less complicated and the need to breed was more prevalent, which meant finding and staying with a partner was possibly easier. However, the factors governing attraction have not disappeared and so are as relevant today as they have always been. If one is clear as to what one wants then the universe will provide. The deepening development of the Tubercular miasm over time has eroded the understanding of this fact. Clarity at the throat is so important because it governs much in the quality of the person and thus the quality of their life and the security of the partner's life. The lips, the tongue, the breath, the voice, taste, smell and the ability to receive sound and love are all used in order to take a bite out of life.

This chakra offers much in the way of insight as to how the dilution of a homœopathic remedy widens its field of action and how the subsequent vibrational wave that moves outward in the pursuit of understanding changes relationships around it. The 'hippie' movement was an exploration into looser structures that enabled greater vibrations, without which we would never have achieved the advances in new structures. These structures are the ways in which we construct our universe and their vibrations are the result of the production of our thoughts. Venus, being opposite to Mars, enables this development as it extends into the astral plane, not by means of exploration but by the act of creativity. It is able to do this by the means of compassion, which is the ability to allow things to come to an end without the trauma of loss, such as the death of anything when the time has come to move on. Venus provides a natural passage from the old and into a new beginning. This is transition, for nothing truly dies and Venus reveals the beauty of everything transformed.

To understand the pure spiritual power of the throat chakra, one has to appreciate its role in all creation, including the Akashic records themselves. It is stated in the Book of Genesis, "In the beginning there was the Word", the Divine Breath. This is the intention from which all was to follow: and all that which has come into existence originated from this intent. Its expression is carried by sound, which as it eventually slows, forms matter. Sound resonates just beyond form and is the bridge between abstraction and the concrete. For humans this emphasis is the intermediary between that which one speaks and the creation of one's universe. One can speak to oneself or others without making a sound but it will be the vibrational intent, so often dismissed, which is more powerful than the written word, which is often used to disguise true meaning. We may be polite or withhold our voice but our truth lies within our intent and should be read by the practitioner. One can work around and be under a constant influence of the vibration of homœopathic remedies but it will be the intent of those taken that Self will chose to utilise. Intent inevitably results in the situation we create for ourselves and therefore negative expression will create a negative reaction. This does not mean to go through life smiling, disregarding the natural reactions to pain, fear and injustice. What it means is to be true to aspiration through integrity in order to attract the means by which one's purpose can be successfully achieved. This may of course involve tremendous change, the frustrations of which will be heard in the words of the patient.

If we return to the notion of incarnation starting at the crown chakra and working down into the conscious materialism of the base chakra, spirit's experience at the throat chakra is imperative in enabling this physical manifestation to be undertaken. Akasha gained at the throat allows the soul to further this exploration by fuelling the blueprint of its physical expression. The soul's relationship to the planet Earth will forevermore, with the use of this energy, be expressed at the throat

Chapter 5 ~ The Throat Chakra

chakra. This is sound, the bridge that enables Self to be of both worlds. If ether is the vibration of the airwaves and Akasha is the spirit of the airwaves, then sound is their intermediary: it connects the body to the head, matter to spirit and life to creative purpose. If the patient has no creative purpose then the throat chakra will be closed. In British society the throat often reflects the frequent levels of trauma accumulated in its people and this has silenced the wishes of many or surfaced as aggression from pure frustration. The energy of this island, in vibrational terms, is burdened with much weight. Trauma destroys the true compassion of Venus, and we are left with a compensatory replacement created out of a broken will. Without balance, Mars pushes Venus to resurrect her dark side. If this creative force turns malignant, this chakra will suck in the life force like a vacuum, which as in the nature of all the chakras means stripping the energy resource of the chakra above and below, leading to mass confusion. Negative throat energy manifests as criticism and arrogance and will push its weight around in order to prove its point in a curious reaction to trauma, it being too proud to resolve things in silence. Such people are propelled through life, driven by thyroid energy that achieves nothing, yet they may face the opportunity to clear their depression sooner than they think by developing related ailments that force them to act. The resultant actions can be life changing but it often takes a considerable threat to health to draw these people away from their apathetic, negative chanter.

Derived from the word Akasha is the word Ankh, the name for the Egyptian symbol that is very similar to the symbol of Venus, a cross with a loop above it.

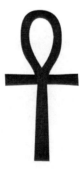

Figure 14. Ankh

To the Egyptians the Ankh was the symbol of life or the 'breath of life', which formed and maintains the universe. This symbol represents the kundalini having raised up the spine and awakened the soul to spiritual possibilities, providing not only knowledge but also, through experience, enlightenment. This is the position of being in equilibrium. The symbol of Ankh was seen and still acts as a magical form of protection when travelling between the two worlds, as does *Turquoise*, a major throat remedy and a stone so admired by the Egyptians for its protective powers. This symbol is the Sun as it pops up over the horizon to bring light to what had previously been dark. It sets in motion that which is great in each and every one of us and creates the strength, through metabolism, to be strong for others. It is the place we teach and nurture our children and the place where they in turn, as we once did, feed their children.

As spoken of in the heart chapter, the accumulation of the four elements in the heart is the root to Akasha, the element of life. This life is immortal and speaks of the reason for existence within the higher planes rather than concentrating on the mortal life of Earthly years. It offers a bigger picture. But one must master the four elements in Self here on Earth before one can use Akasha to explore the higher planes. To the Egyptians Ankh represented being at one with the gods from Earth, which has no divide. This harmony is the same as the pyramid itself, representing the bridge from this world into the next. Therefore, the shape of the Ankh offers much in the way of a blessing, variations of which have been adopted by charities and the like today. It is a link between us and them, a cry for help or the holding of a hand. It is the joining of the head with the body. This link has always been symbolic and was the juncture cruelly severed during medieval practices, for execution by beheading represented the power of the 'head of state' over any inner belief. This sent a powerful warning of the importance of loyalty to the people, the control of which still lingers in British society. Even today and long after the formation of common law, Britain still has the bill of rights but no constitutional rights. It may also be argued however, that this system has saved homœopathy from its demise.

Freedom of speech used to be imperative and an integral part of a community and one in which the House of Commons is built around today. It is so named because previously on common ground, before they were handed over to golf clubs, one had the right to express one's

Chapter 5 ~ The Throat Chakra

grievances without the threat of retribution from one's neighbours which included everybody, as is still the case in the House of Commons today. Anything can be said without the fear of legal or other reprisals, although nowadays, alas, the parliamentary career has taken precedence over any open debate. The purpose of the common which can still be witnessed at Hyde Park, albeit in a very entertaining manner often designed for tourists, was to free the group of control in order that the truth may win out. This is a creative process for it enabled the group to establish an outlet in which it could move and grow without the hindrance of grudges, and enabled grievances to come to the fore without producing festering consequence. Obviously such outpourings on the common were not always true, as they are frequently not in the House of Commons, but this process of expression at the throat centre is still the best way in which to allow the truth to be debated. To a certain extent, the Internet has opened up the possibility of a similar system of debate, it being so difficult to police. But even on the 'net', in theory one is still open to a complicated system of libel laws and because the Web is image based (brow chakra), it is also essential when words and images come together, where the imagination becomes concrete, that these laws protect the vulnerable.

In all aspects of life it is imperative that Self is able to speak its truth. It is its name, the word heard most in life that differentiates it as Self. One's name and one's truth creates identity. It is pure empowerment and it is only through the release of negative karma, that has kept one away from one's truth, that one's name can manifest in goodwill.

In Egypt this truth was held in a different kind of house, the House of Life, which was an attempt to replicate the Akashic Library here on Earth. It was open to all as a meeting place between Heaven and Earth. Magic was used to source its secrets but the layman was equal to the Pharaoh in his contribution, as each soul makes up the strength of the whole. No one was to be excluded. However, all may have been needed in order to receive wisdom but not all were capable. Those in need of guidance or who had lost their way and forgotten their truth would consult magicians or priests in order that the connection to their gods could be re-established. This would also be provided in ritual. This house would of course act as a source of health, advising those of the correct path, of spells and creating prescriptions in which to promote a healing process. The magicians were also responsible for maintaining the security and secrecy of such truths, which if revealed to the uninitiated, would render them in a perpetual state of disbelief and confusion. This inevitably aroused curiosity and also doubt amongst those who sought the knowledge but were not prepared to do the work. Such was the vastness of information accumulated at such temples, and the bureaucracy required to contain it, that corruption was inevitable: but one's truth is not necessarily all truth so it could not just be taken. In order to be privy to such information, one has to learn significance and wield its magic. It was creative inspiration at the throat chakra that enabled this spiritual path to progress through the development of understanding at the brow chakra. The desire to 'own' knowledge prompted an overspill of 'truth' from the House of Life and meanwhile the vehicle of trade developed from the magicians, for they now had a commodity with which to barter. Information is free to all and no matter how those in positions of authority wish it not to be so, it cannot be contained, for the truth always surfaces in the end. Without this infiltration on humanity's behalf the Greeks would never have had the means to establish the Wisdom School. In this school, humanity went full circle back to Adam and Eve, able to feed from the Tree of Knowledge inspired by the Tree of Life.

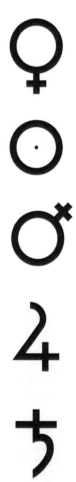

Chapter 6
The Brow Chakra

THE BROW CHAKRA

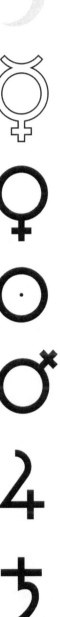

The brow chakra, along with the crown, marks a very large step in elevated consciousness – for here lie the tools by which Self can reach out to all in the cosmos. Just like a door, which is either open or shut, the brow chakra is either open to this elevated consciousness or not. It responds, and is kept alive, by receiving and processing information, which we call thoughts, an amalgamation of living in the physical word and being of the other world (self-conscious).

In the West, thought is kept under tight control by the use of social position or the notion that one is either qualified to think or not. This stifles debate and hinders transcendental thinking. Thought is a faculty that belongs to all – granted there is a talent to it but this may be developed (though it may need to be encouraged). This individual freedom is hindered by poor educational practices that instil fear and perpetuate the negative attributes of a society. Those who believe fact is only something that can be quantified through the scrutiny of logic and by careful testing to determine whether it holds up in the physical world, openly degrade the practice of original thought. There is little interest or support in thought unless it can be used to produce a product. The exploration into quantum physics is still funded on the premise that it will provide us with something that is determinable. However, modern physics has determined that nothing appears to be what it seems when quantified, i.e. as a part, not as a continuum, and so perception is turned upside down.

Chapter 6 ~ The Brow Chakra

As is the nature of exploration, in investigating that which is pushing the parameters of matter, rules that have previously been applicable no longer hold true in the light of new consciousness. This activity is, in fact, an exploration into the history of occultist philosophy, of which the language and concepts between it and science are becoming very similar. The tide is changing, for the physical world is beginning to accept the spiritual one.

There is much that, through the limitations of matter, cannot be tested but can still be known. In meditation, the act of receiving and the way that information is interpreted, is dependent on the integrity of Self and not a governing board. This understanding cannot be obtained by qualification and neither can it be bottled as an instant answer to whatever the question may be, for the solutions are dependent on the awakening of Self, and this is a process. It is for this reason that at the brow chakra there lies a division between the sheep and the goats. It is free thought that divides the two, and it is the source of this thought that is important.

Within the brain lies the greatest mechanism to make conscious that which has been received, but has of yet been beyond human comprehension. However, this does not mean that it hasn't been there all the time waiting to manifest. Some aspects may have already begun but it takes a special mind in an equally unique situation to receive the whole picture. To do this requires an exceptional focus, of which we are all capable. The manifestation of all consciousness has been derived in this way and will be for some time to come.

The virgin birth is a story about bringing in new consciousness. Information is not a private matter and has no business being locked up by a few who pretend to have the group's best interest at heart. Thoughts are a part of the 'Universal Consciousness', so secrets that are kept, in the name of national security say, are in fact a result of global karma and it is the resolution of this through thought and the spreading of information that will bring about a solution. Of course those who are still stuck in the Power School will have a vested interest in making us appear unqualified and stupid. But in truth it is we who continue to mop up their mistakes. Most secrecy is established by our leaders as a reflection of the fear of financial loss, so we allow them to pretend that the world is a place to be feared and not one that is created by our collective consciousness.

WISDOM

At the brow issues take on a global scale, for the thoughts of the group become that of the Earth and the spirits beyond. The brow is the connective point to the other world, for it enables us to see a wider picture, a view of and from the higher planes. This is synthesised through the forming of one's own universe and resonates back out to the world by means of one's own beliefs. These create the waves of wisdom that are attractive to those who wish to learn, to make things better, to undo negative karma and who are searching for spiritual growth. If one has vision, then this spark should be considered within a global context.

Wisdom is more advanced than knowledge for it contains love, which is at the heart of spirit. Knowledge is only a body of information knitted together, which can be used for any means. Wisdom contains that which connects spirit to Divine consciousness, through the soul. It is at the brow centre and through the manas that this connection is made. However, in order that the manas can formulate this reception, a connection between three levels of perception is required, which is the making of the brow chakra. These levels consist of the 'kama' manas and the higher manas, which if not mastered make it impossible to reach the third level, that of the Buddhi.

Having established the function of the throat chakra, it becomes clear that the throat chakra does not contain the manas but acts as a floor pan on which they can rest. The raising of creative energy from the throat centre, in order to find a focus in the brow chakra, is the sign of the initiate. To awaken the brow is to gain high spiritual vision and the understanding of mystical comprehension. This is only possible when the quality of the heart has also been established in the head and vice versa.

Through fear, Self can place great restraint on the development of the manas, especially due to cycles of behaviour laid down in past lives that inhibit Self's belief in its growth. The group also lives by the formation of such constraints, and in the West, the breaking down of systems is essential to the evolving planetary consciousness. It is the development of the mind that is humanity's present pursuit under this stage of our root-race. Now it would appear that thought is driven more by the financial motivation of science rather than a spiritual one.

By pursuing forms and ideas that explain the way in which the universe is constructed, science has begun to recognise energy fields that

Chapter 6 ~ The Brow Chakra

formulate an etheric webbing ('string theory'). This is beginning to yield a vision as to the workings of the astral world. Esoterically, this is the place where Western science is. In the East it is a little different, for action or the desire of the kama manas, has not the same progressive force behind it and therefore still has a close connection with spirit. It is for the West not to run away with itself but embrace wisdom that needs to be incorporated on its route. For instance, great strides have been made to advance surgery in the West with the development of sophisticated technology. However, when surgery is needed in the East, care is taken to avoid cutting through any of the meridian lines running through the body that pertain to organ function. This has a huge significance in not only the recovery but also the future function of the organs, for these etheric channels should not be disconnected. The importance of this is not recognised or understood in the West. In fact, even with all the advancement in technology, these meridian lines cannot even be detected. The cutting of these energy lines also creates huge problems in the overall communication between the chakras. Once again knowledge is important but amounts to nothing if it only produces more trouble. If these connections have been cut in a patient they may require acupuncture, in addition to homœopathy, to rejoin them through the scarring. The case history will reveal this necessity, especially if an organ or the patient is not responding to the prescription.

In the process of expanding thought, the West has historically fed from the East, mainly pillaging its spiritual philosophy to balance its physical philosophy. Information as to the relationship between human existence, energy and Divine reality is now flooding into the West from the East and due to the rapid growth of activities such as new therapies, this understanding is in high demand. But most, if not all of this information, albeit in a different form, has already existed here in the West, suppressed by the greed of a few. The meeting of these two minds reveals to the many insight into that which has been a part of rituals and occult practices pursued by the few since the times of Atlantis. As these induce change they have remained hidden by convention. This is now set to alter.

Like the Sun's daily voyage across the sky, the light of this wisdom moves from East to West and so America formed as a continent in its present state solely to pursue the purpose of developing the mind. It is in the West, through explorative qualities, that the battle as to what freedom means to the individual is taking place. Previously, in the East, this task was undertaken by the guru and was esoteric. Now it is for the group and must be evolved exoterically.

It is no coincidence that technology, gene therapy and the desire to build a super-race has settled on American shores and if the prediction of an evolutionary pattern is correct, then Australia will be next to take up the mantle. This exploration of the mind will pursue the insights of the mystic, but of course in a different manner – one that manifests for all to ponder. This is how the evolution of human consciousness has always been. In Egypt, algebra was a system privy only to the priests and pharaohs and now it is taught as a matter of course in Western schools – though perhaps its significance has changed. Such is the conversion from Divine consciousness to human consciousness, which takes time to go full circle but is the method used by all the root-races. In order to achieve this, the mind must never forget love, which is imperative as an ingredient in humanity's pursuit in building tomorrow today.

THE KAMA MANAS AND THE MANAS

Self has a duty to spirit. Intelligence as vision is inhibited by the ego and its conditioning. The quality of the kama manas determines much in the way of vision, for it is of the empirical mind and thus its roots run deep into the personality. As already mentioned in the previous chapter, the kama manas overlap in a sense with the throat chakra, for they are expressed through feeling and thinking.

When Self became 'self conscious' its manas were born – no Self then no manas. To the Hindus this awareness is known as Ahankara. This term is used to describe that which Self uses to identify what it is, in its entirety. It therefore has a triple aspect by which Self's sense of 'I' abides at any given moment. These three aspects are Satva – pure tranquillity that is rhythm, Rajas – active mobility, and Tamas – remaining 'stagnant' in darkness, inertia. These three aspects of nature together define the nature of human beings and are the three attributes known as gunas. They are that which keeps spirit attached and identified with its body whilst carrying out its purpose. They maintain this connection because they themselves are earthbound qualities. But what is important here is that all three are attitudes of the mind, for Ahankara is of universal self-consciousness. This means the gunas are of matter as well as spirit, for matter is within spirit and vice-versa, both being universal in order for the cosmos to have form. However, Self needs its boundaries in order

Chapter 6 ~ The Brow Chakra

that it does not get lost in universality, or the monad. This is because all is truly the same, individualised only by karma. One has to have egotism and pride in order to remain oneself or have the notion of 'I'. As mentioned before, this is not possible without the awareness of the Laws of Absolute, the three creative laws in which Self can orientate and develop its worldly existence. It is the gunas that make this possible, for they emanate from within but are only states of mind. To the Hindus these three laws, and in a minor way the triple aspect of Ahankara, are symbolic of the trinity of gods: Brahma, Vishnu and Shiva. For instance, without the creative desire for activity that Brahma brings, Self would not have become aware of itself and would not have been propelled into earthly existence. It is for this reason that Ahankara develops through the pursuit of worldly desires, which then perpetuates it into the next higher principle of Buddhi, which is understanding. Such understanding can only be achieved through thought; therefore Ahankara is the essence of the mind. When young, Ahankara, like Self is still developing and thus does not have the limits that growth instils through the experience of caution. Through experience one begins to understand what 'I' means and thus the limitations of life become more important, especially as one life follows the other. However, it must be stressed that Ahankara is not real and it does not really have form. What it provides, through the gunas is the illusion of life in order that as one grows, life appears to have some structure of reality. It is what forms Self's terrestrial manas and reflects the personality, but equally, not being real, it can be altered.

The fact that the illusion grows is due to these three laws of nature – the laws of the Absolute. Once illusion has been stripped, which is the emancipation of the three aspects of Ahankara, along with the terrestrial manas, then the buddhi can embrace the soul with immortal awareness, which is the Monad. When developing Ahankara, it is difficult to recognise its illusion and thus people have dedicated their lives in seeking to construct thought through this recognition. When the separation into Self occurred, so did the first thought – that of the recognition to construct thought. From this supposedly all other thought manifested, so Ahankara is the basis of all thought and to be intrinsically self-aware is to have the ability to tap into universal thought.

The purpose of the higher manas is not to eradicate Ahankara but to transform it by means of purifying the soul. It is aspiration that makes this possible and the vessel is Akasha – only then will it bridge the gap between the higher manas and the Buddhi. The pull of this desire begins at the throat chakra and is driven by the intelligence of existence, which is immortality. For Self to gain a peek at its own immortality is too great a temptation to resist.

The kama manas are filled with delusion that leads the personality astray or is the result of being led astray. The gift of the brow chakra is focus, so contained within it is both the intelligence of 'I' and of course its ignorance. If one pursues that which goes against one's knowledge or does not follow one's truth, then the mind will be awash with contradiction. This is important, for the Buddhi rests on the experience of the manas.

Such is the height of materialism in the West that the vast majority of its inhabitants have to deal with false pride. This underscores our modern sense of 'I–ness.' 'I am this for I own that' or 'I can afford to do this so that grants me power to be who I am.' The Kama manas can contain not much more than a reflection of a material position that creates a way of thinking based on the fear of loss. These are all the constraints of the personality that dull the senses and paralyse the mind. In a sense Ahankara is false prestige. It is the transforming of these desires that is required in order to derive one's sense of Self in the world, which opens up the full faculties of the mind. Nothing is lost, but is evolved into the new. In order to reunite with the Source it is as if one has to de-Self by becoming free from the illusions of the physical world. This is the only possible way to become fully aware as to what it is to be Self.

There are many different systems that explain the construction of the mind. Vedic Yoga ascribes five levels to the mind, but on the whole if all the different boundaries are merged a little, the principles of moving from the lower mind to its upper echelons are esoterically explained in very similar ways. The premise to which they all conform is the movement from duality to unity, without which the mind would not be at one with Divine consciousness. The higher manas are in essence pure mind, a structure apart from any physical context or constraint. It is at this point that the Mahatmas automatically incarnate. It is this energy, or should I say state of being, which is pure mind, that contains the true meaning of the word 'faith.' The intellect contains knowledge that has no moral bounds and thus can be used for any pursuit, be it dark or light. But faith is a component of wisdom, the perceptive tool used by the higher manas. It is this that combats the ignorance of the lower

Chapter 6 ~ The Brow Chakra

mind and prevents one working against the nature of what is already in the process of construction in purpose, thus steering one from forming more negative karma and becoming stuck. Only in the lower manas does 'blind faith' manifest, which is not faith but obsession. This reveals the negativity of the brow which pertains to the energy of its opposite chakra, that of the sacral centre. Faith has much to do with high perception because it speaks with such clarity, being the most central part of one's knowing. Faith is more than judgement, for it takes Self into the realm of Divine reception. Clarity in the brow enables the focus of faith, for ultimately it is this connection, the truth of Self and that of the Source, which produces pure intuition.

The kama manas or the rational aspect of thought can interfere with faith as it does with homœopathic prescribing. Ironically, the notion that faith is important is contentious within homœopathy at present. The pursuit of raising the level of prescribing is surely the reason why we all pursue homœopathy and from which we are able to understand more and thus heal more. This is the reason why the higher mind is referred to as being higher. We have all, I believe, gone against faith at one time or another or simply ignored the existence of it altogether, but this should not be done so lightly, for it involves aspects of telepathy or other means of direct knowing which bypass the ordinary senses. A leap of faith is required for the focus of perception to be sharp. The higher manas have no direct dealings with the physical plane and thus are not corrupted by the indecision that comes through the insecurities of the earthly world.

The purpose of opening up the mind is to look upwards and not be a slave to the intellect, which pulls one down. It is the light of the Buddhi, its spiritual discernment, which guides the initiate towards being able to use faith just like any other tool. Faith is very real and very powerful and when applied to the concentration of the brow chakra it facilitates vision.

As energy moves up through each chakra it undergoes refinement in order to activate the positive qualities of the chakra above. This also happens within the brow itself, for it is the energy of the lower manas that transcend through spiritual growth to provide that which is awakened in the higher manas. This is the process of becoming conscious of what has previously been forgotten. It is because the higher manas are a mirror to the lower manas that this spiritual transformation can take place, as nothing is lost but simply refined to function at a higher level within its equivalent counterpart.

The manas always pertain to free will, which as we know is the same as Divine will. However, Self has the choice of either being driven by its lower attributes or by its higher ones. Both are equally guided by Divine will, so sooner or later the consequence of either will require Self to gather in an upward motion, as with the nature of its Rajas. In the West allopathic medicine fails to recognise these higher qualities and therefore gives no credence to their development in creating better health. Therefore, when embarking on such methods of cure, the patient hands over not only their will but also any higher connection, which could help determine what is best for Self. There is a deep relationship between this communication and the improvement of health. The patient may have lost this connection long before seeking allopathic help and when they finally come to see a homœopath the very nature of the treatment will be to re-establish this connection.

Other treatments and methods that differ from allopathic medicine are becoming very popular because of the power of the higher mind. People are in contact with what they need and are being directed by a higher means within their transition.

It is through free will that the manas have their influence on all the other chakras, for, as previously stated, the aspect of each chakra is within all the other chakras. Maintaining freedom in the brow is what taps into the world of pure thought – that of the higher manas. The karma manas are not free but bound by constraint. It is the higher quality that enables the mind to free itself from physical constraints, and to do this one must have faith in its bounty. It is this aspect of communication that was prevalent before Self was aware of itself – not conscious – having no physical brain and no physical plane in which to ground its understanding.

Through positive as well as negative karma, evolution has brought with it conflict. Essentially karma is all the same, for one has to reach into the depth of one's being to achieve emancipation from it. One cannot be fully conscious in any other way. However, in the manas, a dichotomy of awareness is created between believing something through direct knowing, and that which is inevitably governed by the physical world because it can be seen, touched and judged by means of the five senses. Immediate perception can be a very powerful but also a difficult attribute to have and once again it is a matter of choice whether this is expressed vocally at the throat chakra. This is why the brow chakra is the true place of communication, for it connects the lower attributes with the higher Self, enabling one to hear that other voice and choose whether or not to give expression to it.

Chapter 6 ~ The Brow Chakra

Such communication is what all humans are here to develop. The throat chakra is the intermediary between this voice and that which it inspires to manifest in life. To understand more about this level of communication it is important to look at the way in which the monad interacts above the manas and feeds into them.

Integrity is not only the ability to stick to what one believes is right but also the ability to change when this is no longer the case. Firstly, one has to set a course and stick to it in order to know the outcome. This is the seed, and within it is the whole solution. It is no good to work with the assumption that you won't complete a task, or will abandon it unfinished. To leave things unfinished inhibits learning and the ability to move forward. It is impossible to know the results beforehand or predict what an outcome will lead to in advance. By means of the result Self knows where it is and has also put into place the soul's next step, albeit unwittingly: results inspire purpose. It is for this reason that the higher manas cannot work directly on the body but have to go through an intermediary – the lower manas. The meditative proving of homœopathic remedies demand this relationship in order for that which is received to be of the greatest use to humanity. It requires this level of focus, which needs to be understood by the sitters.

Integrity should bond the pursuit of physical desires with the direction of spiritual ones, for it is integrity that grants vision. The brow chakra is the seer of all and this is why it needs to direct its vision to those higher aspects in order to maintain its integrity, its focus. There is much in life that can cloud vision – essentially the pleasures of materialism. Again the karma manas are important in this discrimination, for they register our experience and aid the memories from which we can learn. However, enlightenment begins when the collection of these thoughts, actions and experiences are placed alongside the spiritual desire to explain why 'I' exist. For this, the head and the heart need to act as one, for the manas can contain all the philosophy in the world, but somewhere between the head and heart will be your truth.

INTUITION

Communication at the brow chakra involves intuition. To ask homœopaths to prescribe from their intuition, the major faculty of the higher manas, which is to perceive without question, is, maybe, to make them insecure. Personal development, or simply the experience gained through prescribing, changes this. Nothing evolves this faculty quicker and more profoundly than meditating on the energy of each chakra as described in this book. To raise one's skills above those usually used to form understanding takes time and support, but it also comes with being a homœopath and the nature of dealing with energy. After a while the invisible begins to take on form, a process that is unequivocal. But what is truly special is the interaction between Self and Divine wisdom, which is immeasurable, for reasoning has no place here.

As homœopaths, we are taught to simply reflect back in remedy form that which is of a most similar match to the symptoms being presented by the patient, in a like-for-like way. It is the 'like' that is important here for the 'like' is energy. With the use of intuition nothing has changed in this equation, for it is still coming through the practitioner. It will only be the justification of the prescription that will be out of the ordinary. The only difference is that this judgement is made at a higher level where it is selected before it has had time to materialise through the symptoms that indicate the prescription to the rational mind. This is more than observation, but observation is required for the use of intuition. It will however, be the rational mind that has to make a decision as to the way in which it discerns the 'like'. This is not the same for direct knowing so the rational mind needs to trust and practise. When we are dealing with these higher sources of reception, knowing goes far beyond the rational. The proof of this lies in the response within the patient and the understanding as to the reason for change.

Using this reception is how information is gained and how it leads to wisdom. This process can be supported further, by looking up the remedy picture in order to confirm the aspect received or to expand on what was previously unseen. This is the relationship with reception at the brow chakra, for in the logical mind it formulates truth. Homœopathy is making materia medica all the time, the point of which is to bring information into consciousness to expand on the breadth of healing. At this juncture, judgement, discussion and argument are all futile. It only wastes physical energy and hinders the prescription. What is important though, is integrity.

To follow Christ is not just to be liberated, but to be united. This means that in order that we too can enter a place that is not simply about the act of following but about having arrived, then Christ must

Chapter 6 ~ The Brow Chakra

be found within. In the realm of the higher manas, the fact that Christ existed in a physical form is irrelevant, for if desired enough, Christ will manifest in Self. This notion has been projected on to a physical structure and evolved as the story of Jesus Christ, rather than as a guide to the path of one's own spiritual unfolding on Earth. To be Christ-like is to be united in the truth of the resurrection. No longer is Self in a state of unknowing, for here lies, in the brow chakra, the chance to glimpse the future of immortality. This glimpse is a respite from need, if only for a brief period, and allows one to unite with the cosmos within.

For the higher mind, the boundaries of the physical world do not exist, only immortal spiritual intelligence. Therefore, compared to such magnificence, the soul is able to ascertain that the true illusion is the physical world. This can only be explained by the means in which the monad interacts here. Like a vine around a tree, the Buddhi and Atman wrap themselves and grow from the soil that is the nutrient provided by the centre of the monad. This happens in the centre of the brow but is also reflected in the heart chakra. It is the place where the orange light of the brow chakra meets the purple of the crown chakra. Energy is pulled into this spot through a slow, corkscrew motion manifesting from the crown chakra that if it can be seen, appears to be a bit like a pinecone. This is the Ayahuasca within.

THE MONADS

It is very important but not an easy concept to understand how the monad interacts within human consciousness. The monad is the seed that offers all possibility, for within it lies that of Divine origin, the Divine spark. The monad has no birth or death, and is ageless, so in human consciousness terms is impossible to define, for it has no space or form other than our knowledge that it exists. It is, however, individual, and pertains to anything within the kingdoms that has a life. Even though through imagery I describe these facets of the brow intertwined within the monad, this, in itself, places the limitation of space and form upon it, which in truth is not possible as it is boundary-free. When it comes to describing the monad, the paradox is that we have to use the limitations of the rational mind, the lower manas.

During incarnation the monad brings with it the spiritual content of the incarnating Ego, providing the layer in which life is not only possible but has a purpose. It does this directly through all the life atoms on every level that make up the seven principles of man. These life atoms of even the lowest realm have been inherited from the death of the previous planetary life chain that created the previous kingdom. They contain the means to carry out the next step in monadic work and attach themselves to the incoming soul. These life atoms are the building blocks for the next kingdom within which are contained the expression of the previous kingdom/s. They are not, however physical atoms which are only used by life atoms as a means to operate on the physical plane. Life atoms that inhabit entities continue to be discarded in order that these entities fulfil their own destiny through reincarnation whilst under the influence of the monadic pull. As already mentioned, some of these atoms are reabsorbed into the planet but the rest that pertain to the higher aspects of mankind return to energise the cosmos and further monadic growth. The monad derives its presence by being what it is, be it a rock, tree or whatever, for it contains a spiritual content – Divine consciousness. As with the Hermetic principle, 'As above, so below; as below, so above', the monad belongs, is equal to and incarnates from the hierarchy of the cosmos. Because of this then, so do we. The faculties that make up Self are in effect a miniature version of the monad itself.

In physical life we construct boundaries. If we are able to reach our higher self and explore our true self, that which is of the monad, then these boundaries cease to exist. What we do find though is the influence of monadic qualities, that of being self-impelled and self-aware, which is in reality truly self-conscious. If Self can ride this wave that extends across the universe, then vision is boundless. It is an important source, for health is maintained by life making sense to Self.

The fifth element, which unleashed the throat chakra and gave forth life, continues to do so using essence, which comes from the monad. This is why the monad is imperative in higher thought, for only when Self is elevated sufficiently, can this perception be obtained. Being of Divine quality, it reveals that which is above the human kingdom. As the monad contains both human and Divine qualities, Self has to loosen itself from the constraints of the kingdom's hierarchy in order to connect with the monad, as have those that have entered the spiritual kingdoms. Presently this is a tall order at this stage of the root-race, as humanity is still having trouble discarding the pull of the animal kingdom.

It is the Earth's development that is subject to the evolution of the ten kingdoms, monadically, but in the form of its life chain. This chain forms

Chapter 6 ~ The Brow Chakra

a circle and is made up of twelve cycles or globe stages of the planet's evolution, which are the means by which each kingdom is established.

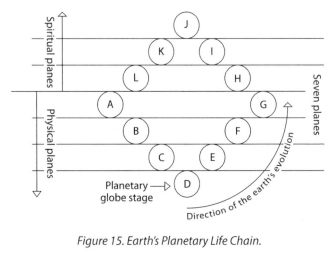

Figure 15. Earth's Planetary Life Chain.

There are seven planes or levels to this chain that are marked in degrees from the most physical at the bottom to the most spiritual at the top. The Earth evolves by moving around this circle, thus gaining its density on the lower four planes (worlds) and then relinquishing it on the higher three (the seven human chakras do the same movement in a seven yearly cycle as they gain consciousness for this is a monadic relationship). This movement between spirit and matter is the method by which the planet Earth evolves within Divine consciousness.

Each globe stage has a further subdivision of seven sections that has to be completed before the Earth can move onto one of the next positions in the chain of twelve. So at each globe stage the planet is rotating through a seven-sectioned development as well as rotating around the chain. The Earth is either ascending into spirit or descending into matter in either its subdivision or planetary chain at any given time. The seven subdivisions of the human kingdom's transformation on each globe stage are referred to as root-races. Each root-race pertains to a chakra on each of the human planes of development. This can be broken down further as each root-race can be divided into seven stages of chakra evolution, there being a point of nirvana at the crown chakra at which humanity rests before embarking on the next root-race, as it does before beginning a new globe cycle and planetary chain.

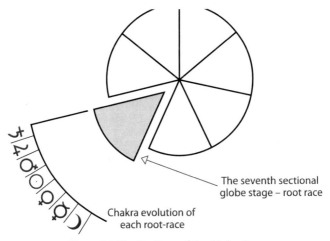

Figure 16. The Sections of the Globe Stage.

It takes one round or a planetary 'manvantara', in which there are seven globe stations where the material work is completed on the physical four lower planes, in order for the Earth to evolve through the 'manifested cycles' (just as with the human chakras). The planet, within its new form, is next absorbed into the spiritual realms (just as in the life atoms) to fully establish its spiritual identity from which the cosmos will also grow. This involves a further five globe stations which will manifest as death and the readying for rebirth. Collectively, the process of evolving through all twelve stations produces the new kingdom.

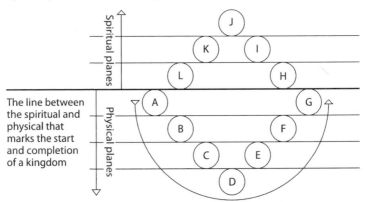

Figure 17. The Planetary Manvantara of the Life Chain.

Chapter 6 ~ The Brow Chakra

Now, because there are only twelve stations to the chain (the Earth's cycle of monadic development), then according to the laws of reflection there should be the same number of stations above as below. But in our model there only appears to be five globe stations on the higher planes to the seven lower ones. The manvantara decree states there are seven globe stations to be achieved before the Earth's new kingdom is ready to be absorbed into the spiritual realms. For there to be a second set of seven, a reflection of these lower planes to the higher ones that makes in total fourteen, on our diagram there has to be an overlap. This misdemeanour is also revealed in the fact that the chain cycle begins at the end of the spiritual planes and at the beginning of the material ones, this being the portal to rebirth. Further to this, being the beginning of something new, this position must contain the ingredients of both spirit and matter in order to formulate itself. So the Earth manifests in both spirit and matter at once, which is the point to the globe station where reincarnation occurs. This is the relationship between the numbers twelve and fourteen, and how intrinsic they are in the manifestation of any resurrection.

The invisible spirit overlapping the beginning and end of the physical globes achieves the equal reflection from the higher planes to the lower ones and it is this that produces fourteen stations from the twelve defined stations. Spirit is in matter and so this invisible factor is that which from twelve forms fourteen. There are in fact two spheres that appear to be only one.

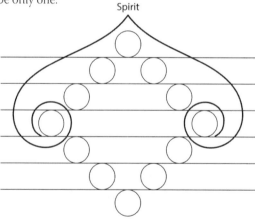

Figure 18. Spirit overlapping matter – a universal image present in many forms to represent the struggle of human existence.

Chakra Prescribing and Homœopathy

On the physical plane matter cannot hide itself, only spirit can remain invisible. Only spirit has the choice whether it wishes to remain invisible or become visible. This may be why the number thirteen is considered to be unlucky for it is a sign of a failed resurrection.

At present the kingdom being developed on the globe cycle, to which anyone reading this book belongs, is the human kingdom and its position presently on the chain cycle is the most physical of all the twelve globes. This human development will not be achieved in the life of a single globe's station but will take seven that pertain to the physical half circle of the chain. Kingdoms can only be produced on Earth within this domain. They then travel into the higher planes where their coarser attributes are refined, just as in the chakra system.

As the monad evolves through the expansion of a kingdom, it takes one planetary manvantara (seven globe lives) and cosmic inclusion for it to be fully embodied in that kingdom before the next kingdom can start to evolve. Hence the monad retains the growth of the kingdom before, from which it rises to start a new chain, which will of course be in a new solar system. As each full planetary chain is completed, then a new cosmic plane is entered. At the end of this the Monad of humanity is emancipated from its physical constraints on Earth and, having gathered within the extent of its riches, starts its long journey in subsequent planetary chains – these new planets being the ones we may know and the ones in galaxies we are yet to know. Perhaps it will be then that Earth is able to join the elite group of sacred planets.

It was Paracelsus, among others, who was aware of the monad within all nature – the connection that all is one – and it was Hahnemann who developed the idea. All is karma, and from the results of actions the monad grows. Therefore every living thing started as an elemental, which through expansion later became an entity. This is important in homœopathy because the relationship between each entity's karma is what is so necessary in its connection to mankind, for we know this connection can cure.

Because of the nature of the development of planet Earth in readiness for human habitation, the monad of any object coincides with the human constitution, for it is part of the same evolution, and life is sustained. Trees create oxygen in order that mankind can breath. It is this connection in homœopathy that we are interested in, and why the remedies we make from substances in our sphere work. People reflect

Chapter 6 ~ The Brow Chakra

this relationship all the time. Just look at the different precious and semi precious stones that each person chooses to wear. Without such a relationship through the identity of each life form in the four kingdoms specifically, the balance, which is Earthly existence, would cease to exist.

By entering the centre of one's monad, it is possible to be in contact with all monads, given the construction of this plane. Each monad (and they are individual) is in fact, a collective single monad – such is the contradiction when we try and apply the logic of a numeric system. It is this connection which enables one to empathise with a stone, to see inside it through its monadic resonance – though one is not a stone! The stone's monad holds the essence of it being a stone but this sense that one is in all things and all things are part of one is the true definition of 'communication', which is probably the most important word that can be attributed to the brow chakra. When one stops for no apparent reason and spots a stone in one's path, there is a reason – communication. This has significance to one's action, not least because one is part of the world and its nice to be reminded of its wonder. But if the example of 'time' is applied as an aspect of the consequence of taking a moment to observe the stone, this slice of time is thus taken out of the day and has a knock-on effect for the events to come. One shares in the significance of the stone being part of one's life. One may kick the stone, an expression of the joy or out of frustration – both communicate. The stone moves, the universe has changed.

It is the communication of each individual monad that is the whole monad as it unfolds, for every object has a soul that carries the spirit of its entity that is in monadic development. It is the monad that draws one to look deeply into the soul of a bird sitting in one's garden, tuning into it in order to try and understand what it is like to be a bird in the animal kingdom. To the human kingdom this capacity for thought is available, so in a sense is the ability to fly like the bird in the realm of imagination. From thought we are able to build the means to do so. All the other kingdoms by the means of facets of themselves provide tools for humanity to use, to help with its advancement. Sometimes all one has is one's own belief to call upon these facets. If this ability to use the other kingdoms is extended, it enables one to completely understand the causes of ill health in people. For it is this ability to extend deep within the connections of the human kingdom or to look monadically, which is the making of our time now – the development of the mind.

Chakra Prescribing and Homœopathy

We are all being asked to join and connect with one another, for this is where communication is building.

To heal is to be honest about whom one is and this means all one's relationships and all that is contained within. This also means the contents of the thymus gland. This level of honesty, the blending of light and dark is very difficult but must eventually be achieved. When we are confronted by what we are, our past, present and future as one, it can be immensely difficult to know how to integrate such knowledge and how to progress with it in order for it to become a positive. If for instance the remedy *Lachesis* is needed the constitutional patient will usually direct the repulsion inherent in this remedy back towards the practitioner in the form of anger, as is the nature of this particular type. But what is needed by this patient to heal deeply is to face their truth: this is what the remedy does. Bear in mind that a patient may need *Lachesis* without it being constitutional and in this case may react differently.

What separates humans is intelligence, and this also separates us from the higher kingdoms. The human monad as an individual (self-conscious) and a collective (universal conscious) refers only to the combination of Buddhi-Atman. The word monad refers to 'One Life' of the kind of unity that is first witnessed at the heart chakra. Although the 'Seven Principles of Man' as adhered to by the Theosophists, do not correspond exactly with the seven chakras, both reflect the difficulty of separating the function of the higher mind and the crown chakra, as is it equally difficult to separate Buddhi and Atman. This is the difficulty we have in creating models to explain that which changed after the separation of Self. As this is in itself a myth planted in an illusory world, it presents the problem of explaining unity through the delusion of our separated Self. We perpetuate this enigma by the very nature of separating things out in pursuit of knowledge. It is, however, the law of the cosmos that all is interlinked, which enables homœopaths to unlock the difficulties of karma. When it comes to 'I' individualising itself, it should be remembered that only our soul in the form of its astral counterpart is fully present in mankind. It is the connection between the soul and the monad by means of a dilution, that is homœopathically prescribed to the patient. This is the definition of a homœopathic remedy.

Without the monad and all the monads that make up Self, that are in a sense children to the one and awaiting further growth, then Self would have no means to make the connections that it does, and the possibili-

Chapter 6 ~ The Brow Chakra

ties to explore way beyond its normal consciousness. Such exploration is a combination of Divine will, intuition and an evolved higher mind.

ELEMENTALS AND ENTITIES

It has been suggested that in order to be able to achieve a higher state the human monad has had to work through the lower kingdoms. All elementals begin their long journey at the lowest form of evolution but not all are destined to be human. There are simply far too many monads, even though spread out over all the differing planes of evolution (including the parallel ones of fractured space), for all of them to fit at once into the designated balance that is humanity on Earth. Only human entities elected will be thrust forward from their state of bliss to enter this planet when needed, as dictated by the construction of the kingdom. In the grand scheme of things there simply isn't the capability for entities of the lower kingdoms to break free of their designated role and neither the manas if not equipped before the next planetary chain. This is not to say though, that all elementals do not undergo a series of initiations before they become permanent entities of their given kingdom.

Monads contain the means to enlightenment because they are Divine-spiritual seeds in which the contents of the higher manas can be passed from one generation to the next. This is not simply by reincarnating, but also via the essence passed from parent to offspring. In pure theosophy, those who had previously done the work, presumably on the higher planes, in order to make our universe possible provided Self with the mind. This suggests that when Self became 'self aware' then the evolution of the mind was already undertaken, and Self was able to step into it, rather than having to start afresh. It appears the first thought of Self was not of ignorance but the beginnings of wisdom.

As time does not really exist then the evolution of this planet is only just starting for some. From being at a place of self-less existence, certain elementals are arising from their cosmic element and only just beginning their journey here on Earth. They are in effect, in evolutionary terms, on the lowest ladder. As potential humans they still remain below the development of the mineral kingdom. However, if destined, their transition through their expanding human monad can be very direct with only a short stay at any transitional stage as echoed in the reduced number of previous human incarnations. This produces what's known as a 'young soul' here on Earth. Placed next to the concept of time, this

Chakra Prescribing and Homœopathy

relates to the manvantara, but the human monad need not be hindered if its movement through the lower kingdoms is relatively smooth.

It is initiation that denotes the kingdom deemed for the elemental, and which kingdom it will become an entity of. So for the elementals destined to be human, this transportation through each kingdom provides the experience needed in order to create human form in all its aspects. They of course have to learn the physical limitations of human existence quickly if the path is to be relatively unhindered. The purpose is to learn, and in the higher mind this extends from being human and thus incorporates the karma of its evolution. Its karma will also then have a relationship with the development of the higher mind of the planet Earth as part of its destiny or the planetary monad.

So there are thought to be seven classes of monad, the human pertaining to one of them. Within each of these is a further seven; therefore there are seven human monads. These are found on the plane of spirit, so the human monad's purpose is the pursuit of this higher enlightenment, or to become one with the Source as the three dhyani-chohanic kingdoms (Archangels) almost touch. Deities have already achieved this and are as co-supervisors of the cosmos. As deities are 'monadically' evolved extensions of oneself (as all is contained within Self), to enter the centre of one's monad via the brow chakra is to perceive the cosmos as they do.

Entities that are human or otherwise, have gained access to their monad, unlike elementals that simply cling on to its presence. Having gained experience as described, the human monad contains within it the essence of all four kingdoms. This is reflected in the atomic structure and the subtle bodies of Self that allow spirit to come and go when required. The more developed the spirit, the easier this is. But the important point here is that humans are of a separate monad to the entities that are destined to remain in the lower kingdoms.

The intellect does not follow evolution easily when explaining the progression of the physical world. One is not a rock and then a plant and so on, as the rational mind would have us believe. Evolution begins in the higher planes of the cosmos and there these elementals are closer to the Source than down here on Earth. Even though consciousness is a process of individuality, it is not physical within the higher planes and so work achieved here is a balance in order that humanity gains a level of completeness or unity with the Source. The illusion is here on Earth and

Chapter 6 ~ The Brow Chakra

Self accesses truth only through the realisation of unity.

Without incarnation, the monad, which hitches a ride with the soul, cannot progress in its purpose, and so elementals cannot become entities. Which entities are destined to be human, as the animal entities are destined to be animal, is determined within the higher planes of the cosmos. Humans evolve through working on facets of these other kingdoms, which they all contain qualities of, but have never been entities of, in the way that an animal has never been a crystal. However, in order to exist, all must conform to laws laid down when at each station of the kingdom. From this, we know that at the start of the next planetary cycle the monad identifies with the next kingdom in pursuit of its destiny; but this is about experiencing these laws, not being an entity of that kingdom.

A human entity has previously been an elemental evolving through the monadic consciousness of the lower kingdoms. It is designated in the higher planes for one kingdom only, and so an entity that has finished with its kingdom, its destiny, is not then lost, but through its monad is absorbed, as it stands, as part of the greater whole, rather than developed into the higher kingdoms. After this absorption, if any spirit is left over, it having graduated on the higher planes to a level seen fit, will enter the realm of dhyan-chohan. This is a term that originated from Sanskrit but is of a universal philosophy. Only those with sufficient monadic experience that have worked through the human kingdom can transcend to the dhyani-chohanic kingdoms, which have also been preordained. Each entity pertaining to a particular kingdom is working in order that all life can be sustained for all things. Every little piece makes up the whole and is significant, as with the balance of the elements that make up life. Without one, all fail.

EVOLUTION

The dhyan-chohan is a collective of all beings that have presently ended their planetary chain and succeeded in reaching the higher kingdoms in order to supervise the cosmos. Here, I will also place the seven dhyani-buddhas under the general term dhyan-chohan or planetary spirits simply for convenience. There are differing evolved levels within the realm of planetary spirits, again deriving from varying aspects of Divine consciousness – spirits in evolution. Of the dhyan-chohan there are fourteen types of Manu. They overlook each of the Earth's manvantara, as humanity evolves beneath. Each Manu emanates as an essence of truth from the higher seven dhyan-chohan that overlook each planetary chain cycle, for it is with the fate of humanity that the dhyan-chohan have been entrusted. This is achieved through the rays of the seven sacred planets as each are responsible for the development of each of the globes of the Earth's chain that make up the manvantara. This is the same as how the chakras work, each acting collectively under the guide of a single planet. Therefore, the seven sacred planets do exactly the same within each of the seven root-races of each of the seven globes.

The Manus are those that give birth to humanity at the beginning of each manifestation – fourteen in all, like a kind of spiritual planetary parent or teacher. They ascertain to what the Buddhists call the bodhisattvas, whose purpose is to save each and every soul and are what humanity becomes after the seventh planetary chain is completed. So the length of time a Manu rules is one manvantara. The Earth is presently under the seventh propagator – Vaivasvata Manu. Remember the heart chakra taught us that humanity is a collective and it can only advance in its planetary chain with all its beings together. It will take the completion of all fourteen Manus before what has been the material basis for the Earth's spiritual development to cease.

Under the Manus' influence and through the sacred planets, the bodhisattvas instil awareness pertaining to a particular globe cycle and it is here that humanity gains the way of thinking that is suitable to each root-race. This accumulates over each subsequent globe cycle until all of humanity has become enlightened. From the word Manu has derived the word 'man' or in other translations it means to 'think'. Therefore the temporary buddhi/mana relationship within the human mind ascends to become part of Mahat – the 'universal consciousness' – and no longer a reflection of it. The soul is then united with its monad. This theme of the previously evolved higher kingdoms and their influence over the human mind continues within its relationship with the Pitris. These dhyan-chohan beings are comprised of either spirits from the previously completed lunar chain, a former embodiment of Earth's present chain, a mother if you like to her son; or very distant ancestors, not related in any way to current living humans. The latter form a bridge from Sunlight to Moonlight, from the Sun, the source of Divine Consciousness to the Moon from which it is reflected to Earth. This is the Moon's role, for although it has finished its planetary chain and so being in a state of

Chapter 6 ~ The Brow Chakra

decay, it having completed the birth of planet Earth as its mother; it still presents an intrinsic part in the growth of humanity. This will of course be elaborated on in the crown chakra chapter but its relevance here is that this relationship between the Earth and the Moon is also met in the dhyan-chohan. The bridge between Sunlight to Moonlight has been made and thus falls upon Earth in the form of intuition, after all we are still only human. It is the task of the lower Pitris, evolved out of the previous Luna chain, to maintain this intuitive connection. Being the result of the Moon's development, these beings are encrypted with instinct so are sensitive to the feeling of Self's entire individual plight.

It is through the dhyan-chohan as a collective that we are able to be born and think for ourselves using wisdom. This is because they are a higher representation of Self and therefore it is they who give birth to our selves as well as all things that are below humanity. They are then the agents of karma. It is through thought or the ability to think for ourselves that the connection between Self and the higher planes is achieved – the monadic connection between all things.

Through its karma, the crystal contains a memory within the monad of its existence, but although containing power pertaining to its kingdom, this is limited. Self may not be aware it is in direct contact with the other kingdoms, but their distribution is so intrinsic to its function that there is no dividing line, hence Self's need in balancing the elements. All function in the physical realm relies on the qualities of all the kingdoms, except the crown chakra, which is not really a function of our existence but of the other existence. This understanding is not rational but is a quality gained and innate within the higher mind and passed down to the tissues and the cells. It is, though, possible to grasp it through Self's interaction with the monad. These are the higher qualities that the crystal, for example, is too limited to experience.

The seven differing human monads are distinguishable at first by their life atoms and, like all things in the cosmos, there is a natural balance depending on the level of human evolution and that which is required by the higher planes. As humans, we are all on differing levels. I will leave it to your imagination as to which level of the seven monads our world leaders aspire. But what is certain is that the differentiation has much in common with the relationship between the higher mind, the Buddhi and the Atman. This triad not only creates the context for the third eye but also forms the root to awaken Atman and the crown chakra. In kabbalist philosophy, this is described as the triad of the top three spheres, forming a triangle in which the monad is contained in the centre. Without understanding these differing levels at the brow centre, it is quite impossible to gain insight into the workings of the crown chakra. But this is the point to the brow chakra; one cannot develop a good crown chakra, only a good brow chakra.

Elementals that have yet to form entities within their respective monads remain invisible to normal human sight. These elementals require monadic consciousness in order to fully make the transition into their respective kingdoms. Having come afresh from the higher planes they emanate down through the dhyani-chohanic planes, but in doing so are passive. The same is true of those elementals that are destined to re-enter the dhyani-chohanic planes, which having returned with self-consciousness, have become active. At the early stage these elementals can only maintain their association with their kingdom through their element. For instance, it is the fire element that governs the development of the Salamanders. They also indirectly play a role in the development of mankind, which is an energetic one and is associated with the connection between the evolution of Earth and the seven chakras.

To understand the seven levels of monadic development we can place them exactly against the seven chakras. The Mahatma can only incarnate at a level suited to the advancement of its soul, that which is received through their monad within the higher triad. The monad enters with the soul, so the seven layers of cosmic consciousness are not only reflected in human development but also in the human constitution. The human being, in fact, is a response to the structure of these cosmic planes, so it stands to reason that each will contain a division of seven monads within, for humans reflect the cosmos. It is the higher manas that focus all in a homogenised whole, so that the universe can be explored. This is the reason why the human monad does not evolve by first having been an entity of the lower kingdoms, but has the means to incorporate them.

The spark is the seed and like all seeds it has contained within itself all that it requires to be – it just needs to grow. These cosmic levels of consciousness, which are the same as the chakras but in a different manifested form, cannot be developed without the development of the previous one/s. Each level or cosmic element gives rise to its own kingdom of elementals on the higher planes and gives rise to or awakens the

Chapter 6 ~ The Brow Chakra

equivalent level here on Earth. This interlinks with the incarnating Ego and its monad, for they travel through the seven planetary planes, picking up life atoms cast off from the end of their previous venture together and from which they can build a vehicle in order to once again function on the physical plane.

The planets enable the monad to guide the soul with the appropriate ray or combination of rays as revealed in one's astrological chart. The raising of consciousness is a planetary thing and because the planet Earth is not one of the seven sacred planets, it not having completed its Third Cosmic Initiation, it is not then at a stage to resonate to the purpose for which it was developed – to reflect Divine consciousness. Hence the influence of the planets acting upon the seven chakras is a means to raise the level of consciousness through the work of each of its spirit-containing monadic inhabitants. All play a part, but due to humanity being the only species to come equipped with the means by which to access the higher mind, it is the task of all humans, every single one, to raise the level of this planet's consciousness.

THE DISEASE PROCESS

There are seven internal monads that correspond not only to the seven human chakras but the cycles of incarnation, for one has to be complete before the next stage can be recognised. In completion, not all of Self's attributes may be the most positive, so one lifetime or many lifetimes may be primarily concerned with altering that. Disease and finally Earthly death (first death) is a process of these monads breaking down, starting in the order in which they were first formed. In the case of the first monad, ill health begins when purpose, the first point to any initiation, is either lost or hindered. When it comes to the sixth and seventh internal monads they act just like the seven chakras, for they pertain to the same influences, and thus provide the reason for death to become known to Self and allow the point to that particular life to enter into consciousness.

The problem with this process is that it is at the brow chakra, it being the command centre, where the acceptance of ill health is first brought to consciousness. This experience, in some traumatic circumstances, can kill as a result of shock, but imbalances that lead to disease mostly start small and grow slowly. So the re-establishing of good health always refers back to the mind. This is because in developing, each one of these monads has to work through the principles of the other six monads that make up the seven in total, as their energies are used to help construct the identity of their own station and thus the function unique to it. So an internal monad does not develop alone but develops at its own station by working within the other six, all being stages of growth. Once again, these monads are separate but they are also one, so have to grow as one. The brow acts as overseer to this, bringing about understanding or acting as a collection point of focus, without which there would be no identity. This also enables a monad to reflect all other monads in order that the universe can be observed.

Thought has to be present for the purpose of change, and this is the reason why all ill health registers with the mind. If Self does not understand the solution or even the cause, it will seek help and track down an understanding in its quest to heal. We know this monadic construction is very similar, if not the same, as the workings and interactions of the seven chakras, for being energy centres of evolving consciousness, they will be an extension of the monad and thus have their own individual monad to identify with.

The constitution is formed around seven chakras that all began as an initial seed of consciousness, and all have developed from one to the other through being a part of one another. Thus, a chakra can be all-encompassing according to its own station; it will pertain to that station energetically whilst being a reflection of the whole. The more we can perceive the chakras as a whole, the more we can tune into the complete picture. This is why major and deep-acting remedies such as the polycrests work in totality on all the chakras, even though it may only be one chakra that gives a good indication for its selection. To be able to perceive the patient in their totality allows the practitioner an understanding as to the place or the position they are in. It makes things clearer as one can get straight to the point. This is the best energy with which to prescribe a remedy, even though confusion is quite normal and even necessary, for it is from this state that we learn. Vision received by exploring the monad is a great challenge but one that can be achieved through reception at the crown chakra. Because the seven human monads refer to that which is way beyond our normal comprehension, it is far easier to account for the actions of their ascertainable counterpart, the chakras. To do this we must first learn to perceive the messages from their tell-tale signs.

Chapter 6 ~ The Brow Chakra

The monad grows through the experiences of Self. Therefore, karma that makes up the journey of Self has differing manifestations, as each chakra undergoes differing influences or reacts differently to stimulus as part of its individual development. They do all work together and at times this process is difficult to isolate. However, each chakra maintains a separate monad and is therefore individual in the development of its own consciousness. Within this structure is contained, we could say, the seven chakras of the planet Earth, of the universe and so on. The monad knows no other pattern in which to evolve, for there is no other structure in the cosmos. But the monad cannot evolve without memory from which the perception of the soul can be built. This relationship is only possible because the seed in which the monad is energetically created is an essence of the Divine Logos. When it comes to understanding the role of monad one has to see it in the form of this essence, of which the human is only a part.

When it comes to identifying at what stage or place of evolution a disease has arrived, allopathic perception is too crude a physical measure. If one has the ability to see auras by the use of the third eye then changes in their radiance, substance and colouring will indicate the monadic roots to imbalance. The pupil of the third eye represents a pool that, instead of being filled by water under the confines of the gravitational pull of the Earth, is full of light held by the gravitational pull of the cosmos. The structure of this eye is porous, so is receptive and absorbent of cosmic light which, using Self as a diaphragm, can be bounced back into the consciousness of planet Earth. It is important for this pool never to dry up, as it is filled from a greater well.

Homœopathy is a process in which essence can be siphoned from matter, administered in matter and used to instigate a healing process. The power to heal is an evolving process, and the next stage will be by using the third eye. Each one of us has the ability to do this, for it is not we who have the power to heal but the power coming through us. The pupil of the third eye is capable of focusing its reservoir of light and directing it to those who are in need of healing. This power to heal is greater than human beings can comprehend at present, although with the right attitude, it is possible to instigate now. On a smaller scale, such healing is already happening as one automatically sends healing light to those in need, through this eye. This is very powerful and induces much change – this is more than simply compassion, this is telepathy. It is the ability to truly see another's pain and to act by sending the appropriate solution via the great Source, just as in homœopathy. This is to tap into the monad of humanity, to decipher the karmic block that is being reflected in the individual's monad and apply the key to unlock it. This is also true of the next generation of homœopathic remedies, for their source will not be in the conversion of matter into spirit but spiritual from the beginning of their construction.

The higher manas are the judge of Self within the spiritual realm. Their role therefore is in discerning explorations in the monadic world, field or plane and this is wholly dependent on what can be consciously constructed. Hence the monad encapsulates the body, soul and spirit, as within it are gathered both the mortal and immortal attributes. This is the same for the chakras, as they hold the cosmos within. It is the collective hierarchy to which the monadic plane is in permanent communication and as this is the way through to spirit, it is thus the soul which interacts between the invisible and physical worlds. The soul, much like the pupil of the third eye, acts as a font, the waters of which contain experiences. Although mesmerising they are only visible because the light of spirit is constantly casting its illumination upon them, just as matter is only visible because of the tiny speckles of light acting upon it.

THE THIRD EYE

The structure of the third eye reflects the relationship of the triple structure of the monad. We have already discussed the first plane of its function, the higher mind. The second plane of its awareness is the Buddhi. This is the universal soul or spiritual soul within man and as this suggests it enables one to build wisdom from vision. What constitutes wisdom and why it is the realm of the Buddhi that is so important in bearing such wisdom to Self, lies in the fact that the Buddhi is nothing, and cannot become active, without Atman. It is the task of the Buddhi to assist Atman with reception.

At this higher echelon of the human constitution, the brow chakra acts similarly to the crown chakra, as is revealed in its glyph, which differs from that of the throat chakra by the addition of a crescent, representing the Moon. The Moon here is smaller than that of the crown chakra and is directed upwards like a satellite dish. It is however, as its relative size and position at the brow centre suggest, understudy to the reception that the crown represents. This is not to demean its impor-

Chapter 6 ~ The Brow Chakra

tance but like a funnel or a lens, it has to reduce light and scale down the vastness of what it receives to create a focus. It is not that the Buddhi simply absorbs directly from the Atman but their function co-exists so that there is a bit of Buddhi in Atman and vice-versa. This indicates how the brow and the crown behave. Because the brow is the place in which that from above is absorbed into that from below, then the energies that work up through the chakras in order to cleanse them behave differently in the brow chakra to the crown chakra. Buddhi is the vehicle of Atman and therefore one cannot be separated from the other, although the brow has a monad and so does the crown.

When trying to explain the monad it is often referred to as being a duad of Buddhi-Atman. This is not technically so until after the fourth initiation in which the son (manas) has been emancipated. This is the method by which the spiritual part of the soul is influenced and can only happen by the means of the third eye. This is the manas, Buddhi and Atman working together in order to expand beyond the limitations of this world. It is the spiritual soul that absorbs wisdom but it is through the quality of focus within the third eye that this wisdom can penetrate the mind. The Buddhi remains functionless unless connected to the manas, as wisdom cannot be gained unless it has become conscious. This connection is that which enables one to know, instantaneously. There is no need for the laborious motions of the lower manas here, for the Buddhi is provided with qualities of love, intuition and spiritual vision.

It is quite remarkable, given the weight of esoteric evidence and centuries of documented spiritual vision, that intuition is not regarded as the means by which to decipher such teachings, given that such teachings depend on intuition for their conception and development. Given the overwhelming evidence for its usage, and the great personal growth necessary for intuition to be embodied, then why is it such a dirty word in homœopathy? Why, given the work required on each chakra to gain the faith and trust in its vision, is it relegated to the level of gambling in some spiritual lottery? Intuition is way beyond Earthly knowledge or the realms of the intellect and flourishes only if one is prepared to listen. This requires skill and dedication, but is work that is designed to benefit all.

Although at present in evolutionary terms humanity is driven by the need to extend the mind, it is important that we understand what this notion means in totality. This is a great opportunity, so why is it that humanity has never been so rich in intellectual knowledge and yet so lacking in wisdom? It is the intellect that so often forms a barrier between Self and the true power of thought. It creates rules and thus boundaries in response to insecurities that in reality do not exist and that inhibit change.

The Buddhi is central to the focus of the third eye, for in part its meaning refers to being awake or 'awakened'. Apparently, the past Chief of the Druid Order, Thomas Maughan, used to describe people as being something like the 'walking dead' if this attribute was not in operation. Here again the manas, the Buddhi and the Atman cannot be separated for this higher triad, when well developed, is the means by which enlightenment can be gained.

One of the quirky positive balances of the way in which miasms are a positive, or protective, influence as well as a negative one, is the way in which the sycotic miasm forms a siphon in the brain by which the reception of the crown can be limited before absorption at the brow. If the division between the lower and higher manas is too wide the manas will not be sufficiently conscious to be able to cope with the influx that a charged crown chakra creates. This is often the case with psychic reception. Without the congestion of the sycotic miasm hindering or filtering the flow of intensive crown energy, what it has to reveal could drive the recipient to madness, were their manas insufficiently developed. So the manas develop as the grip of this miasm loosens. This is also true when working on this centre during meditative practice, for the candidate has to be ready. Homœopathic remedies pertaining to the brow chakra may be needed from the initial consultation. However, usually neither the brow nor the crown is the place to start, for spiritual initiation begins much further down the chakra scale. First one meets Mercury's father – Jupiter – and by the means of his thunderous bolt of heavenly consciousness, one is first inspired before one finds oneself in the melting pot of quicksilver.

Trying to achieve too much too soon can also be true homœopathically-speaking. The use of the new remedy *Orange*, the colour of the brow chakra, is a remedy best given only when the patient is sufficiently spiritually integrated. This integration is similarly important for those who are developing their perception as they attempt to see auras or entities, or are clairvoyant in any way. One needs to adjust to receiving such information.

The sycotic miasm has another quirk that reverses the negative aspect to its congestion: because it prevents so much information from

Chapter 6 ~ The Brow Chakra

being received, it can be extremely discriminative with what has been absorbed. Hence the sycotic homœopath, instead of being overwhelmed by a barrage of confusing symptoms, can be a very specific prescriber with just a few. The same is true in identifying aetiology, for patients often cloud or have lost the cause of their problem. As part of this paradox the sycotic miasm can lend itself in supporting extraordinary powers of vision. This miasm can also provide help in leaving one's body to explore the other world, although it may well hinder the retrieval and instalment of the fruits of these travels from becoming grounded in the material world.

In the light of what we understand about their relationship with negative karma, it seems strange that positive qualities arise as a result of these miasms. Again, we have to escape from the notion of good and bad, as there is only consequence. Therefore, the way to move forward will always be provided and spirit will choose that which best suits its circumstance. It is as if the miasm itself creates a possibility or the means by which Self can heal, lessening the significance of its influence in life. Perhaps the miasms themselves provide the platform on which to work through negative karma. Or miasms are the inevitable result of the development of the human kingdom under the structure of the cosmic hierarchy. Either way, the act of being a homœopath is not simply to spot symptoms but to understand the role miasms play in poor health by pushing the patient, through experience, into making choices. Expanding on such wisdom and allowing it to inform your prescribing based on an awareness of where the patient is at on their long journey, is totally reliant on the strength of the third eye.

If Buddhi is the centre of one's perception, the place on the forehead just above where the eyebrows meet, then it is here that one concentrates one's focus. It is also the centre of telepathy, of universal consciousness, where one's own consciousness is also a part of all of the others. When it comes to channelling this consciousness, this can only work through Self. What is received, therefore, has an unbreakable link with the work and circumstances of the instrument. It is the energy coming up from the base, meeting that which enters from the crown, that becomes united.

I have spoken of the role that the kundalini plays in entering each chakra so that it may be filled with light. At the brow chakra something quite different happens, illustrating the endless importance of the third eye. Kundalini energy is ever the mechanism by which one can reach as far as possible whilst remaining a spiritual being on Earth. The kundalini rises up the spine to the head and travels over the inside circumference and down to the point of the pituitary gland.

This is why the crosier or the shepherd's crook is often seen being held in rituals, their shape replicating this movement, emphasising the need to focus at the brow chakra. It was the shepherd who was led by a star or in other words, was able to stimulate the vision of the third eye, seeking the insight to be co-creator.

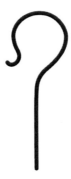

Figure 19. The Crosier.

The pituitary gland marks the point where the ida, sushumna and pingala come together in one spot, and are unified before separating out. This amalgamation also happens at each previous chakra but at the brow chakra the result of this meeting produces a very different outcome. Here, the unity where the three strands meet reflects, and is the power supply behind, focus. The three strands of kundalini then separate here, for it is the pituitary that marks the last stop in the human physical domain and where 'reason' of the intellect can go no further. The kundalini has to undergo this deliverance so that the sushumna can transcend and thus venture forth to the pineal gland, it being the place of the making and thus matching of the energies descending from above – Cosmic Fire.

The subsequent cross formed at the pituitary gland by the separation of the three kundalini energy lines is known esoterically as the second crucifixion, the first being the incarnation on Earth. This is the place that Jesus reaches out for during the last supper in order to further his aspiration to become Christ. The food of the supper represents the last

Chapter 6 ~ The Brow Chakra

relinquishing of physical need, no longer relevant after this transformation. This is only possible in the human kingdom, for what separates mankind from the animal is an upright spine or the pole of the crosier, which enables the sushumna to connect from the earth to the sky, vesting the power of authority through mankind.

The light that the second crucifixion creates is the lamp that provides vision when all may seem dim. The two eyes of the animal and human are light receptors and create form by receiving reflected light bounced off minute particles that we call matter, but this of course is not the object itself; it is this reflection that produces the illusion of space and thus form. The third eye deals with no illusion other than that of the Tamas. Therefore the third eye is able to receive a different form of light, one which could be described, as the term 'The second crucifixion' suggests, as Christ within the human being. This is only possible if the candidate is ready for its reality.

In Christian iconography, Christ is depicted on the cross above which is a plaque inscribed with the letters: 'INRI', which is an abbreviation of the Latin 'Ignis Natura Renovatur Integram', meaning 'Fire incessantly renews all of nature'. This fire is that which has the means to transform everything. Cosmic Fire is the spiritual matter of the cosmic vortex; it is the means by which the word of the cosmos can be received and passed on to mankind. It also destroys or renews all in its path and thus is in constant dialogue with all the monads including the planet Earth as a totality. As the source of renewal, Cosmic Fire is thus the director of fate. Through the reception of its presence, the clairvoyant is not only privy to the past but also the present and the future.

To the Hindus, raising the kundalini slowly through the chakras, a bit at a time and starting at the base, with the use of this Fire, enables the three major knots of the body, the Granthis, to be undone. The last knot is the Rudra Granthi, which is situated at the third eye. As this knot dissolves, it releases the soul from the confines of the five elements, so that the physical limitations of time and space no longer have any meaning. However, this should not be confused with a dream state, for this new awareness provides the vision of infinity, which manifests in a downward direction as wisdom. This transcendence is a doorway, a rite of passage to the crown chakra. Energies can then flow upward to the crown chakra, which has no physical basis; this conversion has to be made in order that the brow and the crown can come together.

It is important to note that at the brow chakra one is still not free from the essential qualities of the Gunas that make up the fabric of nature and are essential within consciousness itself. Without access to these qualities the crown chakra would contain no means of existence to us, and thus would not be accessible to the soul. Being essentially desires, but cosmological desires, the main attributes of Shiva as the Hindus see them, they determine manifestation for the dark as well as the light, which are both blended to the same outcome as one another, as are the Gunas. It is the blending process that as humans we pay particular attention to. Therefore the Gunas remain the same outside the confines of materialism as well as within, and thus form the glue of the cosmos that enables this connection to be made. They are conscious and thus lend structure to Self within what would otherwise appear to Self as a very formless cosmos. In a sense, the energy of the homœopathic remedy *Thuja Occidentalis* acts in a similar way to the Gunas in revealing the nature of the miasms in the physical world.

When the kundalini hits the pituitary gland it divides, and the ida goes off to the left and the pingala to the right. So to the left goes the cool calming lunar energy and to the right the vitality of solar energy. They then descend back down to the place from which they rose, in a spiral motion. The sushumna, being the most important energy form running through the human constitution, connects that which enters from the base with that which enters from the crown. It is this that enables one to channel. This is a profound connection, the join in the circle, the current between Heaven and Earth. Being of pure mothering or Divine feminine creative power (fire), sushumna directs all of the other energy systems in the human constitution. So all of the subtle bodies are shaped by their energetic connection to it.

Once separated at the pituitary gland, cosmic fire travels upward to make this connection. It is this division of the kundalini at the pituitary that makes the form of a cross, the innate symbol of enlightenment that marks the true meeting of human consciousness with that of the Divine spirit.

The symbol of two snakes twisting up a central pole has been adopted and presented in different forms, but its origin is that of the caduceus.

Chapter 6 ~ The Brow Chakra

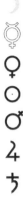

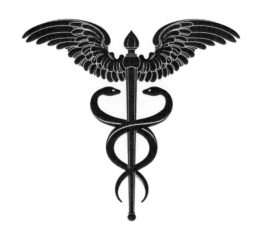

Figure 20. The Caduceus.

The Greek god Hermes, later to be named Mercury by the Romans, carries this cross, for in the caduceus there is unity between the upright motion that signifies the active and the horizontal motion, which is the receptive or passive. This unity is required for the function of the third eye and mimicked when observing the patient, for one has to be passive to receive and active to prescribe. This relationship can also be found on a major junction of the human spine. The seventh cervical vertebra is the most prominent vertebra and can be found by drawing an imaginary horizontal line from shoulder to shoulder, forming a cross with the spine. The point at which they meet is known by acupuncturists as the Dazhui point or Du-14. At this point all the yang energy of the body meets after it has been gathered, before being sent to the head. So this is a point of extreme fire – fire too extreme simply to enter the head in its present state, for if it did inflammation such as meningitis occurs. In order to make it acceptable to the head this fire has to undergo a resurrection, revealed in its formation of a Tau Cross.

Moving up the neck from the point of Du-14, the next seven vertebrae contain only one acupuncture point, which is situated just below the first cervical vertebra – Du-15, as Du-16 is positioned outside these seven vertebra between the skull and the first cervical vertebra. Du-15 is a very important point, for it acts as the doorkeeper (Venus) from one world to the next, keeping out energy that is insufficiently refined and giving voice to that which is. It also acts as the form within what appears formless, a point from which we can still perceive energy in order that it may be analysed. Du-16, on the other hand, is the point that can be considered to be the centre of the formless.

As the Chinese do not use numbers to describe acupuncture points, Du-16 is known as Fengfu in Chinese philosophy – the Storehouse of the Wind. This is the point from which the rising energy is converted to yin in order to enter the head; the cosmological equivalent is leaving this world and entering the other. Wind to the Chinese is the means by which energy can pierce through from one world to the next. Therefore, in having this ability and by not being visible (which is why it is stored within the formless Fengfu), Wind is considered to be of spiritual content. Only by acting upon the material world does it become visible, as witnessed when wind blows dust from the floor. This notion of the movement of energy from form to the formless and vice-versa is illustrated in the shape of the Tau Cross. Visually, the vertical (active) of this cross does not extend above the horizontal (passive) but we know it's there, for it is described as a cross and not a 'T'. So its invisibility is telling us something is different, something has changed. This is by the means of Wind and therefore the resurrection of fire is complete when it is no longer yin or yang within the realm of the formless.

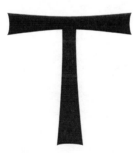

Figure 21. The Tau Cross.

The two sets of seven - the visible seven and the invisible seven, as found in the human spine and in the structure of the universe, are of the highest fundamental spiritual significance. It is essential to understand the importance of the role of the two sets of seven in the journey of the human spirit and therefore the journey undertaken in this book. This will become clearer as the book progresses, but for now, both sevens enable the transition of fire and of course represent the freeing of physi-

Chapter 6 ~ The Brow Chakra

cal constraint when entering into the other world. The seven vertebrae of the neck and the invisible counterpart represent the route into this other world, from matter into spirit, just like the seven chakras of which they are an integral part. The point Du-14 represents a border to this. All the major acupuncture points of the body are, in fact, borders to something. They are all points that pertain to resurrection, for they act as portals providing significant change. Therefore, if Du-14 is stimulated, it helps to awaken the pituitary gland by the exchange of this fire energy (kundalini).

This relationship between the need to balance matter with spirit is also true of the evolutionary failings of Christianity. Whilst over the years matter has battled to gain prevalence, the symbol of the cross has thus been transformed by having Christ in the physical form of Jesus, being nailed to it. This changes the significance of the cross from that of a symbol of a state of being, to one that signifies the re-enactment of a physical event, so becoming object-ive. The true meaning of this state refers to the control that Self has gained over its emotions (ida, the Moon and its feminine attributes) and also the achievement in mastering its strength of mind (pingala, sun and the masculine attributes). Only after these are united can the freed spirit transcend. So that which is being crucified is one's ego.

In Christianity the unification of this division between mortality and immortality is represented as an equal-armed red cross bottony (trefoiled), signifying the right to sit on the throne and reign over one's kingdom.

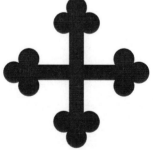

Figure 22 The Cross Bottony.

The cross is red in colour to signify the blood of Self, the bridge between who we were, who we are and who we are going to be. This is much like the Rose Cross adopted by the Rosicrucians, and it is within this symbol that all their philosophy is contained.

The position within the forehead at which the Kundalini separates to form the shape of a cross is often depicted in paintings or statues as the head of a serpent or a flame. It is also known as the horn of the unicorn. These images not only symbolise freedom from physical bondage but also the process by which this can happen. By protruding through the dross of the manas, the rubbish from daily existence that fills the head is burnt away, like the dissolving of the Rudra Granthi. New remedies pertaining strongly to the brow chakra will also act in helping to clear this dross such as *Moldavite, Copper Beech, Earthworm, Clay, Hazel* and *Sequoia*, to name just a few. Here the energy of the kundalini reveals more of its quality. Its fire, force, light or whatever term chosen to describe its energy has been raised above that of the five elements and is now able to resonate with that female energy, which produces the building blocks of the cosmos. It will therefore only resonate with that which is of the same quality, and, as we know from the destructive part of the female creative process, it will turn over the soil of the mind in order to aerate it with fresh perception.

It is said that the function of the third eye is dependent on the pineal gland. This pineal is both the point of action, independent from any other gland, and also the place of origin where previously it was the form of the third eye before the process of materialisation took it into the human body. This is not true. This idea may have arisen because in Hindu philosophy the pineal gland is known as the eye of Shiva, or sometimes just referred to as the third eye.

It is proclaimed that Shiva is everywhere; this is nothing if not vision. Its vision pertains to both the etheric and astral but here Shiva relates more to the process by which the third eye acts as a vessel, in which sushumna is liberated. The third eye in this sense is more like Brahma; residing in all and so receptive to all. This comes back to the fact that the initiator needs to be ready in all faculties in order that the third eye can accommodate vision. This is only possible in the mutual development of the pituitary and the pineal gland or the brow and the crown chakra. Only when working together can the sushumna make the relevant connection in order to enable one to tune in.

The third eye thus has an important bearing on the development of soul consciousness and thus the cloak in which it is clothed – The

Chapter 6 ~ The Brow Chakra

Causal Body. This body is formed by the conjunction of the manas and Buddhi or love and mind, the head and heart as one. For this reason, it is the bearer of soul consciousness. In relation to the realm of matter, it is not really a body yet its aura is visible to those who can see it. This aura is produced by the growth of a flame that is fanned by what may be considered as the good in each life, reflecting Divine life. As all is good, then its radiance may be considered as a barometer of Divine vibrancy.

In kabbalistic philosophy, the human soul corresponds to four planes – the Four Worlds, from which the Tree of Life can be divided. These are not to be confused with the four kingdoms which lie in the realm of the lowest sphere Malkuth (our material world) but are of course fed by that from the highest sphere Kether. The lower three worlds recognise that the soul has creative barriers that shape choices when things get too difficult, or when the soul is faced with impossible obstacles. The higher mind pertains to the third world and thus the faculty of reason ceases to have meaning beyond this level. All four worlds are expressed through the mind in the realm of thought. To achieve mastery of these lower worlds, and this is a karmic question, means to utilise light, for the fourth world is the realm of 'Emanation', which is spiritual in content and filters down to action in the physical world. The causal body is supplementary to this fourth world, where its role in reincarnation is directed by the tasks of the lower worlds. Thus once the soul, in its pursuit of initiation throughout its long cycle of reincarnation, has progressed through the fourth initiation, then it is said that the obstacles of karma have been freed.

Alice Bailey taught that there are nine initiations but like the Rays, we now know there to be many more, spanning way beyond our present comprehension. Everything that forms a body undergoes initiations, hence the British Isles like any other country that has a border and thus an identity, will have had and will continue to have initiations, as it evolves. All life forms are produced by them and are also a consequence of any mistakes in evolution. They are also a means by which one can transcend the current modes of thinking.

The beginning of an initiation can be brought on by a crisis. Next comes the need to work through what has been perceived in order to respond. This is the principle behind all change and what emancipates us from miasmatic bondage. In the fourth initiation, thought having been changed, the initiator has become the monad, having given up the material life for a spiritual one. This process applies to all creativity, regardless of its significance, so is the same for an idea coming into manifestation as it is for Self during its resurrection. There is no need for a causal body after the fourth initiation, for the fear that is associated with this body's existence has transcended out of matter. There is no further use for its illusion. Feeling is no more, just simple, pure initiation or death and rebirth of the next stage. The spiritual bond is so strong that the command of the Ego is no longer required and neither is reincarnation. One is now in a position to do one's work for humanity from the higher planes. All that we are is either a build-up towards or a response to these initiations. Therefore all that happens to us contributes to their outcome. It is a very, very long road before this outcome but the series of initiations provide the means by which to cleanse the monad, for it is the monad that makes Self aware of the next incarnation.

The causal body is the spiritual overcoat that is concerned with that which rises up from the personality to fit that which is entering from the higher planes. Essentially, the limitations that perpetuate the myth of duality, have no place here. So that which rises up from the personality has transcended, to match this overcoat. What there is and what the personality believes there is are two different things. The two meeting this energy is what forces the causal body to radiate from within. This light is the vehicle of expression for the soul and is why the causal body is often referred to as the 'Temple of the soul'. This light builds and reflects the quality of the soul to those who can read its aura – and also to others regardless.

Here on this plane, the consciousness of one's purpose in evolutionary development can be found. Although often referred to as the abstract mind, it is hindered by the limitations of the lower bodies, but the important thing to note here is the causal body is constructed by the monad. How this ties in with the beginning of self-awareness and the formation of what was to become the syphilitic miasm is that the origin of one's own monad is the result of one's voluntary exile in order that humanity and the solar system may evolve. Whereas on the lower chakras this may be perceived as an act of altruism, here it is revealed as a pact with the Divine.

Perception changes depending on the level one is at, and so how something may appear through the energy of one chakra will appear differently when kundalini has awakened a higher one. To build up one

Chapter 6 ~ The Brow Chakra

chakra has a positive effect on all the others. The purpose of kundalini is to have all seven cleansed and working together in harmony to present the bigger picture. This is about transformation, where nothing is lost, just altered. Change brings things together, it unifies, and unlike stagnation, it does not keep things apart.

Being the immortal part of man, the monad is the part of Divine power that creates the spark, which instigates individual life. This life remains connected to the Divine, otherwise the individual would cease to exist. It is the monad that encourages the Ego to incarnate in order to evolve. Thus the separation into Self was the doing of Divine will, which by necessity suggests that so too was the resultant formation of the syphilitic miasm. It would seem that the Divine insists at times that humanity has to work against the light so that change may come about, in order to gain Divine consciousness. This miasm would appear to be a pact between man and the Source, so that in order to be conscious one has to have, at one's disposal, all types of tools in order to instigate creative purpose. Problems seem to arise the greater the division between the Ego and the monad.

This bolt of cosmic energy, the monad, which creates a crisis within the Ego, also induces a desire to resolve this crisis, and if it pertains to the lower worlds, this can only be played out down here on Earth through reincarnation. This crisis will, of course, manifest as a miasmatic collective when in nature. However, it is the syphilitic miasm that offers a crisis of confidence of the highest magnitude, creating the deepest of obstacles for Ego to push off against. Only this desire would cause it to leave its state of bliss and re-enter the depths of the despairing struggles that are the physical plane, for like attracts like in order to induce change. This desire, which is in reality to connect with the Divine, is instigated by the monad. Only through exile can Self develop within the three aspects of monadic essence, these being the means to develop its intelligence as received from above (The Holy Ghost), the relationship that creates love-wisdom that we know as the son (Christ) and the power of Divine Will (The Almighty or Father).

To take this notion further, Self is thus the Breath of the Father. This breath is the spirit that forms our entity from where the monadic triad is cultivated in the pursuit of purpose, under the guidance of fate. However, it is the aspect of the Holy Ghost that offers Self the opportunity to evolve, through the development of consciousness. From its very beginning, Self began its quest with an unforgettable road map.

This map is like a star, as from its birth it has contained all the means to manifest in nature, and this is the reason why homœopathic remedies made from all can heal all. All differing energies are, in essence, a part of this Divine spark and therefore of the highest spiritual resonance. The point of dilution in homœopathy is this resurrection, from matter to spirit, in which understanding and a heightened perception provides homœopaths with the means to tune the energy of nature and appropriately stimulate all the planes of the human constitution. This is to work on and with the essence of the Divine spark, and to me is the reason why homœopathy is a spiritual pursuit. It is also the reason why the syphilitic miasm is part of cosmic fire, to further cosmic creation.

In life one has to reconcile consequence, and that enables the monad to build that of the Divine within oneself. This is about refinement as well as development, which is another way of expanding on the qualities of the spark. The monad remains largely uncontactable to us because Self has yet to rise and the monad has yet to fall to the plane where the structure of matter and Divine consciousness are the same.

Cosmic Fire or Shakti (if we consider her to be the origin or power behind all existence including Brahma, Vishnu and Shiva) pertains to the monad as well as being the constituent of the kundalini containing both male and female polarities. It is the pure energy of light, and in the brow Cosmic Fire is unified. This can be seen as Shakti ascending and Shiva descending and the meeting of the two. Therefore Shiva is attributed to the crown chakra. It is this relationship that enabled Self to step into a mind already developed on the higher planes.

The source of cosmic fire goes back a long way, beyond our reach. So the means by which we describe its existence is also very limited, as with the monad. Much that is seen by the third eye manifests eventually as action, and this may in relative human years be a slow process. Even though what has been received may not be understood, it affects the mind and creates a change. We use this anyway, as we make decisions without knowing where the guidance has come from.

Like exercising a muscle, the more the third eye is used, the more it becomes of use and reveals secrets when concentration is used. Its vision, as is the nature of tapping into this fire, brings clarity to thought before it reaches the throat chakra to manifest through the vibration of words to create form.

Chapter 6 ~ The Brow Chakra

Cosmic fire, the Supreme Mother of the Universe, has its role to play as constructor. What grants the third eye vision is the awakening of the pineal gland, which is the gland of spiritual perception from which Self gathers the purpose. It is the pituitary gland however, that directs desire in order that this purpose may manifest in form. This is the means by which the throat chakra and the thyroid gland supports the inner vision of the third eye, for in all psychic reception a channel is required to enter this world, and of course into the heart.

The third eye is at its most liberated when the head and the heart are in concordance with the throat. The human voice is required to echo the voice which is received, however convoluted this may be. In astrology this relationship is known as the 'Eye of Taurus' – the bull, whose constellation is said to be able to decipher Divine voice. The pituitary is of a lower resonance to the pineal gland, hence the division required between the ida and pingala and the sushumna or the division between Earthly spirit and Divine spirit.

The third eye is used as a means of focus. It is not the place in which clairvoyance is obtained, but understood, which in itself is no mean feat. Just like the receptors of solar light – the two visible eyes – the third eye is a receptor of images, but these images are both solar and cosmic in their making, so clarity is important, for the lower can hinder the upper with meaningless clutter. Images pertaining to the interests of the personality, and deciphered in the lower manas will inadvertently feed the mind, or clog the pituitary, and inhibit the reception of higher vision. Whether or not this happens depends on what Self concentrates upon. Light is propelled at Self all the time, and self constitutes both light and dark in order that we can differentiate the light. So discernment is required, so that we know the difference between what is feeding the ego, and what is feeding the soul. The better the use of this judgement, the sharper the focus of the third eye, enhancing the Buddhi's power to perceive. This is self-fulfilling, for the greater the clarity, the better the judgement. This also breeds sensitivity, which is why the use of the third eye is imperative in understanding karma, for, in a roundabout way, it is the mirror of the soul. It reveals to us all that we are, so therefore, all that we have been. It is during meditation that the third eye reveals Self's secrets to Self. It also comes bearing gifts, an opportunity for the Cosmic Fire to incinerate unwanted images and so cleanse the blood and distribute health to the cells.

There are seven Hermetic principles, a few of which have already been incorporated in some form within this book. They make up the Egyptian Hermetic philosophy, said to be the root to spiritual healing. The ideas flourished after having been bestowed on humanity by the Egyptian god of wisdom – Thoth. The second Hermetic axiom and the most commonly quoted: 'as above, so below; as below, so above', formed the basis of the Greek Hylozoism. It refers to all the forces of the universe, packed with the activity of conscious life that are working through the life of each human – they being a microcosm of this cosmic whole. This is the means by which Divine consciousness is interpreted within the many facets that make up the human constitution. We look for and make a judgement, for we know from what our monad tells us that the soul is more important than the personality. So it is through the lower planes that one can unravel the mysteries of the higher ones.

The first of the Hermetic principles or the first world if you like, states: 'The all is mind; the Universe is mental'. This refers to the limitless awareness available to Self or Ego in the infinite creative mind, which is the cosmic root of all things. Put these two maxims together and they reveal that all acts through Self, whether conscious of it or not. All existence is based on consciousness, so the work we do on the lower manas enables vision on the higher manas, lifting the veil from the unknown to the known. It is true therefore, that mental control is imperative in spiritual growth, for without its clarity one cannot receive enlightenment.

All souls on Earth differ in age and experience and thus in their make-up. In order for them to progress they need more than bliss to react against and on Earth they surely find it. In doing so they develop will-power. This battle between feelings is played out in the lower worlds, forming integrity. Integrity is an important link, for it is the reflection of one's word, that which makes form. In the lower worlds obstacles act in order to prevent one from keeping one's word. If one can stick to one's word, then subsequently more negative karma will be freed as a result of discovering outcomes. This is not simply about being wrong or right, it is about the judgement of one's word, which is the experience that creates integrity. Changing one's mind without knowing the outcome of the original decision leaves Self vulnerable to more negativity.

Integrity is a powerful tool in the soul's battle to combat fear. Another of its tools is memory. Within the safety of the Ego's bliss on the upper realms, the soul has the security to reflect on all of its past experiences.

Chapter 6 ~ The Brow Chakra

This is removed during incarnation but the record remains in the unconscious and is expressed through the maintaining causes, beliefs and the patterns to which we all adhere. Change involves becoming conscious of these causes and by having the deep desire within to be free of them. When one is aware of something it does not remain the same as when one is not aware of it. What has changed is the reaction to it. If the opportunity is taken, then memories also change, having been falsified by the repetition of past actions. Memories are not written in stone but are merely a form of perception. One may learn a poem word for word but what it means can change. This is the same for any spiritual text, as it is not what is written that is important but the way it is read. It can only ever be relevant and have context in the here and now. Like a mantra, it is the energy that it evokes that is important and so its resonance can only change that which is present. We all see and perceive differently so our memories of similar experiences are all different. These differences are the making of individualism and emphasised by the ego. Memory, in the biological sense, deceives Self, for it is fluid and is open to emotional responses.

Memory is the record of day-to-day experiences, which in this life make up what Self can identify as 'I'. Trauma of any kind, especially the most invasive, will encrypt itself into memory and can remain locked in the being for the length of this lifetime. It is the soul's task to unlock this, hopefully in one lifetime. It is because these memories are transient and the subject of influence that homœopathy is able to release trauma. Although transient, they can be extremely stubborn when accompanied by a lot of fear.

Memory is a thread that runs from life to life, forming a bridge between the higher manas and the Buddhi. The illusions of physical existence can be changed when homœopathy speeds up karma. Memory is a process, a faculty required between being conscious and not, but is, like everything else in the universe, never fixed. However, Divine thoughts, memories that emanate down from the Atman to the Buddhi, are those that create homœopathy and not that which can be changed by it. This source of intelligence, although beyond ourselves, allows us to be privy to it through imagination. Again, this is a process of ascending planetary consciousness meeting the invisible descending Divine. These memories are what should guide our actions.

At the brow it is relatively straightforward to act seriously when under the influence of such energy. The challenge can be to incorporate fun, for such revelations demand a great deal of focus, but fun is a creative necessity. At the brow humanity finds it difficult to justify this fun, for, as with comedians, there can be a thin line between it and tragedy. One has to understand that fun is an important factor in purpose, for fun is also a serious business. Fun and one's ability to chose it over the pressure of serious matters is healing. It can be the most difficult of challenges when trying to develop focus, but as in meditation itself, the more one concentrates the harder it is. Fun is a powerful part of freedom. Even at times of deep crisis, of a healing crisis, never forget your sense of humour. It prevents the heart from becoming sucked into the head.

For the philosopher Jung, the amalgamation of duality was of constant interest. He believed there were four ego-functions that made up one's construction of reality. One of these four, and the opposite to thinking, is feeling. The other two opposites are intuition and sensation. From his findings, one begins to understand the role of imagination, having an interactional relationship between the functions of the higher triad.

Part of wisdom is to have the imagination to see. This is to have the ability to focus the imagination so that the mind is able to deliver into its own consciousness that which forms the structure or picture that has been received. Imagination in its Divine sense is necessary in order to see the unseen. This may be the female counterpart that is creative, of which creative imagination is an important attribute. To use this form of imagination is to recognise the role of Shiva as the destroyer of all things that have ceased to be relevant. As this is a process of destroying what has already manifested, it pertains to the female and thus acts through Shiva's counterpart – Shakti or Parvati – in order that Shiva can evoke the new. Much in the same way the harvest is not only about bounty, but is an opportunity to review the changes one could make.

Imagination and trust are very closely connected, and both are necessary. All mystical content, be it wrapped in religious form or any other, essentially harks back to the same source, for they all speak of the same thing. Enlightenment is a process and cannot simply be given in the form of a lump of information, for it is the work that is important. Before embarking on this journey, one requires the imagination and then the trust, for this road is long and demanding of both time and effort. This is necessary for progression and so change, but right at the beginning it takes imagination to plant the seed and trust to germinate it.

Chapter 6 ~ The Brow Chakra

The brow chakra, more than any other chakra, presents the opportunity to change the cycles of the past in which Self gets stuck. Here the mind, and with it the limitations of the biological brain, acts as a barrier to insight, but being barriers, they can come down. Revelation comes at a price and one needs to be ready and prepared for what will be perceived in the form of altered states. These feed down and adjust the lower chakras as they are integrated, building wisdom and placing Self back into a new comfortable position. Perception is the tool that becomes sharpened – as sharp as Saturn's scythe. It is used to dissect significance, for here even the slightest thing will reveal the reason for its purpose, all having relevance and adding to the wider picture. This is something we healers are trying to perceive.

There is of course imagination pertaining to the lower mind, which is quite different and the result of the dross of memory that leads into the realm of fantasy. A dose of the remedy *Opium* or *Calcarea Carbonica* can bring people back out of an illusionary dream state, which some may say is the only means to cope with modern living, and also helps to clear the fog that is preventing the activities of the third eye. This realm of fantasy takes form through the personality in the kama manas. Basically in this state, who people think they are, their behaviour and aspiration cannot be further from the truth. Patients who, for one reason or another, have built layers of compensatory behaviour, present themselves in this fantasy state or it may be that they are simply suffering from congestion in the brow chakra which is, anyway, the result of delusional desires. Inoculation is both created by and also creates delusional desires that separate the connection between the pituitary and pineal gland.

The third eye is also destroyed by the use of pleasure drugs, the result of which creates much frustration and later deep anger in the psyche. These drugs lead Spirit out and away from its body by destroying the connection necessary for its return. They can also blow open the aura, letting all manner of things in, which will not make spirit want to return. In a fantasy state, patients can also be proud and aloof but at the same time lacking in principles. They can be cunning and manipulative in order to get other people to do the things that they are avoiding. Avoidance is a lack of focus. As a consequence, these people play emotional games. They can also be rash, making decisions without clarity of thought. These are all attributes of a poorly functioning brow chakra.

To live one's truth does not take exceptional confidence or courage; it should be a natural state, as truth is life and one's purpose is pre-ordained. But it still remains an interesting question as to how much of who we think we are lies in the realm of fantasy and how much its consequential behaviour is blocking up the kama manas and clouding the third eye. So to use the third eye, imagination is imperative, but this imagination should be stimulated by the pursuit of reality.

Thought is not possible without the creative process of both imagination and memory. It is the making of the soul. To search into the past and to resurrect past karma may jog a memory, for our psyche is that of our collective past. It is that collective past or the consciousness of one's evolutionary development that makes up the Causal Body. The soul, in its totality, can thus express itself on the causal plane through the causal body. The causal plane is the Buddhi of the higher triad and it is through the Buddhi that the soul is expressed.

If possible, the Monadic-Ego reunites before incarnation, there being little purpose to evolution if Ego does not have the desire to expand on the good given essence that the monad is – Divine Fire. The soul, whose task is to act as the vehicle for spirit, houses its manifestation in the causal body, which connects the lower constitution of mankind with the higher realms. It is through the soul that the monad works its destiny. Consciousness is passed through the soul, and the soul evolves through experience. However, the centre of consciousness is the monad; the soul always remains the vehicle for experience and thus the past is reflected in it.

To not be 'awake' means that Self, although innately connected with the monad through the soul, is not connected consciously, so the soul does not develop with the experiences that await from the connections coming up from the personality and down from the source. Being immortal, spirit uses the soul to make the connection from the immortal to mortal attributes of Self, from that above to that below. It is this connection that fuels the Buddhi and without which the soul cannot radiate or dwell on the causal plane. Wisdom and the aspiration to it, which is integrity, will be lost. This is the reason why every homœopathic remedy works in some form on the brow chakra, and they all aid the process of transcending through spiritual fire.

Chapter 6 ~ The Brow Chakra

THE PITUITARY AND THE HYPOTHALAMAS GLANDS

The Hindu name for the brow chakra is ajna, meaning 'to command.' The pituitary is supported by the hypothalamus, for its function is to act as control centre to physical life, governing the function of the other endocrine glands. For this reason the pituitary is known as the gland of persistent effort; to achieve this it is reliant on a good blood supply, which if hindered can result in insanity. It has in structure two lobes that extend from a stalk much like a sycamore seed. This is why the new remedy made from the *Sycamore Seed* works wonderfully on the regulation and pathology of this gland and helps to correct and balance the whole of the endocrine system.

The pituitary gland is usually the first gland to indicate that there is an endocrine problem and its sensitivity is due to minute movement of the lobes as they respond to the flow of the constitution. Without this regulation, all of the body's chemistry would take a wrong direction. This flow can be hindered by restriction in the growth and movement of the twenty-two cranial bones that make up the skull, especially the sphenoid bone, which is prone to locking due to birth trauma, head injuries, dehydration or dental braces. Each time dental braces are tightened then the subsequent pressure needs to be released from this bone by the means of a visit to the cranial osteopath. This also applies to all the other causes of constriction that may be associated with inhibited function of this gland. Homœopathic remedies will also be needed in conjunction with the osteopathic work to loosen these structures and allow the lobes to pulse their rhythms once again. These rhythms are also influenced by the hypothalamus via the hypophyseal fossa that channels emotional content into their path.

It is the cerebrospinal fluid (CSF) that protects the brain, its glands and stem from damage by acting as a kind of cushion. The spinal column is not fixed to the brain in the physical sense but ends at the medulla oblongata, a swelling of liquid medium that prevents a rigid junction and which will give if this joint is knocked, absorbing the forces of impact. Of course there is far more to CSF than simply acting as a fluid buffer. It directs and supplies nutrients and hormones not only to all cells, but also most importantly to the brain and its endocrine glands, removing toxins in the process.

The sphenoid bone, moving its wings to the rhythm of the breath in the process of cardiac reception, works like a diaphragm in the head, pumping CSF around the brain and around the whole body via the central nervous system. This gentle rocking also stimulates thought by the rhythm of reception that promotes focus and understanding. This timing coincides with the absorption of prana into the body and up to the brain, in order to stimulate the participation of thought, and explains why too much study depletes the spleen. Congestion of the brow chakra locks the movement of the sphenoid bone causing more congestion, so it is imperative for this bone to have free flight. Too much fat in the diet will not only contribute to this congestion but also to the subsequent fogging in the third eye. Patients with blocked sinuses, ear and Eustachian tube problems will most definitely have a problem as a result of trauma in this area.

The two lobes of the pituitary are known as the posterior and the anterior. Between these two is a cleft or intermediate lobe. These two lobes act as two distinct organs of differing function. The anterior lobe secretes hormones, which by means of the thyroid, governs growth and the reproductive system.

The pituitary, as a single unit, is the direct link to one's past, present and future development, the source of which are the three seed atoms that produce the dense, etheric and astral bodies. They remain housed in the heart where they can be charged with the greatest supply of oxygenated blood. It is from this possibility of growth that the embryo develops these three bodies and subsequently all forms of human development are directed through the pituitary gland. In this aspect it is the anterior lobe that takes up the influence of the tubercular and the psoric miasms.

The posterior lobe is, in effect, a protrusion of the hypothalamus or the alta major centre, where the spine meets the cranium and where the nervous system meets the endocrine system. Through the hormone ADH the fluids in the body are regulated, so the balance of the water content of the blood, as opposed to the level being excreted by the kidneys, is maintained under the guidance of the posterior lobe. These hormone levels adjust to the rhythms of sleep and also increase in response to a nervous system overburdened with emotion. They also provide the means by which a woman lactates after childbirth.

The word Hormone comes from the Greek meaning 'the force of being'. These physical fluids are the means of miracles and can powerfully dissipate ill-health. It is easy to see why the posterior lobe takes on

Chapter 6 ~ The Brow Chakra

the influence of the sycotic miasm, while the pituitary directs the constitution. The cleft in the middle that joins these two lobes is where the syphilitic miasm builds up. It influences not only the balance between the masculine and the feminine in Self but also the balance between emotion and reason. It also inhibits the proper growth of all the organs and related forms. The pituitary gland is the realm of the concrete mind, where, under syphilitic influence, the truth can be distorted. At this place, the 'control' centre, there should be no division, but only unity. It is the syphilitic consequence of our past that creates a division, as it appears in the cleft, and the greater this karma of deluded truth, the greater the division. This is also the division that connects, or more often separates, the two halves of the brain. Here again, there should be unity, especially in their communication.

The brow chakra at root is about communication, of the left and the right and of the higher planes to the lower (the cross). The left half of the brain receives thought in the form of the conventions of the rational. The right's thought process is far more intuitive and concerned with the alternative structures of thought under the influence of the pineal gland. The two have to co-exist but the syphilitic miasm breaks this link in order to remain hidden. So through its desire to deceive it creates two poles of opposition that, in actuality, need to be united.

Over-activity of the pituitary gland in childhood leads to over-growth and early maturity: giants are produced in this way. As adults, over-activity generally produces a heavy appearance with coarseness and thickening of both hands and feet, and it is in the skull and facial features that this thickening is most obvious. The personality is also affected, leading to a more forceful initiative and intense way of living, the kind seen in American cities. This is because the pituitary has command over will.

If the pituitary is directive then the pineal gland is receptive. This relationship is of interest at this stage of our present root-race – which is concerned with the development of the mind. In the West and especially in American society, the emphasis is on reason, which is a polar opposite to the practice of belief. So with this in mind, the combination of the ida and pingala is like East meeting West. In the West at present, the purpose of life is to develop the mind and that means to become more conscious of Self. To think is to perceive oneself or to see how one is perceived. This has the effect of sharpening the mind. The problem arises when young souls incarnate into such a sophisticated situation and this in itself may be the reason why the pituitary becomes over active.

Under-activity of the pituitary results in dwarfism. There may also be symptoms of hair loss and the laying down of large quantities of fat. Poor memory and a dull mentality will result. These people are thus opposite in many ways to their over-active twin. There is lassitude, timidity and the belief that one is a failure. These people simply can't think for themselves and an inability to finish the task is a sign that the life is draining from this gland. If people are made to feel like this at any stage in life by any overpowering force, then the pituitary will reluctantly accommodate. There will also be an aversion to sex.

There is a strong connection between the creative force induced during sexual activity and the increase of pituitary secretion that stimulates the brain cells. Sex has been used in the past, as it is today, to increase perception. It is the sex act that triggers the energy of the kidneys, which is sent to the brain and heightens awareness.

Sex, or the energy it induces, stimulates the connection of the opposite polarities in Self, the passive and active or the female and male, which are both within Self but operate unconsciously. This energy causes the polarities to unite at the pituitary gland. Jung named them the anima (female) and animus (male) and to the kabbala they are represented by the active (right) and passive (left) sides or pillars of the tree, as is the same in the outer two meridians of the kundalini. The act of falling in love involves the intermingling of these opposite polarities within Self and between partners. If this is a very powerful connection, not only will there be a special level of intimacy but the dynamic of push and pull, of projection and reception which constantly builds, will enable the relationship to be raised and joined at the pituitary gland in both partners. If this happens then a psychic connection develops between the two lovers, for we already know this unity is not limited by the bounds of time and space. This is why even when apart they are still connected by their unified aura.

This balance also indicates how the hormones secreted by the pituitary keep these male and female aspects in-check, for like the outer pillars of the Tree of Life, these polarities can be reversed so that the active and passive aspects in a man or woman change. The fact that there are two aspects to this in Self, can produce a man who is active in his female qualities and passive in his male and the same can be so for a woman,

Chapter 6 ~ The Brow Chakra

often producing an aggressive female.

The emotional response to trauma or negative past patterning will, through the pituitary, have a determining effect as to the circumstances in life that shape one's identity. This fragility can undermine Self, which is beset on a daily basis by images which are pumped into the pituitary and which can, like Jupiter, confuse Self in regard to what it thinks it wants, with what it really needs. As already revealed by the way the miasms interplay with the pituitary or the command of the Self, there is much here to manipulate one's truth. When I was a child of about six years old, there was a competition at school to name the prince and princess of my class. It was inevitable that the two who most resembled the archetypes of these fairy tale stories won. Alas we know from the story of Samson and Delilah that beauty, whilst captivating, soon fades. Samson forfeits his stamina by being enticed by something transient. It is interesting that in the kabbala, the unity of these two sexes at the pituitary gland is known as the 'marriage of the King and Queen'.

The union of Shiva and Shakti, the ida and pingala, are the masculine and feminine principles that need to be consolidated in Self, and it is at the pituitary gland that the two reach a place of reconciliation. The pituitary contains the measure of both our male and female lives and balances the feminine and masculine aspects, as well as allowing understanding of these energies, for the male represents the un-manifested and the female the manifested. Beyond this point they are devoid of positive and negative polarities.

These polarities are the twins of Gemini, the seeds of germination that holds the duality of opposites as one. The sign of Gemini gives much astrological insight into the function of the pituitary gland, as, along with the brow, it is ruled by Mercury, the planet of knowledgeable pursuits. The pituitary gland creates for the brain and nervous system the greatest of alchemic possibilities – to be in absolute control of Self. This is possible when the positive, male current of pingala joins the negative, female current of ida, thus creating the inspiration of Gemini, which is about liberation as well as relating. It is by the means of these two forces coming together that expansion (the physical manifestation of which is at the sacral centre) can occur. This amalgamation of fire and water ('vapour') is refined to its purist constituent, intellect and love, the heart's emotion with the rational mind, producing wisdom. It enables one to decipher true meaning.

The conscious act of maintaining focus at the brow centre connects us to the pituitary gland and enables the personality to be eliminated from perception. It is this ability that liberates thought and connects us to the truth.

The pituitary is evidently very important, for it is tucked deep into the vault of a bony structure in the skull, offering a level of protection not seen elsewhere in the body, other than perhaps the throne of the sleeping serpent of kundalini. It has the appearance of a red pea, in size and structure, but this can fluctuate depending on the morality of the person. Images of misdemeanours can weigh heavily on its form. Meditation on the brow chakra exercises and so enhances its function, improving focus. In so doing, much fear can be removed, which quietens the nervous system, for it feeds into the hypothalamus, where the brain meets the spinal column and thus the nervous system. Images that have formed memories, which may well have been hidden from the conscious mind on account of being too painful, can be released here during meditation. Dying also involves the discharge of these images, returning them to the astral plane in order that one can start afresh. By this instantaneous resurrection and then by the process of forgetfulness, the soul is allowed to die in peace. These images of painful memories are retrieved in reverse order, the most vivid or pressing coming first. Memories pertaining to past lives as well as those retrieved as cosmic memories, or those from visits to the higher planes, also need to be left behind – which can be confusing to those who witness the death, especially if these obscure memories are released vocally. They will sound as if from another world, or completely unrelated to the dying person. Allopathic drugs can interfere with this process, but the homœopathic remedies *Ayahuasca, Arsenicum, Purple* and *Amethyst* can break through their grip and reinstate the process.

It is because the human brain is the connection between the material and the psycho-spiritual, that all this weight has to be discarded. Self is not fully aware of its mortality, for if it were it would not need to reincarnate.

The hypothalamus is responsible for homœostasis, so is very much concerned with equilibrium especially after emotional reactions, such as anger, pleasure, pain, depression and hunger, and therefore with the physical response that accompanies such emotional arousal. It instigates changes necessary in calming the nervous system, especially from the effects of a full range of emotions. Blood pressure, or rather the means by which its flow can be increased to the muscles during

Chapter 6 ~ The Brow Chakra

exercise as in the case of fight or flight, also lies within its portfolio, as it acts directly on the adrenals.

The hypothalamus is situated at the point where the brain connects to its stem, located at the top of the spinal cord, and is one of the body's major methods of regulating the rhythms of hormone production around the light cycle of day and night. It thus guides the soul into astral travel during sleep in order that the dense body may be repaired. Esoterically speaking, it forms a triangle between itself, the pituitary and the pineal gland. This triangle or pyramid is very important to spiritual reception but again relies on the unity achieved at the pituitary, the master gland. When the hypothalamus resonates with this triad it fills the whole brain with light, activating the temporal lobes that are required in the process of pulling exploratory thought processes into memory. Once the cosmic fire connects with its source it burns cold, and the hypothalamus clears the pathways that enable the distribution of the waves of pure thought. It is this gland which is the centre for psychic reception.

The hypothalamus has much to do with memory which grows through emotional responses and thus because of its relationship with the pituitary, it can con the pituitary into repeating nasty habits, holding back Self. As new information is received in the brain, it is the hypothalamus that determines whether a logical, methodical response is required, or an immediate response, such as that of fight or flight. Either way it is the memories of past emotional responses that set a system of predetermined reactions, which have been instilled through the experiences of learning. These determine how the mind decides to respond to such information and will inevitably continue the cycle of fear if there is patterning that is the result of painful memories. This is also true if Self has not been encouraged to respond as an individual, and hence the response goes against Self or Jiva, one's individual consciousness: but any response, be it positive or negative, becomes established by that which we call conditioning. The more positive one can feel about new experiences, especially in the field of learning, the more the mind can develop. This has recently been referred to as the importance of 'Emotional Intelligence'. With too much stress, the mind goes blank, but because the hypothalamus stimulates the adrenal glands, it can generate a positive relationship with pressure when Self feels safe. Again a sense of fun is required. If Self is incarcerated by habits then this will reflect in the emotional body, and symptoms of dysfunction that pertain to the hypothalamus will result.

Often, to change for the better the way in which the hypothalamus functions, one has to take a chance. Basically, one has to form new memories of positive experiences in order to change those which suffocate the soul. Rituals or meditative visualisation techniques that enable Self to use the power of the truth gained from the higher planes may be needed to replace those that have beset one's path. These must be made by Self, perhaps under the guidance of another, but not put there by another.

Because this gland distinguishes between night and day it counts these cycles in terms of structures that are provided by memories. This is not simply to counteract the changes in bodily needs that are determined by the ageing process but the means by which time can heal outmoded cycles. It sends pulses of positivity to the organs of the body so that their physical and spiritual content can become enriched. Electrical charges in the atmosphere and radiation created by the microwaves of mobile phones seriously interfere with this process and with the communication between the pituitary and the hypothalamus gland. Thoughts need to be earthed, so the connection from the brow to the base chakra can also be lost through such interference.

The brow chakra, and the base, have a strong relationship with time through the way memory bounces off Saturn, as this planet remembers everything in order to remind Self that a major factor in gaining positive experiences is to maintain stability. Hence there is a relationship with not only daily but also life cycles, and this communication can also determine life expectancy, it being tied to the Lords of Karma and the three creative laws. Also, the registering of ill-health in the brow chakra marks the point at which ill health can be changed into wellbeing. This needs focus and vision and on a physical level, serotonin, which maintains concentration in the function of the cerebrum, and with which allopathic and pleasure drugs interfere. These create doubt, and destroy focus. Self-confidence is very important in the healing process.

The pituitary gland is a very powerful gland and when used to control memories and emotions, the influence of the hypothalamus can be both positive and negative. For instance, the mind hunts for energy and distributes it to where appropriate for strength in a given situation. If an organ is weak or missing, the rest run around to support its need as directed by the pituitary, via positive impulses from the hypothalamus, and this is a very necessary and positive process.

The negative side to the relationship between these glands comes in the form of the control of natural expression. If we take the spleen as an organ, and recall that its function is destroyed by food additives such as colourings and preservatives, a child who is fed such additives will express reactionary behaviour, as he or she is still uninhibited enough to just go with this response. As an adult one learns to suppress this reaction, so, denied an outlet these toxins inevitably continue to harm the spleen. Further, the adult believes that as it has control of its reactions to these chemicals they are not doing any harm. This innate reaction to things is what is lost when the pituitary gland is conditioned by negative hypothalamus function and it is this control of emotion that needs to be addressed by the homœopath, alongside the poor organ function. This may be interpreted, astrologically as the point of Scorpio – the ability to use the power of control only when it is most appropriate. This is for the pituitary and the hypothalamus working together to learn in a Scorpio way, through reincarnation.

The homœopathic 'like' that is needed here to readdress the balance between these two glands will be one that reflects what is happening in the brow. The notion of like curing like has been around a lot longer than homœopathic prescribing, as has the wisdom pertaining to the function of the brow chakra. In yoga, high blood pressure is mainly associated with an overactive mind. This produces a build-up of pressure on the pituitary and thus on the hypothalamus. To alleviate this a weight is applied to the forehead. This can be remarkably heavy, so is best applied by experienced practitioners. The external pressure alleviates the internal one by dissipating or finding an outlet for the stuck energy and the mind is subsequently soothed from its harmful activity, thus calming the nervous system.

MERCURY WAS A THIEF

According to Greek mythology, the conniving Hermes (Mercury), as legend has it, was conceived in secret and gestated, born and then wrapped in swaddling bandages in just one night. Within no time he fully exploited his clever, shrewd and cunning attributes by stealing half of his brother Apollo's cattle. In order to become an Olympian, he sacrificed two of the cattle and divided them into twelve parts (signs of the zodiac), offering eleven to the gods of Mount Olympus. In order to cook one for himself he discovered how to kindle fire (the spark of Gemini intelligence). He then returned and replaced the bandages to disguise his guilt.

During his return journey he made the first lyre from a tortoise shell but this was witnessed by his father Zeus (Jupiter) and so his ruse was thwarted. An argument ensued between his parents and Apollo, during which Hermes played his lyre to soothe the situation. Apollo was so impressed he exchanged the lyre for the cattle that had been taken, for this is a reflection of the Hermetic talent for foresight, thinking several moves ahead. Music was so important to Apollo because he could see the way it ascended to the vibrations of the heavens.

Hermes next developed the flute and on hearing it, Apollo knew he needed it and approached Hermes to exchange the flute for his Caduceus (figure20), or Kerykeion, as it was known in Greece. This was the means by which Hermes obtained his twisted staff. It was Hermes' father Zeus who recognised the positive aspects of his son's qualities and their potential. He first directed them towards commerce. This is how Mercury became known as a merchant, as the name suggests.

There is of course more to this story. Being dissatisfied with remaining in his cave to count while his half brother was seemingly bathed in material wealth and adulation, Hermes thought: if my father is to ignore this injustice and my brother not see his own reflection, then I shall risk my honour and take what is rightfully mine (the dichotomy of the Cain and Abel story again). This sense of injustice presented Hermes with the desire to explore beyond Olympus and again, once recognised and under the direction of his father, he sought out justice regardless of personal discomfort. This is in part why it was really Zeus who bestowed on him the caduceus, for within its power lay the scales of the natural laws of justice.

When Odysseus was still mortal and had been kept on Calypso's island too long, Zeus sent Hermes to rescue him. He was equipped with magic sandals that enabled him to fly, so that he could transport himself with ease and materialise wherever he was needed, an attribute only previously possessed by the higher gods. He was also given a hat, a helmet providing the level of protection not dissimilar to that surrounding the pituitary gland. Thus Hermes became the messenger of the gods, his full purse representing the wealth of personal insight: but it has to be remembered that his messages, like the metal of mercury itself, are

Chapter 6 ~ The Brow Chakra

not solid but fluid, and thus elusive. No sooner have the messages come together, than they have slipped away again into their separate parts, often reacting to the resistance to their reception. Like all thoughts that become concrete and later become rules, they are only as worthwhile as their relevance permits. It is Mercury who acts as a barometer to this.

Later Zeus, in an effort to liberate his lover Io from the one-hundred-eyed giant Argus that had been ordered to enslave her by Zeus' jealous wife Hera, enlisted Hermes to play music, until each one of Argus' big eyes fell asleep, in order that he could behead the monster. As a gesture of pity towards her loyal servant, Hera removed each eye and scattered them over the tail feathers of her favourite sacred bird, the peacock.

Two things in these stories about Hermes are important here. Firstly, the representation of flight by those that are given wings. To the Greeks, to have wings signifies that one can lift thought up into the heavens. Wings give flight only after one attains a balance between love and will. Therefore, whenever this is represented, the wings are always placed below the forehead, as on the Caduceus. The peacock symbolises the pituitary gland in its ability to see from all those eyes but it also represents pride, the negative attribute of blinded vision. When worn at the front of a hat, turban or headband, the peacock feather represents the path from the pituitary to the pineal gland.

Through the refraction of its colours, the peacock is often used as a metaphor in describing the means by which the unseen becomes concrete during meditation within the brow chakra. Because of this connection it has become a symbol of immortality, or more precisely, of the immortal soul.

Each chakra has a symbolic bird that signifies it raising itself to its highest state, for each chakra has a higher and lower level. The winged feet of Hermes also allow him to mediate between the physical and spiritual worlds. To some cultures the migration of birds was seen as a route to the Milky Way, these birds being in search of its stars which number more than grains of sand held in the Earth's deserts. Stars first appear at twilight, the point at the pituitary of unity between night and day. To be conscious of this significance enables the human soul to do the same. The peacock tends to fly only at night, up to the trees, which perhaps symbolises the energy of the stars being directed on to the Earth.

Hera (Juno) created the Milky Way by spilling her breast milk

– such is her creative purpose. Part of the Milky Way is a constellation known as Pavo, meaning peacock, a large constellation lying to the south of Sagittarius and so named because of its beautiful tail. Its influence on humanity is said to be longevity, time given in which to focus one's changes.

The symbol of the peacock is found and used in Sufism, denoting the point at which unity nurtures duality. To the Hindus the music of the heart expressed through the head is represented by the peacock. Shiva is said to dance like a peacock, which must refer to perception through the movement of the sphenoid bone. Shiva also wears this bird as a brooch, an emblem presumably to the one immortal soul.

To the alchemists, the colours of the peacock's feathers became the perception of beauty that accompanies the road to renewal and resurrection. We know gold is symbolic of the sun and silver of the moon, but long before chemical divisions were laid out in the periodic table the alchemists had only seven base metals with which to demonstrate their talents. The base metal that pertains to the brow chakra is of course the quicksilver of Mercury. The speed of Mercury enables it be the mirror of all the planets, just as the pituitary is mirror to all the other glands. Thought is a collective of all the planets of the universe manifested in the single planet of Mercury. This is alchemy, by which the wand of Hermes turns lead into gold or the karma of the soul into spiritual enlightenment. It is the staff of life or death, to be 'awakened' or not, as it rules the pathways of the mind as well as the Earth. It is also the speed of perception – that leads to vision.

All vision comes through Self. It may be the highest cosmic consciousness but its relationship is through Self. It therefore has a connection between when, where and why Self is doing the receiving. It is the responsibility of Self to allow this to happen and to adjust to its demands.

Alchemy came into its own in Egypt through the work of the Hermetic Philosophers. Thoth not only gifted these principles but also the written word, which enabled communication to be taken up by the Greeks, the result of which was the Wisdom School. It was later adopted by the Byzantines and then by the Arabs, from whom the Spanish took great pains to retrieve it. In the search of immortality these original thoughts on transmutation were laid down in the writings of the Tabula Smaragdina, the Emerald Table of Hermes. Another

Chapter 6 ~ The Brow Chakra

version is that Abraham founded alchemy, and its secrets were laid down in the kabbala. What appears to be certain is that the succession and growth of wisdom remains constant, the movement from the East to the West, and from this long tradition homœopathy is an important extension into the new age.

Concerned with the development of wisdom, Greek society was very sophisticated but, in relative terms, it was not long-lived. To understand why, one needs to look at the relationship between Zeus, Apollo, Hermes and his son Pan – and of course Pax.

Apollo represents the heart and Hermes the head. Apollo has been seen as the god of wisdom but then so has Hermes. Thoth, in fact, is thought to be the first provider of wisdom, so who is it to be? Well the answer is none of them. It is the goddess Athena (Minerva), who sprung from Zeus' head and set about housing herself in Athens.

The lightening bolt that Zeus possesses, like all lightening, is five times hotter than the surface of the solar sun but Athena had no fear of it. Therefore Zeus was able to trust her judgement. Like Zeus she needed to be able to communicate to mortal beings. The solution to this lay in the trade between Hermes and Apollo. Remember Hermes is an expert merchant – the head needs the heart in order to create wisdom. In spiritual pursuits, the head and the heart must act as one, the joining of the ida with the pingala, as witnessed when representatives of the mind and the heart come down from the dhyan-chohan to instigate the next root-race. Apollo gifted Hermes the caduceus but this was under the influence of Zeus in order that he and other gods could metamorphose into the serpents of the caduceus and seduce mortals with their attributes. This is the same as that bestowed upon Aaron's staff in Egypt, he being the high priest that marked the start of Mosaic dispensation. At first the splendour of the wand was unbeknown to Hermes and in return he had inadvertently married the head with the heart by trading music for it. Music was the method through which the heart could express its love while the head pondered. It was this relationship that was ignored in Egypt and led to the transformation of Aaron's staff from that which could receive Divine Will to that of a deadly serpent which administered it.

Greek civilisation was built on the secret wisdom of the immortals, revealed to them by Hermes as their Herald. In doing so the Greeks lit the six candles of the Menorah but they neglected the seventh, the internal flame. They excelled in physics, philosophy, astronomy, mathematics, music and medicine but at the expense of the amalgamation of the seven – spirit. They failed to take heed of Hermes's golden wand, the symbol of unity. So Hermes provided a son, Pan, in which the 'all' could be expressed. Pan, who is often associated with fertility, offered the means by which his grandfather could fuel spiritual awakening in the brow chakra. It is fertility that offers a time for reflection at harvest time and thus the opportunity for change as the old becomes the new. As things turned out, one group controlled the rest of the population by creating a religion which suppressed the means to emancipation. Because of his sexual connotations and hoofed feet, Pan thus became the image of the devil and something to be feared, when in fact he represents conscious freedom.

By using the name Pan, we are entering into Roman territory. The Roman god of peace, Pax, does not get much of a look-in when it comes to deities worshipped by the Romans. Mars takes centre stage. The Romans inherited the continuity of Greek society and culture on breaking its political independence but what a sorry state it was in spiritually by then. In its short life the Greek empire was besieged by war but Athena was determined to make Athens her throne. She bartered for it by planting an olive tree, a symbol of peace, competing with a horse, the symbol of war. The gods, pleased by the olive, chose this but the mortals didn't listen and hence Minerva spent the reign of the Roman Empire trying to keep Mars from completely destroying Pax.

So what was the second point to the Hermes story? Well, in order to save Io, Hermes had to enter into the darkness of the Underworld (which can be thought of as Earth if we consider that by being here, we are already dead and our body is our tomb). He carries his wand as a means of guidance and his dubious past provides the credentials that enable this rite of passage, leading mortal souls through the Underworld in death. His speed enables him to manoeuvre around all that obstructs his path. He appears at difficult junctures, at crossroads where one part of the journey has ended in order to allow for the new, as at the time of spring and autumn. This gift is guidance in the form of inspiration, ideas granted by the wand of Merlin (who is also Hermes, as is Ulysses). All of life's connections are under his guidance. This is the nature of Gemini, for it is fascinated with duality and thus the reconciliation of the dark and the light. It is from this reconciliation that we are all able to benefit through communication, for it is here that Self gathers its rights. This is why the brow chakra is used for making connections in its never-

Chapter 6 ~ The Brow Chakra

ending pursuit of the whole. The Caduceus is symbolic of this pursuit, the human mind in tune with the cosmic mind. This is the responsibility of Self, and it is this that determines health, a notion perhaps forgotten when this symbol appears plastered down the side of an ambulance merrily racing to the scene of an emergency.

Originally Hermes was depicted as a phallic god of fertility. This fertility was about trade and having the goods to trade with. By means of the lungs the cells become oxygenated and through the spleen the kidneys nourish the lungs – thus the mind can be energised. It is for this reason Gemini rules the lungs in order to maintain thought. This trade is also about opening up links, and therefore travel. In ancient Greece there would be a phallic statue at every crossroads, reminding the traveller that the flexibility of an open mind raises this energy, in order that it can manifest as intuition. Hermes resides where the four paths meet, north, south, east and west, the centre of which is the second crucifixion. It is this point of focus that routes the channels of the mind and its decisions are reflected in the pathways on Earth that map out one's life.

Hermes offers the rite of travel, both on and off the Earth. His father is Jupiter and they are opposite one another in the chakra system but, when working in harmony, they are an indication as to how the expansive qualities (Heaven) can come together in a single destination – 'All roads lead to Rome'. Mercury inherits his father's aspiration – the lightening bolt – but here the electrical impulses are far more refined, so by night he can process these subtle impulses of the higher realms as dreams, and by day focus their input on constructing purpose.

Being the god of thieves, Mercury is accustomed to deceit and deception, so is best equipped to deal with the dark as well as the light of the underworld. He is able to deliver frightened souls by tricking them into seeing the truth of the underworld – the illusion of emotion. So it seems Mercury obtained these powers by being a god who does not behave like one. It may be this that enables him to be an intermediary between immortality and mortality.

The nature of Mercury, as in the fluid metal which is its namesake, separates here, there and everywhere and then reunites seamlessly by keeping its own counsel as to the nature and destination of its travels. He understands duality and the subsequent need for unification and in doing so he has examined both. An emphasis on the one polarity, be it either side, without the desire to unify, is the perpetuation of the syphilitic miasm. Mercury is anti-syphilitic, for he cannot keep from making a Divine connection. His truth is guised in jokes and jests that assist one or the group through their fears.

By focusing on the brow chakra, the clarity of focus is dependent on the level of change required. Mercury does not allow Self to do more than Self is ready for, at least if he can help it. He balances the ida and pingala, but it must be stressed that this is only a balance as nothing more can be achieved at the brow chakra. However, without this, the brow would not create the platform required for progression into the realm of Life Spirit. The planet Mercury receives from the Sun seven times more light and heat than the Earth. It is this light that, through the pituitary gland, provides Self with the chance to free itself from the limiting patterns of the past, for this light reveals that there is universal order in the cosmos of which one's mental development is a major part.

Chapter 7
The Crown Chakra

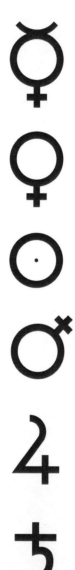

THE CROWN CHAKRA

Welcome to the crown chakra, a very special place that has taken great dedication and transformation to reach. I say welcome but this is not to confuse the fact that the crown chakra is in operation from the moment of birth. However to explore this centre consciously, or rather to explore through it, is one of the greatest gifts known to humanity.

In homœopathy, many methods have evolved in order to make the act of prescribing easier. Structures, rules and patterns are all devices that are used to aid perception. The repertory is a tool said to simplify remedy selection. However, the use of probability in homœopathy is very limiting. There has also been the development in recent times of electro-magnetic based devices or diagnostic 'boxes', that are said to produce the precise prescriptions without having to go through the human process of making a decision. This is to put such instruments above human perception. When it comes to the crown chakra, which comes gift packed with the rest of the human condition, all I can say is 'shame on these claims!' Why use a box when we have within us the most extraordinary mechanism for retrieving answers? This portal of a thousand petals that is the lotus flower in full blossom, is receptive to a degree that makes these 'boxes' appear like trying to hitch a ride on the back of a gnat.

You may have already detected by the tone of the previous paragraph that the crown chakra is not simply a place of bliss, which it is so often described to be (in various books, etc). For sure, if one is karma-free, then this would be a state of permanent nirvana, but as

Chapter 7 ~ The Crown Chakra

human beings we aren't, and the Moon can bring up much in the way of rebellion here. This place is not of the physical realm, and can create quite a storm in the psyche as the two forces (bliss and maintaining causes) try to interact.

The crown chakra emphatically indicates the extent to which somone is 'connected', and this should be noted when the patient comes to visit. It is most important in chakra prescribing to assess the level of spiritual connection, an assessment that seems to be absent these days in the West. This chakra provides the brow with the knowledge that furthers much healing.

The patient who is determined that they cannot be helped, making you wonder why they have come to see you at all, will need their crown chakra addressing. But the fact that they have come at all offers a small but significant glimmer of hope. Alcoholics, cannabis smokers and allopathic drug users all have blockages in the crown that inhibit Divine connection, which in turn prevents the acceptance of who one is. When Self is broken at the crown, then death is inevitable without spiritual nourishment. When this chakra is blocked, one finds it hard to justify what is happening in the physical realm. This is because what is happening is the result of the difficulty created by these blockages. How does one come to terms with painful life events if there is no internal or external connection to anything else, leaving one feeling victimised? This connection needs to be established on some level before healing can occur.

One has to recognise that it is only from within that suffering occurs – therefore, it is only the desire of Self that can create a change. In refusing to acknowledge this, allopathic medicine serves as a crutch, obscuring the fact that all the connections that facilitate healing are contained within.

Just as the base chakra is concerned with physical embodiment or being in one's body, so the crown is concerned with connection to the higher realms. This may evoke in some minds the image of being a puppet on strings but in this connection we learn there is far more than this to being human. In recent history, the West has paid little attention to this connection, though it has tried to vindicate itself through the practice of visiting a particular building on a Sunday. Although entering sacred ground, the only real participation in many churches seems to be in just being there. This site is actually meant to provide the means of transcendence from the confinement of the physical world, as was the

Chakra Prescribing and Homœopathy

use before the present landlords. This opportunity is all-encompassing, like the crown chakra, and so traditionally, rituals have been designed to slowly unlock this potential on such ground and not try and achieve this transcendence all at once. It is clear then, that when working on patients with blocks in the crown, this chakra is not necessarily the best place at which to begin. In this sense it is much like the brow chakra. It may be where the sense of separation lies, and will eventually need addressing if any lasting help can be sustained, but other chakras may need to be addressed first, to further stability in the patient.

Work on this chakra heightens receptivity. All perception becomes intensified and if developed, everything will attain significance, which is very useful when practicing homœopathy. Therefore, there is no need to use a homœopathic repertory, as the prescription will present itself if one pays attention. In its awakened state, the crown chakra makes all things significant, constantly bombarding Self so that one's enlightened perception can enable the higher mind to make sense of it all. This will not be possible if the significances are not noticed in the first place or put down to coincidence and ignored. When a patient comes to see the practitioner, it is this significance that reveals so much. It is a reflection of their energy that presents more of the story to the practitioner, through the receptivity of a heightened intuition. This can reveal itself in many ways; I once visited a homœopath and droplets of water, just like tears, ran down the vase from the stalks of the cut flowers. The more developed the crown, the more these indications will speak to one, just like learning a new language. What is required is trust in order to learn the new vocabulary. At the crown, the notions of space and time are entirely different, so one reacts more clearly to events, seeing their significance. As this communication heightens, one becomes accustomed to its constant presence, and this bestows remarkable guidance and clarity in prescribing for others.

At the crown, one has reached the top of the spiritual triad within Self, that of Atman, whilst still remaining of Self in a single incarnation. This can only change when all karma has been resolved; when no longer is the individual's monad detached, a witness to Self's endeavours. At this chakra, Self enters a pact with the will of the monad, and from this state all becomes one, the Spiritual Will or the supreme conscious observer, which extends far beyond the limits of the psyche. It is the highest celebration for the monad, for the individual cannot become more complete

Chapter 7 ~ The Crown Chakra

—yes, complete – a part of all existence without having left the Earth.

The crown centre is a paradox. It is Self in all its completion whilst simultaneously transcending individuality. Being there is also the result of the third initiation that Self has embraced within human existence, subsequently mastering its mind and all its lower aspects. One is, therefore, ready to develop psychic ability or strengthen it if it already exists. The crown chakra provides the ability to see the unseen and receive directly from those in the spiritual realm.

The act of the crucifixion of the ego is that which transcends Self through the fourth initiation. Here one can appreciate the toil one has gone through. It all becomes clear, and through that which is now received, one is finally in contact with the complete picture. However, if the crown chakra is unable to facilitate this, more work on it will be needed. Hence this chapter will oscillate between the development of the crown chakra through each lifetime (reincarnation), and that which can be achieved once the work is complete (karma free). This is similar to the significance of the second crucifixion, for within it lie two transitions, the first being that of the fourth initiation, which the man Jesus mastered in his quest to achieve Christhood. Christ is the Divine expression that was the forerunner of Jesus, the aspect that subsequently became unobtainable in a physical form and so evolved into an archetype. At the same time as Jesus succeeded in his fourth initiation, Christ succeeded in the seventh initiation, and was initiated into the Hierarchy. Hence Jesus, having begun to access Christ within, was now able to receive and understand Divine judgement without any of the sway of Earthly doubt.

In looking at the crown chakra, it is wise to perceive it with these two aspects, the latter of course, being the most difficult to describe and comprehend as language is as yet inadequate. To become Christ means that one must endeavour to master the seventh initiation.

The fourth initiation only pertains to the Buddhic plane. Even though the initiate has moved towards a new connection, there is still reliance on the connections of the lower worlds and thus one has to learn to trust this new higher world – or more to the point, to live on the planet, but by the gifts of the crown chakra. This is new light, which connects to no element or physical compound, and which can take you by surprise, underlining the importance of having worked on all the chakras first (and especially having a good connection from the crown to the base).

Chakra Prescribing and Homœopathy

To understand this light one has to understand the various aspects of the physical Sun, all the way through to the aspects of the Logos of the cosmic Sun, which ironically will be explored further in the Moon section of this chapter. The significance of the second crucifixion should not be underestimated or passed over, as it resonates so strongly with the vibration of mankind. This is the hardest of all initiations for, as already discussed in the previous chapter, it involves the dissolution of all worldly karma. This of course means being free from all miasmatic influence, but the price to be paid in achieving this is to free oneself of all worldly influence. There is one great obstacle that is a major obstruction here – the syphilitic miasm. Its making is the very nature that is prominent in the crown chakra and is responsible for the vast extent of blockages that cruelly obstruct this centre. It has a strong relationship with the third initiation – Divine destruction – which humankind tries its utmost to avoid, resulting in the experiences which, however slight, build over many lifetimes, making Self feel worthless. The sense of separation is devastating at this centre and feeds down into the physical body, causing mental chaos which at first may lead to crankiness, and later a descent into insanity. The mental chaos is the result of what the physical body cannot absorb. Dis-ease is created by chaos in any of Self's bodies. Hence, it is unusual for cancer to attach itself to insanity. This is the syphilitic miasm at work.

The seventh initiation is very relevant with regard to communication at present, for light on the lower spheres here on Earth is currently being divided and used by technology to further the telecommunications industry. This started with electricity and has progressed by means of the nuclear route. Microwaves are currently being used on the planetary plane with little awareness as to the wisdom being evolved on the seventh plane; these, like all other forms of radiation, are very dangerous to the human constitution. Only the evolution of this communication will prevent the levels of harm generated when radiation is used in this crude form.

The relationship between the seventh initiation and the seventh cosmic plain, of which the crown chakra is a microcosm, has evolved through an obscure connection to do with the use of light in the emancipation of suffering. This has been necessary in creating progress for the incoming Aquarian age in which a greater interaction is a priority. This means that by the way the crown chakra instigates the conversion of reflected information, the work in communication down here

Chapter 7 ~ The Crown Chakra

has to catch up by replicating the work achieved on the seventh plane. Humanity at present is stumbling through this initial stage.

Those planetary Hierarchies that have evolved from the seventh plane are currently working to communicate to us how to develop healthier modes of communication. The message given is that at present our methods are damaging, even killing people. Souls are now being born that are armed with more tolerance to these dangerous levels of radiation as a process of protection. However, even they can't entirely screen out their effects. The physical levels of light frequencies are dangerous to us, for at present we are nowhere near to mastering their use.

The crown chakra at least provides the means to understand this and offers the means to change, for this is part of its function. Through the Moon, the ruling planet of this chakra, the gift that it presents to us is the differentiation of light and their frequencies, but not as a filter, for the rays of all the planets are reflected here. Yes the Moon is considered a planet although it revolves around the Earth and not the Sun. This is because it is the ultimate Lord of Time within the Earth's progression through its chain and although one of the seven sacred planets, its movement is distinct from all the others. It is to time what Christ is to karma (solar) – head of the Lords of Karma. Although dying and slowly relinquishing its power to the Earth, as reflected in the degradation of its status being no more than a satellite in modern times, its influence is that of the 'death' of time. In the crown chakra this equates to re-birth, hence the Moon's maternal reputation.

The Logos or Brahman emanates seven rays, of which the seven chosen planets are a lower embodiment. It is the frequency reflected by the Moon, which is important here. For instance, the light of the winter solstice, the darkest day, provides a focus on what little light there is, underlining how special it is and subsequently bringing the hearts of people together in order to share this experience. This understanding of light will be the kind of vibration that will lead to devising methods of communication that enrich the soul and not harm it. It is this level of communication, where the heart meets the crown, that is present at Christmas.

Through the crown chakra it is possible to glean information on all the initiations, even though they have not been undertaken. Such is the power of insight given at this chakra, for its receptivity makes so much possible. This is what it means to be in the heart of the monad of which the seventh initiation is an expanded version. From the crown chakra, one is only an observer, but the experience of this expands human consciousness, so that the monad may be reflected on Earth. This is achieved through the Atman. Atman is Self in all its completion, which is more than the soul, and is often referred to as being even greater than the spiritual soul, so that of the Divine Soul. It is the sum total of the human entity, including from whence it sprang. This interaction or the 'part' which is universal selfhood is that of the Father or Absolute. The Atman is one drop of the great well of consciousness, which is Brahman, the Father, or the Absolute. But that one drop contains it all. Spirit that has transcended matter is the source of true consciousness. It is that which is available and provided by Brahman.

In a sense Atman is the Divine lifeline that enables Self to be Self. Atman is known as the 'Self' because it is the consciousness that enables individual existence, which if not supported by the whole, would cease to exist. It is this spirit in a person and its various levels of resonance or obstruction that the homœopath has to assess. So the spirit within each is the one spirit within all, the super-conscious memory, the illuminated consciousness, The Holy Ghost, which is female, for it is the mother of the second birth, this birth being the gateway to enlightenment. This is also why the crown chakra places the greatest of focus on the inadequacies that Self feels, for here shortcomings are highlighted by the extended group spirit, from which there can be a mighty exclusion if separated through one's negative karma.

Very few human spirits gain the privilege of being able to exclude their karma when working on this chakra, therefore inadequacies, struggles and any forms of syphilitic-induced history will feel intensified here. Much in the way of deep karma stuck from many lifetimes can start to shift when working on this centre and so can be very unsettling, manifesting as dilemma upon dilemma. This can appear to be extremely confusing and scary, for these changes are not under the domain of the rational mind and seem to come from the complete unknown, but are in the fact the result of the depth of our karmic fears. But these are aspects that surface in order to be released – much like the way a homœopathic remedy can intensify the symptoms before they clear. Therefore, if allowed, the consequential changes can lead to the most profound of life transformations. The same is true of the startling clarity and the accompanying imagery that one is witness to when this centre is open. This can be alarming, when what one thought was reality is seen to be

Chapter 7 ~ The Crown Chakra

illusion, and vice-versa; thus, much preparation is needed here. This also creates change in the world, for what was previously seen as reality will no longer be so.

When one is privy to the group spirit of the cosmos within, then perception of the world changes and new consciousness is gained. This is the consequence of this chakra being open. This change of course will also have a knock-on effect in one's personal life, and that can be difficult. Up to this point, one has been directed by the Lords of Karma via the members of the Karmic Board, and choices made from one's own free will adjust accordingly. One believes that there is choice and control over destiny but in truth there is only one's fate. At the crown chakra it is obvious that this is so. To be hit by this consciousness creates a new awareness – that of Divine choice. No longer is one steered through the rudimentary decisions that life presents believing that they belong to Self. They all have significance and are the result of Divine will, for there is no other.

In the physical world, will relies on the mind to make sense of it so that one can direct one's life in the pursuit of freeing personal, and subsequently group karma. This direction comes with being conscious and open to that which is received, even to the very fine things. These insights grow; they are seeds of wisdom and thus start very small. Once they have been implanted in the physical world they take shape and attract weight. It is difficult to get the balance here between the two worlds. Many have been worshipped for this, and in the East gurus are still a means by which to access the other side. The only true path is for this direction to come from within and if trusted, honed and developed by the homœopath, prescribing can then take on a spiritual significance. Deep syphilitic karma inhibits this connection, or at least tries to, and it is this challenge that makes many determined to master this level of prescribing.

The world of our existence, which is the name and the energy of the Earth, like all energy that has its seed in the spiritual world, works its way down into physical manifestation. Beyond the physical realm, this energy is not of the same word and does not act by the same means as it does in the physical world. It does, however, interact with the light forces so that the lower planes are a reflection of the higher ones.

Initiations continue on the higher planes long after physical emancipation, but negative energy does not exist there as it does in the physical realm; this planet and its outer layers are the means by which cleansing takes place. Negative energies hinder reception from the other world, but such reception eventually will create positivism and raise consciousness. That which was unconsciousness is thus given life, a form, for it has been sought in the physical realm and subsequently all will adjust accordingly. Dark forces act to try and prevent receptivity, and so those who receive via the crown chakra require protective mechanisms, which ensure their safety when opening up and leaving the protective shell of their auric field.

That which is beyond is not necessarily easy to explore, for it not only reflects that which is in our world and so can be dense and awkward to negotiate, it is, unlike our world, not under linear manipulation. Even though these constraints exist, it is important to escape from the notion of them in order to overcome them. Once again, it is only human fear that limits reception and thus perception. It is the truth which has ultimate power and which can transform both customs and character. It is this level of enlightenment that brings about change so directly. This change can be difficult to bear for the human being, and of such a powerful nature that its impact cannot be softened even by the buddhi, the bridge between Atman and the manas. Again, preparation is of the utmost importance both when meditating on the crown and in working through its consequence. Coupled with this should be the ability to judge as to when it is most appropriate to open up the crown chakra. Such awakened states should not be embraced just anywhere and at any time in everyday situations; one must be discerning as to when and where such awakened states are sought out. Being a very open state it requires respect in the form of a private, peaceful and secure environment in order to guarantee the utmost protection. Holy ground where one will not be disturbed is the best place for this. However a secure familiar place which has been properly cleansed, purified and consecrated, with a door, will be adequate. This should be the same when meditating or performing rituals that evoke the energies of any of the chakras. In addition to this, whilst meditating on the crown chakra the soul becomes very much accustomed to this wonderful tranquillity and can be reluctant to shut down – but it must. When meditating on the crown, hours become seconds within its timeless bliss, a feeling which, if induced by a powerful meditation, can evoke a state that cannot be compared with any other Earthly state.

The consequence of working on the crown chakra is the contradiction of being aware of the other world integrating with one's known world

Chapter 7 ~ The Crown Chakra

whilst continuing one's daily activities. Within this unsettling experience there are varying degrees of difficulty, which seemingly arise through one's simple daily interactions. It's as if way in the background there is a theme going on that can only be expressed and developed through the next action that Self either makes or has to respond to. This theme is where one stands in the universe and so feels as if one's past, future and present endeavours are all being addressed together even in the simplest of actions. One is confronted by the whole whilst only dealing with a piece. It is a frustratingly problematical process that is, paradoxically, ultimately pleasurable. Self can feel addicted to it but nevertheless it is hard to maintain a grasp on reality, or a grasp on anything. One does feel carried though and if one can relax and trust in the flow it will result in what is meant to be.

So the Atman is the complete Self, embracing all its lower forms that extend down into the personality and which are linked to it through the Buddhi. Decisions are either made from below the line in the personality or above, from the point of the higher Self – but either way these decisions will take on form. Therefore, the Atman comprises that which is form and formless in Self which, in the true sense of the word, is all form. This connection that the Atman has with form is considered to be close to the aspect of Brahman, the Divine love within all. There are no higher levels to Brahman for he is of all levels; hence there are no hierarchies other than the illusory ones made by man's ego. If that of the Divine is in all things then hierarchy does not exist, for Brahman cannot exist, for he is existence. He is neither a beginning nor an end. There too is no beginning or end for the Atman of Self – the undying soul. To make a decision from one's lower or higher Self should be the same, for they are equal in the sight of such love. It is not possible to look beyond existence, as it is finite, there is no more: looking only manifests that which exists, as what is truly infinite can be found within. Atman is the Divine monad within, and thus all the kingdoms have an Atman in order that they may thrive. Atman is both the impersonal Self, and the personal Self that has transcended up through the chakras. It is not simply the individual soul but the Supreme Soul and thus it is present and continues to designate the meaning of Self through all reincarnations, for the two are the same. Atman's making from transcendence furthers Self's understanding as to what it is. This can only happen by being honest and by recognising oneself in all one's completeness. In doing so, one recognises the negative aspects, respects them and heals them by integrating them as positive attributes. Atman knows no division between the lower and higher attributes, the male and female attributes or any other Earthly divisions.

The four elements are important when it comes to understanding the workings of miasmatic activities in the body but at the crown, no such elements exist, so how can a syphilitic influence manifest? The answer lies in light – or rather, where there is light there is dark. Light on all levels is sourced in fire, but on this level it burns Self in a different way than the physical manner with which humans are obsessed. It is here at the crown chakra that the ultimate battle between light and dark, which is their unification, can be won or lost.

The Atman has been depicted as a halo, the light that shines, which denotes the combination of the holy trinity: the light of the Son, Father and Holy Spirit (Mother) combined. Saints are distinguished by their wearing of the halo, having achieved here on Earth that which merits this prestigious state.

The three aspects (the three schools: power, love and wisdom) that have formed conscious human development throughout the fifth root-race have enabled humankind to use the triangle created by the three aspects of the kundalini which peak at the point of the pineal gland. In esoteric representation, this triangle is seen as resting on the top of the head, within the centre of the thousand-petalled lotus.

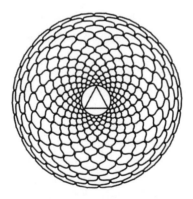

Figure 23. Thousand-petalled lotus with Equilateral Triangle.

It represents the landing pad of receptivity, the circle shaved by monks and other religious followers in order to facilitate its flow. This triangle

Chapter 7 ~ The Crown Chakra

holds the key to transcendence: the Son, the Mother and now finally the Father all united. Without the Logos of creation – Brahma, being the first, then there would be no second -Vishnu, the preserver of reality from which sprung the seven, the parentless, and these would have no place of expression without the third – Shiva, the destroyer of illusion. The Buddhists have no room for this or the Atman in their original philosophy, for their belief does not extend to any pre-existence other than what they would call Self. Atman, as seen by the Buddhists, is the consequence of ignorance, ultimately self-defeating, the cause of all misery in the world. For the Buddhist the concept of a Divine quality is not quantifiable.

As a consequence of the subtle arrangement of the higher triad, the crown chakra is very sensitive to trauma in childhood or any violence that creates great shock, anger and fear. If not dealt with properly such trauma creates a block in one's connection to the Divine.

During the years leading up to the age of fourteen, Self is moulded by the great forces of completion, which need a beginning and an end in order that all that lies in between can develop. Hence a damaged crown has a dramatically adverse effect on the base chakra. One requires faith and trust at both ends, in the Earth and the Heavens. As these two are in an opposing balance to each other, each will reflect the other's disharmony. Trauma, especially if repeated, creates breaks in the chain of the child's sense of harmony, which causes great confusion, especially if the child perceives such trauma to be the norm. Remember, the level of subsequent consequence that is perceived at the crown is heightened whilst working on the crown and Self will avoid such consequence if it is felt too great a gap to bridge. The need to evolve and heal through such consequence will be lacking with unawakened spiritual chakras or the base and the crown in disharmony. Therefore if no support or help is offered to a child in this situation, then he or she disconnects from their spiritual purpose. Past life experience will often be the reason why one draws such a situation to oneself. The homœopath has to be aware of this when treating trauma, as its roots may go back a long way.

Trauma accumulates in the form of division within the crown chakra, the division attributed to the syphilitic miasm, which deepens the further away one is from the Source. Such blocks in the crown chakra create despair. Addiction is mainly the method chosen here to alleviate the despair of separation and the feeling within oneself that the universe has turned its back. Such addiction may present itself in any form

– addiction to allopathic or recreational drugs, or to alcohol. These are very serious, for it is at the crown chakra that one is most vulnerable to blowing holes in one's protective aura allowing negative energy to infiltrate the soul. The consequence of this can render Self inactive, unfocussed and begin a downward spiral into despair. However, it must be considered when endeavouring to expand upon the potential of an evolving crown chakra that even the repetition of buying a morning newspaper can be an addiction.

Karma can make living in the modern world extremely difficult as well as immensely pleasurable. The difference depends much on being connected at the crown chakra. Love comes up from the heart in order that it can leave through the crown, so that one can make contact. It is the route back to the Source in which we have our origins. To be separated at the crown is the most painful and unjust of all forms of human existence, for it makes it impossible to complete and so to express one's purpose in life, killing aspiration.

In Kabbalist philosophy the sphere that pertains to the crown chakra is Kether. The study of Kether does not, however, contain the complete image of the Divine, for it is only seen as one of the ten Sephiroth. To take away this complication of the crown chakra being all encapsulating but of a single place, Kether is also known as the 'simple point', the place from which all is revealed. It also suggests that because we know Divine will is ruthless, this 'simple point' is not the place from which Self should be lost.

When one is meditating on the crown chakra, an eight-pointed star offers the utmost protection. Not only does it encompass the four quarters but also the four diagonals, which are equally as important in any cycle. This is true of the agricultural cycle, on which our survival and the yearly calendars are based. One would think the eight-pointed star had special relevance to the base chakra, which it does to a certain extent, but one has to realise that the crown is the base in reverse. So for the crown this symbol provides much protection; this is why traditionally it is positioned resting just above the head, as an instrument of intuition, a half-way-house between the crown and the eighth chakra. It also forms an extension to the triangle previously discussed which lies in the centre of the thousand-petalled lotus, for the eight-pointed star has evolved from this triangle, therefore it is more than the coming together of East and West. In fact this star provides all-

Chapter 7 ~ The Crown Chakra

encompassing protection. The shape resonates to the inner structures of cosmic fire and subsequently can dissolve all things that are not of equal measure – a tool for the most enlightened aspirant.

Astrologically, the cross, superimposed against the Star of David, produces the eight-pointed star or, as it is known, the 'Star of Bethlehem'.

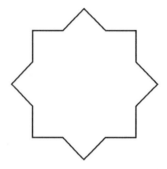

Figure 24. The Octagon – Star of Bethlehem.

This shape can be mapped and revealed on an astrological chart, reflecting the formation of the planets that ushered in the 'birth' of the last Piscean age. This marked the beginning of the new and present twelve sectioned planetary cycle as seen from the Earth rotating on its axis and thus moving through all the constellations of the zodiac. The completion of this full cycle is known as the Great Sidereal Year – approximately twenty-six thousand years. Each one of these years enables the Earth to grow and brings about subsequent change within each root-race. The Magi were informed of the new beginning by this star composition, for this group of priests was deeply involved in matters of the crown chakra, and very knowledgeable in astronomy. The new remedy *Frankincense* is connected with this sacred capacity of being receptive and guided by the crown chakra. Christmas is a very useful time to take this remedy, for it awakens or deepens one's connection with group spirituality. The Magi could read the constellations and studied their patterns, for they knew how they impacted on every human life. They understood the importance of interpreting the affects of the constellations, and used channelling, as well as the rational tool of mathematics, to do so. They were responsible for receiving what was essentially the beginning of Christ entering the seventh initiation. Hence the Magi were one of the first groups to be privy to the purpose of the new energy, and thus the opportunities of the Piscean Age.

The seventh initiation refers to the coexistence of Christ entering the cosmic hierarchy and the knowledge of the event being manifested down here on Earth. The eight-pointed start is the sign to this. Within it, when the star's form is simplified to that of two shapes – the diamond and the square, the meaning of this coexistence is revealed.

Firstly, the square represents mankind, the building block, Jesus.

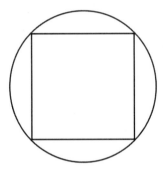

Figure 25. Circumscribed Square – Microcosm on Earth.

When the rules of the 'golden section' are applied to the square (mankind), the golden rectangle is formed. This is the doorframe, the starting point of one's journey, and by stepping through it that journey begins. The golden section, which at first sight appears a simple mathematical equation, helps to explain what is of great mystical proportion. It reveals the natural progression of life and so resonates harmony and instils the calm reassurance of possibility.

It is this central theme of growth deriving from the building block – the square – that provides insight into the close relationship between the golden section and the Fibonacci numbers. Both sequence of numbers reflect that which is being carried out on the higher planes but in physicality. However, growth on Earth is under the domain of mankind, hence the square, and thus these growth patterns are seen in nature revealing that each kingdom is here for the benefit of mankind and also under its control. Therefore what the golden section and the Fibonacci sequence are both incorporating is that the growth of humanity is the growth of planet Earth for the benefit of the higher planes.

Indian, Jewish and Arab scholars were privy to the knowledge of the sequence of Fibonacci numbers long before they bore his name. Originally

Chapter 7 ~ The Crown Chakra

the sequence was used within sound, being passed down through the mystery schools, as sound is the making of matter. Metaphorically, this sequence of numbers plot the pattern in which life can extend itself, from which we are able to look out, forming one's point of view. This is the doorway or portal from which we can leave our confine. It is self-providing, for as a repeating pattern it builds the means to escape, to transcend. The spiral, the pattern created by both the Fibonacci numbers and by the golden section, is the cone that connects the brow to the crown chakra.

The diamond on the other hand, the second shape within the eight-pointed star, represents the journey after having passed through the doorway. It is formed by the ascending and descending triangles passing over one another as one leaves the confines of the restrictive world of matter and communicates directly with the spiritual world.

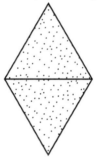

Figure 26. Diamond formed by two Equilateral Triangles.

The point to the crown chakra is that one gives oneself over completely to the spiritual world. When one receives from the spiritual realms the descending triangle is pulled to the ground in order to be earthed. Those ascending conscious forms driven up by the force of kundalini make their way into the spiritual world and thus an exchange is made. Self reveals its offerings and accepts the offerings from the spiritual world. So at the heart chakra, when the seven chakras are balanced in the material world, then these two triangles form the Star of David. However, when one transcends the physical plane, either by jettisoning physical existence for good or by psychic reception at the third eye, then these two triangles form a diamond. To do this for the purpose of psychic reception, one relies on the quality of the lower organs and the upper endocrine glands, for it is they that have to establish the reversal of exchanged consciousness.

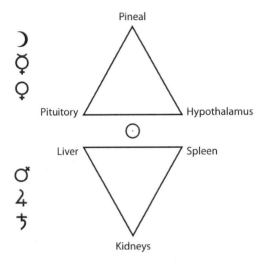

Figure 27. The Exchange of the Ascending and Descending Triangles.

To do this for the purpose of psychic reception, one relies on the quality of the lower organs and the upper endocrine glands, for it is they that have to establish the reversal of exchanged consciousness. This is why lower psychic ability can only be advanced if the liver, kidneys and spleen can sustain the training and much work has to be done on the lower four chakras to achieve this. If they are weak, then there will be only limited activity, if any, in the third eye. As one gets stronger and the third eye more exercised, there opens up the opportunity to use three methods of receiving information that relate to the three corners of the triangle resting on the top of the head, within the centre of the thousand-petalled lotus. One either absorbs a spirit on the higher planes and therefore information is imparted and repeated from the experience as in direct knowing, or one repeats what is spoken by a spirit on the higher realms, or one enables a spirit to communicate directly on the physical plane via one's denser bodies.

It is the blood of the cross that creates the inner structure to the diamond. Blood fuels the right of humanity to gain Divine Wisdom. It is not especially the mathematical relationship that is important to highlight here, though the relationship between the diamond and profound calculus is fascinating, known and exploited in decorative patterns for thousands of years; neither is it that its outer boundary formed by the internal structure creates two triangles, as mentioned, an upper and lower that

Chapter 7 ~ The Crown Chakra

also contain the numbers that are the symbol for Universal Harmonics. It is that these outer boundaries energetically resonate to the number eight. On the Tree of Life eight is the number of Hod, the Sephiroth that is the intellectual and abstract mind, both of which have to be mastered before the substance of the cross is ready for the seventh initiation.

The invisible inner constriction of the diamond is lost to the defiant form of its boundary. The boundary of the diamond is born out of the same dynamic as the figure eight, for the number represents the infinite, having no beginning or end as illustrated when it is written, the pen can simply never stop. Here infinity is both horizontal and vertical, flowing out from the axis of the invisible energy lines (cross), but this energy is halted by forces acting upon it that create the boundary of the diamond. These boundaries represent the remaining restrictions placed upon the soul's journey and the internal angles of the diamond, the inner constriction of the soul. As the circle represents spirit, then the diamond is that which lies between the circle and the square – the superellipse.

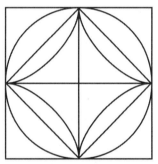

Figure 28. The Superellipse.

Hence it is with the blood of the cross, humanity's journey to a greater being, which is used to navigate into its newfound form after the fourth initiation. However, it is not until the seventh initiation that one's spirit is Self and Divine as one, as entered in the book of cosmic hierarchy.

Eight is the number denoting the order of the celestial world here on earth. It is the power that one needs for one's journey. So in placing the diamond and the square together, Self becomes one with the celestial world. Once here, the initiate is no more. As with sound, the eighth note is the same as the first in a seven note scale – just of a higher resonance. Hence the number eight creates the structure to which many temples pay homage– heaven on Earth – and this provides much security when leaving one's body, the purpose of building such places. Therefore, it can be surmised that the route by which the seventh initiation is achieved is the eighth chakra, to which the star of Bethlehem gives much protection.

The purpose of the Magi involved sending the message as to the next step for humanity. Now, thanks to the spread of knowledge and a wider interest in developing consciousness, humanity is more in tune with the beginning of the new era, the Aquarian Age, which is understandable for it is concerned with brotherhood. However, not all are ready to share their individuality. The Magi did not disclose the whereabouts of Christ, but spread wisdom to those who were ready, those who were initiated in the power of spiritual receptivity. The Star of Bethlehem represents this wisdom and offers much protection when leaving the physical domain behind for a while. This is the star of Christ within or the sushumna reaching up to regain its contact with the cosmic fire of universal spirit.

It's not often that the crown is associated with the dark quarter that is winter, but this is the route by which one returns to one's spiritual home – the time known as Christmas. This time of year is also an opportunity for those spirits who are stuck or are no longer needed down here to return home. The energy of the crown chakra facilitates such movement at this time, for it is the light in a darkness resulting from the lack of sunlight. The Moon is dominant here, and as its light is always in a state of change, adaptable and very profound, it offers the possibility, like the stars, for lost souls to navigate past the maze of obstacles and dark dead-ends, upwards to where they truly belong. Such souls have been separated from spiritual love. This centre can spur the release of those souls overwhelmed by physical attachments and those that may be resting within one's aura, or festering in a particular chakra.

The crown chakra is like an overseer – able to view the bigger picture. It can facilitate great change in the other chakras, for a part of itself resides in them, that which is Divine guidance. Being of both worlds, it provides the means by which these souls feel safe to move on through the love of the crown chakra or Christ (the limits of our universe on the road to nirvana). This love differs from the heart's love, for it is free of consequence.

The Divine connection at the crown unleashes that which is above the rational mind, being far greater than that considered generally in the scheme of things. At the crown this works both ways as much can rise up from the depths of the constitution and may well be released in the

Chapter 7 ~ The Crown Chakra

form of hidden entities. A crisis or shock within a chakra can manifest entities that are an accumulation of stuck energy; these will only be found in the particular chakra that matches and enables the entity to thrive on its qualities. This is also true of entities that enter through a broken aura, as they are attracted to a particular opening, though this usually pertains to a general weakening of all the chakras. Patients with these entities acting upon them will find it very hard to distinguish between reality and fantasy, as they are interfering with the connection made at the crown and subsequent flow through the chakras down to the Earth. This will be reflected in the flow that is life. It should be noted that not all these entities are negative and some have come to help to resolve stuck energy. One can contain friendly, kind and useful entities, but if that isn't how they are, one may well find oneself adrift in this other world, driven by another soul's fear with no protection – a very scary experience.

Without the notion of separation between the two worlds, be it any two worlds distinct from each other, the soul is laid bare to terror. Patients who have not been sectioned, but cannot make this distinction are seeking this particular kind of help. Others may not be in such an extreme position, but the purpose of a strong reception at the crown chakra is to release the kind of fears that have denied Self its true desired connection. This is why it is imperative to close down properly by re-entering one's body and sealing one's aura after any meditative practice. For one to roam the Earth safely, one must be in one's body.

This centre is Divine guidance, and even though at times this may be hard to assess, being outside the realm of everyday human perception, it all comes down to a matter of trust. This is the stuff that the modern world likes to iron out, as it prefers control and predictability. When working on the crown, what may appear bleak is in fact a Divine opportunity. Information received from the crown chakra about a patient regarding such an opportunity can give the practitioner a dilemma; having made sense of this information, should they pass it on to the patient or just allow the patient to work through it? This is made harder if a deceased loved one or ancestor delivers this information. However, what is imperative is the making sense of this information and this is necessary to the growth of homœopathy, for its roots and survival were due to a few who kept its magic alive by themselves being magicians. In recognising Divine opportunities, they were not only able to perceive new levels of healing provided by the crown chakra, but to steer homœopathy forward on to its new course. This takes vision or spiritual guidance of a timeless quality. Therefore it is up to practitioners to push the levels of perception in order that all at least have a chance to help themselves.

With the pressure of conformity brought upon in a modern society and the restrictive perception of the Western medical establishment, homœopathy has had to comply with many stringent rules in order that it may become acceptable. This hasn't supported its need to cover the wide spectrum of the human condition that this book discusses, or the scope required in helping patients in the modern world. Prescriptions that are first obtained at the crown chakra and then feed their way down to the rational mind, do so through inspiration, and pinpoint that which is at the centre of the problem, creating a richness of healing. The irony is that it was within the secret chambers of occultist philosophy that homœopathy did not only germinate but was kept alive, when convention didn't want to know. The investigation into these chambers is continuing and from this comes the ongoing development of homœopathy – because it belongs to the systems of energy medicine, that when understood create growth. Doubt is the greatest threat here, for we all still have our weaknesses when receiving from the crown.

Working with the crown chakra really emphasises one's doubts, as the differences between Earthly existence and that of the cosmos are revealed. To become conscious changes things forever and this is true for the prescriber as well as everyone else. One's own development produces a better prescriber and this does not necessarily refer to arbitrary, business-orientated pursuits that lack any spiritual content, such as the need to build a portfolio! The greatest portfolio you will ever have is in the head. Why waste time in converting it to paper, when one's energy should be used for the purpose of its development and not its justification, i.e. healing people? This is another poor attempt at trying to get energy to conform, and a reflection of this carcinogenic age, one that puts comfort and fitting-in before risk. If something is maintained purely because it is easy, it will lack struggle and therefore produce heavy consequence that leads nowhere.

The more difficult something is, the lighter the consequence. This is true when drugs are used to induce alternative mind states. Rather than

Chapter 7 ~ The Crown Chakra

doing the preparation needed to explore states that can be reached without drugs, one takes the quick option and is propelled further than one is ready for, which has great consequences. With spiritual faith, having a connection at the crown chakra and the means to receive, places the burden of development away from the rational course. This is where the prescription should manifest from, as the spreading of trust is both historically linked and imperative to the nature of the people of the British Isles. Working on the crown chakra changes one's perception forever and thus one's prescribing, which should not be held back. Doing so engenders the clarity of the third eye.

During the middle ages, in England, the crown chakra of the country was entangled in the crown of a single leader, just like the high priests/priestesses and pharaohs in Egypt. Their crowns were meant to be symbolic of who had achieved an elevated Divine connection.

The crown was initially configured with fourteen points or made of fourteen pieces and later jewels cut using geometric shapes that hid within a fourteen-pointed star were worn. This shape represents the extent to which the king has achieved spiritual unity. This position exoterically enables others to become enlightened, which is why the man Jesus was a teacher. In the past in ancient civilisations to be king was not a matter of gender. The esoteric counterpart to the king's position, or what could be considered going on behind the scenes, was the inner council that guarded occultist wisdom, the foundation of all esoteric and exoteric knowledge, whose members numbered fourteen. This number refers to the seven double letters of the Hebrew alphabet that refer to the seven sacred planets – the visible seven and their invisible counterpart from which this wisdom is entrusted.

The first seven sounds of the double letters of the Hebrew alphabet are called 'hard' and when written, are indicated with a dot (solar). The second seven sounds are soft, so when spoken require a different form of breath. Both sets of seven working together, as intended, relate to the process of exploring and returning, of the inner and outer world. The double seven letters, along with all the letters of the Hebrew alphabet, can be separated into three groups, forming a triad that reveals the very nature of the structure in which reality (the cosmos) is created and, with Self as co creator, is maintained.

Of this triad, the seven double letters form one group that represents 'time' or the steps to the initiation that are the descent of spirit into matter, and the ascent of spirit at the expense of matter. In no chronological order, the second group of this triad is formed by the three mother letters which represent 'space', much like the three Gunas that enable evolution by binding spirit through the soul to the body and from which all illusory material manifests. These three letters also reveal how the three principle Hindu deities, the Trimurti, operate in the world of matter, each representing an element of earth, water and fire. This makes it easy to see why these three letters are referred to as being 'mother', for within the Hebrew letters are the secrets to human existence – how one harnesses knowledge to create one's own universe. If we were sufficiently enlightened then these twenty-two letters in the form of knowledge can construct all that has manifested in the cosmos. So, being that the universe is found within, the correlation between Self's freedom through the creation of the cosmos is held within the triad of the mystery of these letters. When one writes, not only is there expansion through new ideas but also exploration of cosmological secrets within.

It is from 'space', that the three then subdivide into the seven that represent the different manifestations of space that denote 'time'. Thus the third group in the trilogy of Hebrew letters that encompass the twelve simple letters refers to the astrological signs that shape Self in its quest for individualism since its separation. These are all the 'souls'. So from the three and then the seven – the twelve evolve. This triad within the twenty-two letters can also be taken to mean the father, mother and their descendents or the 'principle', 'contrary principle' and 'balance', as in the three principle Hindu deities – the primary law of three. This would also apply to the three mother letters if seen as energetic cosmic potential before manifestation and then after.

In human spiritual evolution, it is that which is 'contrary' that interests us, the light and the dark, as it enables transcendence. However, its study is always in relation to the other two parts of the triad. No triad can function without having an aspect of the other two within itself, being three differing expressions of the same thing. Hence humanity builds its universe through the struggles of light and dark in order to create balance as decreed by the source. Even all gods have two sides. The letters of the Hebrew alphabet and the triads within reveal the nature of humanity's quest within the duality of spirit and matter; for being the same as the gods but just more in matter, we

Chapter 7 ~ The Crown Chakra

use the knowledge of the construction of the cosmos to deal with our manifestation in order that we can undo the grip of its karma. As the Great Egyptian pyramid teaches us, to be earthbound is to die and to transcend is to be born. It is the Moon that provides the understanding to this and the process establishes wisdom. So the triad within the Hebrew alphabet teaches us to be king, priest and prophet.

The meaning of 'time' in association with the seven double letters refers to the relationship between the base and the crown chakra, both being the two major gateways of life that the soul can perceive and occupy. The Moon represents the opening to that which is evolutionary in the cosmos, so instead of the influence of 'time' being that of the physical existence of Earthly karma, it reveals the creative process that is the cosmos, to which, of course, physical existence also adheres. What is deemed to be 'time' is the development that is one's interaction with the cosmos, which for Self, not being karma free, is yet to fully come.

The vibration of these fourteen sounds of the seven double letters of the Hebrew alphabet evokes the Fourteen Stations of the Cross, the 'fourteen precious things' in Hindu mythology. These stations are steps where the suffering of the sacred life force represented as Jesus by Christians, coincides with the desire of Christ to succeed, depicted as cosmic fire. This suffering is dependent on one's karma. Hence the fourteen stations resonate with each chakra, seven via descension and then consciously via ascension. This process also illustrates the seven positive and seven negative ganglionic powers of the sympathetic nervous system.

However, for the soul, the Fourteen Stations of the Cross begin at the point of physical birth. Hence the soul ascends up the seven physical steps in order to progress in the seven spiritual ones. It is at the crown chakra that this intermingling with the spiritual world is completed. Hence the eighth station of the Stations of the Cross is known for the communication with the 'daughters of Jerusalem' – those of the spiritual realm. At the third station it is personal will that Self tests, at the seventh station it is Divine will. The seven physical steps are a reflection of the seven invisible ones that have already been shown to Self in its descent into matter but have been forgotten. Because Self then ascends the physical ladder to the crown chakra, the spiritual is thus absorbed by the actions of the material ascension.

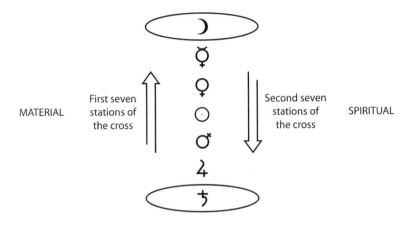

Figure 29. The Amalgamation of Spirit into Matter.

Like the base chakra that acts as a mirror in reflecting spirit up through the chakras of the material world, there too is a mirror situated at the crown chakra to reflect spirit down through the chakras though via the spiritual world. This mirror is the Moon and this double reflective structure has to be so, for it is the heart chakra that is the centre of our universe and around which all revolves. This means the spiritual counterpart is founded by working backwards from the crown chakra to the base.

Chapter 7 ~ The Crown Chakra

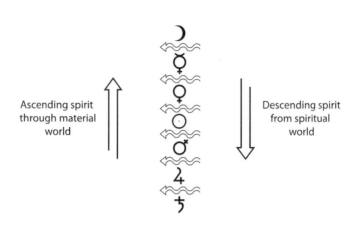

Figure 30. The Means by which Spirit Amalgamates with Matter in order to be Emancipated via Consciousness.

So the fourteenth station of the Stations of the Cross represents the spiritual base chakra. But because this spiritual counterpart can only truly resonate on the higher planes, this is where in the cosmos it will develop. This is the same for the way the Earth evolves back through the astrological cycle during its Great Sidereal Year, for it is spiralling upwards.

At the crown chakra, the configuration has gone full circle – from the spiritual base to the physical base, returning to the spiritual base once more. Numerically this means that the whole is the result of completing the two in order for there to be a third. This is the one plus two, which we know to equal three or the double that results from dematerialisation, which becomes the many. Therefore, once having returned to the crown chakra one automatically embarks on one's journey up the invisible seven planes or chakras of the cosmos, for it is being present in the crown chakra that creates this portal. One cannot have made it to the crown chakra without having been a part of the seventh cosmic plane. Hence if we take the Egyptian pyramid to represent the physical aspect of this transcendence up the seven chakras, there must also be a further pyramid underneath it that is mirrored at its base and an invisible one mirrored above it at its peak or 'simple point', forming a triad.

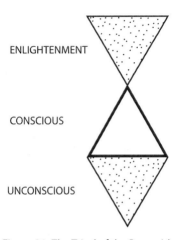

Figure 31. The Triad of the Pyramids.

The Fourteen Stations of the Cross are very significant, for they refer to the number of stations that require mastering in order to first obtain the key that is granted to unlock the door to Christ. With this key the unknown can be sought and the invisible be explored. With Christhood within, one is then ready to take the next immortal step above heaven. If all fourteen stations are evolved in a single lifetime, then one obtains martyrdom from which miracles are derived. This number fourteen coincides with the inner council where a representation of the twelve apostles (the mind) plus Paul and Jesus reside. Again, Jesus is not to be confused with Christ here, which is why the fourteen stations are marked by the Fourteen Beatitudes.

What is required at the crown chakra that gives insight into healing is at least an understanding or perhaps a quest into the enlightenment of the fourteen stations of the cross. These are principally the same as the fourteen body parts of Osiris that Isis resurrected, as the Virgin Mary did with the stations in hope for her son (gave birth to potential). In Hindu metaphysical systems, they are referred to as the Chaturdasa-bhuvanas, the fourteen planes or the seven lokas and seven talas of creation. It is through these stations that one is able to free oneself of the pain and suffering incurred over all one's previous lifetimes.

The fourteen stations are metaphors for what we carry, and that which requires discarding as part of human existence. But what is important here is the experience of each station as lived through. This is how they enter into one's consciousness, and those who can receive their guidance and understand their significance will be invited to move further down the path. Once through this final door, and having mastered each step, the concept of suffering is flipped into the 'fourteen stations of joy', from which ultimate freedom is obtained – the Holy Spirit free within nature. Once this is achieved, one no longer is bound by the confines of physical existence. However, this does not quite end the process of reincarnation, as there is more to this task.

If death occurs before the fourteenth birthday, the cycle of life has yet to be amalgamated by the fourteen yearly junctures that enables Self to recognise itself as an independent ego (chakras develop on a yearly as well as seven-yearly cycle). This in chakra terms is nature laying down the physical foundation to life. This comes about through the establishment of the fourteen Stations of the Cross but by the means of spirit fixing itself in matter enabling life to flourish. In creation, if something is spiritually correct then nature will sustain it. Therefore, if this has not been established before death, Self is not equipped to begin another cycle, not having fully established the present one. So the soul can be found waiting in limbo for the arrival of its next opportunity to reincarnate and finish this existing life. This necessitates a suitable ancestral opening in order to complete the original life and in a positive sense, enabling it to go over the years already completed, which should make for a stronger beginning, undoing the reason for death.

The resonance of the two multiples of seven creates a stronger sense of unity, for it has doubled and thus completed, providing a higher quality of potential, the world of spirit and matter as one. The phrase 'in the beginning', is used to start the Book of Revelations, and refers to this point of potential. It is all beginnings, which Self places before the next step on its path towards reaching a position of bliss. One has of course come from a state of bliss, so it can only be wisdom that the initiate can contribute to the greater whole. The number fourteen refers to the core of this transcendence, forever being in a state of change.

By its very nature, when a ritual is performed, its structure remains the same but within this there is room for experiment. This is because through what it evokes, a new form of consciousness is released that causes its content to change. Nothing, if repeated, will ever produce the same result. This is the same for homœopathy, and do not let any governing body tell you otherwise, for from this awareness the greatest breakthroughs in healing have sprung. Those who partake in this wisdom have enabled homœopathy to live, heal and continue doing so, despite the changes of the times and circumstance. In the pursuit of materialism, the convention of modern living may try to burn the soul out of Self, but those who are on a spiritual path remain so for the benefit of the change that is taking place.

The 'Double Holy Seven' is so-called because having reached the crown, one begins the second set of seven, which becomes a double vibration of its original. At the crown, one is completing one cycle and beginning the next but they are, in fact, part of the same thing and thus one depends on the other. This is the invisible pyramid that sits on the visible one. In Christianity this is symbolised by a descending dove, as depicted in a large painting of the 'Black Prince' in Canterbury Cathedral, presumably testimony to courage. The dove can be seen above the horizontal arm of the cross, thus replacing the top half of the vertical arm – the Tau Cross (figure 21, page 271). The fact that this top section of the cross is missing is symbolic of that which is not material, so therefore signifies the immortal in the cosmos, to which man is closest, being the most consciously developed in the physical world. This image of the dove above the Tau Cross illustrates the importance of being able to enter and leave the immortal world. This is the portal that is the crown chakra and from the pull of the base chakra (the first crucifixion) the soul is materialised and then resurrected in the form of the ascending Eagle, a cycle of fourteen stations. The purpose of ascending up the seven chakras enables the soul to remember that which was forgotten in the unconscious descent enabling spirit and matter to be infused in new consciousness. As a result spirit can evolve a loftier position on the higher realms raising the level of its mind in communicating to those within this new position. Of course at the crown this can also be taken away by Self using its mind in a way that is not deemed to be of any use to the higher beings.

The same principle is reflected in the lightning bolt within Kabbalist philosophy, as it will only strike by being earthed.

Chapter 7 ~ The Crown Chakra

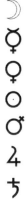

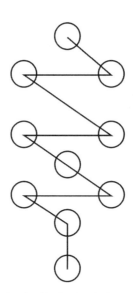

Figure 32. The Earthed Lightning Bolt on the Tree of Life.

Thus the connection is made at both ends enabling the soul's journey to begin back up towards the crown chakra. An example of gaining enlightenment through the balancing of spirit and matter can be found in the life and the reason behind the death of Thomas Becket. He not only had to renounce his own connection with the material word but also, like all the Bishops that preceded him, used his material wealth as guise to try and protect the teaching of the true mystical inheritance. Within the churches and cathedrals all over Britain and Europe there remains physical testament to this spiritual purpose, exposing Christianity's true mystical past relationship with the fourteen stations. In such artefacts, writings and of course the silent whispers, the true centre of Catholic or Protestant belief is revealed, that of the power of reincarnation.

Recognition of reincarnation was central to the church's spiritual beliefs that took a turn for the worse in the twelfth century as the theologians took hold. They were determined to take humanity further into the world of materialism in the name of personal rather than spiritual sanctitude. They gained influence by using the doctrine of the Seven Deadly Sins as their weapon to sideline the importance of karma; which generally has been the motivation in the West ever since.

Originally, the Seven Deadly Sins referred to the attributes of the planets and their relative chakras and were an insight into esoteric balance – not actually being sins at all and having nothing to do with guilt. Is it a sin for a chakra to be out of balance? Sloth, for example, would have been attributed to the unawakened crown chakra. Before this misrepresentation, the Church was a place of refuge for those who had incarnated with a purpose to evolve the planet spiritually. These souls, these children of destiny, were highly-evolved, and the priests of the time, privy to the purpose behind their previous incarnations, naturally drew them to their teachings. This is the meaning of the word candidate. The role of the priest and those associated with the inner sanctum of the fourteen was to evolve the quality of the planet by raising the quality of the souls within it. The progression and safe keeping of the teachings was the priority.

This apprenticeship through the Church was to end when power shifted to the monarchy, and thus a bloodline was developed to represent the 'chosen one', replacing the 'many' and from which ordination became a symbol of control. For the priests, the chosen one referred to a soul that was open to the teachings, and that had an evolved crown chakra, thus able to assist in the expanding of consciousness. Under the deepening control of the monarchy, in order to continue occultist practice, secret groups sprang up that were often made up of members of the Church. Of course, the theologians tried to increase their grip and used torture in the process. Secrecy has always been an important part of occultist activity and in the case of the Knights of the Templar, sadly became the justification for their downfall.

The philosophy behind the process of assisting the evolution of souls has extended into the modern world through techniques of personal development programmes and various groups. It is even beginning to mix into the world of business. But the real work is difficult and requires great change and dedication, in order to raise consciousness to the level where spiritual love resonates in the battle of light and dark. All these teachings evolved around the knowledge of the chakras. There was great receptivity, and tremendous importance was placed upon the precise reason and purpose for each incarnation of these children of destiny. The candidate would plot their soul journey, and uncover the purpose of their current incarnation, in order that there be as little conflict with personal will as possible. This is precisely what the Jesus story is about. Teaching the development of receptivity and vision is central. Jesus represents the awareness of what has gone before, and the

Chapter 7 ~ The Crown Chakra

next step, by being in the present. This can only be provided by reincarnation. This is why it was considered so important by the old masters to support the evolved souls coming through, for the good of humanity – for this is what is delivered through the transition of the Double Holy Seven. At present this support is insufficient, as there is a lack of spiritual perception in a world where money comes first. We need to do more for these evolved souls that are required in our time, and this in part can come through our homœopathic practice. At first these souls may not come packed with light, their depth having often evolved from the darkest of backgrounds. This is syphilitic in origin but the paradox here is that such travels can produce an evolved crown chakra, it having laboured to make such investigations possible and so enabling the soul to arrive safely in its next position.

Being an extension of tribal leaders, the first kings were not naïve to such teachings and neither was their motivation to be leader of one country without spiritual input, of which knowledge of reincarnation and karma was a major factor. They aspired to be the 'chosen one' and used many forms of manipulation in order to provide Divine justification for wearing the crown. In effect, Kings would graft this idea onto their bloodlines by means of reference to reincarnation. Images and stories appeared that gave significance to not only their present life in royal succession but also to previous ones, often placing them as prominent characters in major religious events.

At this time, it was important for royalty to establish its destiny as well as its spiritual credibility. This meant (and as these images were intended to show), that they had the means to broach both worlds. This attracted followers who were prepared to give their lives for the monarch, and this is still very much apparent today. These depictions also put royalty in opposition with religious leaders, such as the Pope.

The royal leaders pursued the mystical teachings of the Church, as this provided justification for sole rule. What was recognised by them and church leaders alike was that such teachings held power. If they could control these teachings (and there were plenty of Bishops and church representatives who were happy to oblige), then they could control and select all positions of power. Hence the relationship grew between the Church and those who claimed the Divine right to take the throne, which could be misconstrued as the amalgamation of ancestral and personal karma.

These royal descendents did of course underestimate the power of the crown chakra and the true meaning of being King on Earth. Having destroyed the structure of the fourteen guardians in an attempt to replace it with a single figurehead, conflict would from then on continually arise between the Church and Crown, which is really the battle between spirit and the state, of Heaven and Earth – hence Becket's death on sacred ground. The true meaning of the word 'King' is to be in command of a sword of unified chakras, from base to crown. This is the harmony that brings spiritual peace to all people: the kingdom of heaven.

To be King is to sit on the Divine throne on Earth, which as described in the Apocalypse of John, is surrounded by twenty-four elders (The Dragon Court here on Earth which elects the Pen-Dragon). Each elder wears a crown of gold and each has the same significance as a priest. Written within the passage of the seventh church – Laodicea, John writes, 'listen to the Spirit and understand what the Spirit is saying to the churches.' The 'churches', seven in all, are representative of the seven chakras and the twenty-four priests act upon us in order to help with this listening. They are the twenty-four orders of priests, the twenty-four families and the twenty-four hours in the day. Hence having the ability to manifest this number on Earth is to obtain guidance from, and be in the centre of, the Universal Source, symbolised by a twenty-four pointed star.

To represent being of the Universal Source, royalty would place the present King's mark or crest in the centre of such a star as a statement of the kingdom's grandeur, marking the boundary. This star is also a celebration of the twenty-four books of Tanakh (Hebrew Bible), the written manifestation of this guidance here on Earth. The priests gave way to the knights, for only the King could represent God, and thus the Knights of the Round Table were in evolutionary terms the closest equivalent to the circle of elders. Hence the Knights Templar designated themselves as protectors of pilgrims en route to the Holy Land. What was truly under protection, though, was not directly the Holy Grail but the knowledge of the group of fourteen (inner council) – the Double Holy Seven, the Knights having placed themselves also within its progression. Their demise was part of the denial of reincarnation, so much that had previously been done by ritual and teachings was relinquished to authority, 'Divine' authority, down here. In the case of Becket, wealth

Chapter 7 ~ The Crown Chakra

and prestige became the guise in order to continue occultist teachings, but when these were stripped away, his soul did not relinquish, certainly not to the temporary state of an earthly death.

There is much written about spiritual development in relation to the fourteen stations of the cross, of which the fourteen beatitudes of Saint Anselme and Saint Bernard give an insight. These are a breakdown of the journey, the junctures which lead to a blissful paradise within. They are represented as the seven beatitudes of the physical human existence: health, beauty, agility, force, liberty, pleasure and longevity, with the seven of the soul: honour, power, security, joy, wisdom and friendship, and concord. The presence of all these ingredients in the character marks the obtainment of sainthood. Hence the number fourteen is a holy number signifying the completion of a cycle, though not necessarily the completion of one life. In addition to this, the number fourteen relates to the two opposing cycles of the Moon's nodes, and directly to the fourteen ascending lunar days of the north node. The descending and ascending nodes together make up a cycle of twenty-eight days, which is also the maximum number of degrees between the Moon's most northerly position to the celestial equator and its most southerly. This is a reference to the immortality of the Moon and the Earth, as this number refers to that which is completed on the higher planes – the twenty-four elders plus the four corners of the cosmos.

In cosmology, the structure of the cycle of fourteen can be seen working its way down into dense matter in the form of the fourteen Bravais space lattices. In its solid state, matter comprises atoms that form patterns known as crystallites. Other than the fourteen lattices, there are seven groups of crystal systems that are found in three-dimensional space. The repeated pattern is known as a lattice because it is defined as a series of dots in space, hence the comparison to structures in the universe. None of these points are random, but are identical to one another in their collective environment – just like patterned wallpaper. These points are not atoms, nor do they comprise material form; hence they are an abstraction. The lattices can only be observed by mathematical language, for they are markers of the etheric body, but as they govern form, so the inner hidden structure is revealed in the outer visible form.

Manipulation of these patterns has been used by industry for some time, and of course for a lot longer by healers. The shapes that are formed replicate ancient structures that have defined effects on us human beings. Science has found ways of using the intricacies of these systems in order to produce complicated circuitry – by applying electrical charges or light to them. Interestingly, when light is applied to these structures, much can be revealed of the relationship between the Moon and the Earth.

Reflection and refraction can mirror an image or information from one source to another, much in the way that some remedies are made using crystals as a medium between the source and the alcohol. Information is transmitted and implanted from one plane to another. This is exactly what happens with the lattice, for it is nothing more than a repetition of information. It's like a Russian doll scenario, in which the external form reflects internal structure. Such patterning is very common in the mineral kingdom, which homœopathy has siphoned and used to great effect.

At the heart of the electronics industry, silicon is used to store information. In the advancement of technology, where more and more information or data needs storing, new crystalline structures are being devised and grown. This is in direct correlation with the expansion of human consciousness. Without the understanding of such structures, this new growth would not be possible. This demonstrates how the crystal matrix can be manipulated by light. Crystals are now being used to produce holograms, an interesting extension to the question 'what is reality?', a question which the Moon, lying between this world and the other, has been posing since the beginning of its collaboration with Earth.

The three periods outlined at the beginning of the Gospel of Matthew signify the genealogy of Jesus from Abraham, which is said to be three lots of fourteen generations. This is a reference to the period required for the blood to undergo cleansing, in order that at the crown chakra one can reach a position of transcendence. This is to be blameless – free of consequence, the ego cleansed of ancestral as well as personal karma. This can only be achieved through aspiration that burns away karma in order that the candidate is sufficiently free of all Earthly constraints.

The belief that only when the soul has lived a pious life (Divine balance of love) three times over, is it then liberated from the cycle of incarnation came up from the training of the mystery schools. This in reality is three times fourteen generations. This is the completion of

Chapter 7 ~ The Crown Chakra

the Double Holy Seven ('Holy' referring to the three or triad) and the significance of the resurrection, for to find Christ, Buddha, Krishna, Osiris or Yahshua or whatever name applied to this manifestation, Self has three attributes to master – three lots of fourteen. This is the same as the number of names mentioned by Matthew – forty-two – that are, in fact, divided into three tiers or levels. This means to accomplish the Double Holy Seven, the form must firstly be determined, which needs to enter into consciousness in order for its Divine format to be recognised within, which is its purpose. In Matthew, each name represents one of the various stages of significance that need to be achieved here on Earth in order to complete the triad. Each name is a code, which can be deciphered either by studying each life, or by using numerology, or esoterically through its dual meaning. The best way of decoding this information is to receive insight via meditation. Either way, each stage still remains to be achieved. One can use this insight to ascertain whether a particular station has been established. Each station being worked on will, however, show its significance in life when Self is ready, as ordained by the Lords of Karma. This progression can be seen as being a bit like the invisible points on the scale of homœopathic potencies in which there are significant differences.

In Matthew, the three generations are not meant to signify a chronological representation of historical events, however it has been observed that they do coincide with certain dates when the lunar calendar is applied. This may be because each of the forty-two steps contributes to the whole or The Double Holy Seven in its completeness, the ultimate goal achieved at the crown chakra. So when each is put together they resonate to the number forty-two which also best fits the configuration of a mathematical lunar structure both materially and spiritually. This is obvious when one knows the spiritual connection between the number fourteen and the cycles of the Moon in relationship to the crown chakra. In the bible, Matthew's list of generations leading to Jesus differs from that written in the gospel according to Luke. Many reasons have been pondered for this but as already explored in this book, Matthew's list refers to the metaphysical means to follow Christ – the means to bring one's incarnation to an end, whereas Luke's is supposed to be the physical counterpart, the forefathers of Jesus from Adam not Abraham. Here again is another example of spirit and matter coinciding in the same thing.

Abraham was named 'father of many nations' (ideas) from whence kings could be sprung in order that the three sets of fourteen, the triad, when resonating collectively result in the final retribution from the need to reincarnate. The retributive soul will never need to grace planet earth again unless called upon in order to bring a vital message on behalf of humanity. This message may be fleeting or take many years to deliver but it will not be induced, nor will the vehicle be provided by a conventional birth. The secret to achieving this freedom, which all souls pursue, is in the establishing through knowledge of the seven worlds that is Self within the cosmos.

Abraham's seed represents the deeds that are planted in the name of the good of humanity, there to germinate even when all seems barren. Each of the forty-two stations is undertaken with the notion that Abraham's offspring represent the right and wrong road from which we learn and which result in the 'many' or descendants – shaped by consequence. This is the nature of the Holy Double Seven, for the lessons that are learnt are equal to the way in which one has arrived at each station. It is, however, the eventual outcome that is important. Hence it was Abraham's second son and not his first that was the inheritor. In the modern world this inability to make and accept mistakes whilst pursuing perfection is the result of having been overridden by syphilitic values. These produce more, rather than less negative karma and perpetuate the cycles that inhibit growth in each of the soul's forty-two stations.

In the pursuit of three pious lives it is not enough to simply curtail the consequence of one's own actions but, as the word generation implies, this is achieved through what can be done for others and those souls to come. Hence until Jesus reached the crown chakra, he was still servant to his people before finally being able to unite in Divine service. War, the result of Abraham's two opposing sons, is waged within Self until the lessons of the next station can be achieved and one comes closer to the three junctions of emancipation which divide Self from the Divine. Therefore, mistakes are necessary on this journey and cannot be avoided. One can, however, avoid learning from them, thus halting the journey's progression and rendering this emancipation impossible.

In no small measure, the yearly growth patterns, which adhere to the seasons of the solar calendar, can be divided by the succession of the Moon cycles that apply directly to the triad of The Double Holy Seven.

Chapter 7 ~ The Crown Chakra

The starting point when applying this calculation begins with the fourteen-day cycle of the waxing moon, added to the fourteen days of the waning moon, and then finally again to the fourteen days of the waxing moon. Put more simply, fourteen days to the full, to the new and then to the full Moon. Each differing Moon on each differing day of the forty-two days represents a new name or mark of significance that makes up the generations of the yearly cycle, the emancipation from the cycle of reincarnation but in miniature. This means each new day brings the chance to change the pattern of negativity; the repetition of stuck ideas; the rules of our ancestors and that of our own past lives that inevitably hold us back. Each day brings the opportunity of independence. Of course this does not in itself represent instant success but presents, through the forever changing focus of the Moon, the possibility of success. This is the meaning of 'time' within the triad that is the creative structure of reality. It is also the reason why some homœopaths choose a six-week cycle between prescriptions.

In biblical terms it is generally considered that between twenty-three to twenty-five years span a complete generation. This figure multiplied by three lots of fourteen amounts to roughly a thousand years, a figure presumed to be the time distance between each reincarnation. This is the number in which the Earth adjusts to the number on the planet at any given time and is determined by consciousness – each soul's quest to complete the three sets of fourteen generations. Each name on Matthew's list represents a point of understanding, a juncture of thought that is learnt and passed on to the many that are known as the offspring. This is the means by which we love, support and help one another to move on collectively. It is also the same for an idea, for it has to adhere to the same process by replicating the triad in order for it to be released into earthly existence, it being the reflection of Divine in humanity.

Ideas on a smaller scale are the making of completion in each step on Matthew's scale; hence each step also has forty-two parts to it before one is free within the crown chakra of one's life. One part is not necessarily mastered in a single lifetime, let alone the completion of one of the Double Holy Seven's steps. If it is deemed impossible for one of these sub-parts to be awoken or lit in a single lifetime, death can be swift, allowing the process to be reserved for when the circumstances of completion are more appropriate. Remember there is no room for waste in the universe. It is the higher cosmic planes that feed the purpose to these junctions and although their premise, remit or vibration remains the same, their relevance due to the purpose of the soul is always changing. Therefore, this flexibility allows the incarnated soul to always be at one with what needs to be done at any particular moment. The success of this depends on whether this focus is met by Self. This is the same with the parameters of a homœopathic remedy picture or any energy source defined by the hardened boundaries of its own existence. The patient's need for the remedy or the remedy's relevance – the reason behind the prescription, is always in a state of change according to circumstance. Each one of us is doing each of the forty-two sections to the forty-two stations of the triad of fourteen as best we can. There is no set format for success.

The first generations of the forty-two names on Matthew's list lived much longer than what we would consider to be a normal life span today. This span of time relates to the amount of energy in reference to the number of reincarnations or the amount of time that may be required to complete a single station consciously. Self is required, by the cosmic planes, to reintegrate and can only do so by fitting. Hence the time spent in the presence of these planes between reincarnating has much to do with this fitting. We make a guide of a thousand years but this of course is Earthly time and has no bearing in reality to the time spent in the higher realms. So what may be recorded as a thousand Earth years is not a true measurement or definition as to the dimension that is home between incarnations. This measurement is roughly considered to be when the planet Earth is ready for the soul to return and the soul is ready to return. Therefore, the time necessary for the next stage of the soul's progression or the new beginning also relates to Matthew's three times fourteen generations, as is the ongoing developing cycle of Earth. So the time set for reincarnation also depends on the correct level of consciousness of the soul. It is now possible to understand what is meant by the word genealogy, it being the similarity between successive generations and the space created for Self to reincarnate into the appropriate generation, which is dependent on the soul's readiness.

Reincarnation presently is considered to be far shorter than a thousand years, at times even only a matter of days, as the levels of trauma and lack of spiritual growth in the modern world deem this frequency to be more necessary. The soul enters the chain of the generation that best fits the work already achieved and the work to be done. This is depend-

Chapter 7 ~ The Crown Chakra

ent on which of the three runs of fourteen the soul resonates with. It thus takes any time up to a thousand years before this opportunity may arise again but it must also be considered that this is not necessarily taken. In order to make a full study of the patient at the crown chakra, the homœopath has to speculate as to the number of reincarnations the patient has achieved and the frequency, both within regularity and level of advancement. By developing the crown chakra, one releases much in the way of healing the past, present and future lives of the forty-two stations. This is precisely what those who undertake rituals seek to achieve.

The figure forty-two, when reduced, amounts to the number six; comprising three – the triad of the Double Holy Seven, plus two – the spiritual within the physical of the stations, which stems from the one – the Source. Hence the number six in numerology represents Venus, the first planet to encapsulate Self in spirituality. This is, as we know, not simply that from which we originate but also from whence we return, the meaning of the word evolution. Each one of the triad represents the mastering of the invisible pyramid or the amalgamation of all seven worlds in their triple aspect. Each part to the triad is significantly different, but together and by the means of initiation, they enable Self to integrate with the seventh cosmic plane (the cosmic plane's number is greater the furthest from the source). However, this integration is still only of awareness, as one represents Jesus here and not Christ. The cosmic planes are made up of three upper planes and four lower, so by leaving the confines of earthly existence, Self can be absorbed into the first rung of this ladder. The purpose as to the emancipation of the first three sub planes makes sense in numerology, as this brings the power of the Supreme Being within reach. Three is attributed to the planet Jupiter, the king of the gods or supreme god, the planet of growth, interaction and thus of genealogy – the ancestral line. Here we can begin to understand why this line is interwoven with one's destiny on Earth and how it makes possible the soul's journey from it.

Jupiter is the lower octave of Venus and it is from the energy of Venus that some of the new souls are being propagated to enter the world, in order that humanity can raise its vibration to that necessary in the Aquarian Age. These children need to be recognised for the contribution they can make, but sadly for some this is not forthcoming and they find themselves excluded from the transition that is obviously not yet ready for them.

Generations speak not only of change but also tradition, from which Jesus, being a teacher as are all the forty-two names, was able to preach. Tradition or the 'boundary' contains the power required to bring in new consciousness, as it holds what has come before, and this is the same for meditation. Through the weight of insight, fresh things are provided and that which no longer holds water can be discarded. When working with the crown chakra tradition is imperative, for it establishes safety in order that most benefit can be gleaned from its use whilst being of this physical world.

Tradition and ritual are a means by which to enter the other world, as was represented by the Feast of Dedication at the Temple of Solomon. Not surprisingly, being a cycle of transcendence, it lasted fourteen days: seven days of dedication and seven days of feasting. In this time the temple was both purified and consecrated, the amalgamation of Cain and Abel, and readied for its purpose – to gather together all spirituality to be housed in one chest, the Ark of Covenant. This is to have Divine love here on Earth. The number fourteen when reduced makes the number five, that of Mercury and the place of focus for such love – or the head and heart together. It is the reception of Divine love that the brow chakra should be focused upon, so that the brow and the crown can co-exist in harmony. Strictly speaking, Mercury represents the heart within the brow chakra – the two having come together to absorb Divine love. It enables this messenger to process that received at the crown chakra, as it is at the crown that he is guided by the gods.

It is said that the Ten Commandments are placed in the Ark, and these relate esoterically to the ten Sephiroth on the Kabbala tree. All emanates from these ten but all is also contained within them, as is the same in numerology. Whenever a figure has more than one digit these can be added together and reduced to a single digit. This is why in reality a number never gets beyond the number nine as ten can be reduced to one, which starts again back at the beginning, and so all returns to the Source, the number of creation, the root back to the Divine. This is why the tenth sphere represents the non-material on the Tree of Life, and why there is not an eleventh sphere to represent the abyss for it does not exist, as its hidden quality is the illusion of existence. Whenever nine is added to this reduced figure, it will always reduce back to its original number. Therefore, one cannot go beyond it and remain in the physical. The numerological importance of the number nine is as the jumping off point that divides matter from spirit. Hence the figure ten is always one (I or 1) plus spirit (the circle) or one's relationship to spirit. It is this relationship that St. Bernard knew to be so important, and St. Augustus knew to be so precious. This is why the number ten is considered 'all embracing'; nothing has existence beyond it, for it marks the beginning, the first of all, or the start and the end. The 'All' is mind, the mana – Buddhi, and the crown the viaduct for the brow. This connection is enshrined between the brow and the crown chakra; without an open mind that is ready to receive there is no deep level of reception at the crown that can call itself Divine.

The brow is about assimilation and crown is about reception. In Britain, this wisdom was not written down but passed on through ritual, concerned with the whole spiritualised Self, rather than simply the intellect. Rituals have been a part of enlightenment for thousands of years, for they change the body molecularly (the connection from crown to base chakra) in preparation for a greater reception of higher energy. This has a direct correlation with homœopathy, for the receiving of Divine light at the third eye relies on physical, emotional, mental and spiritual receptors being of one accord – a task homœopathic remedies are in tune to assist with.

The Ark is also said to contain Manna, or 'a grain of heaven'. It is the seed from which Aaron's rod grew, as a symbol of the sequence of creation and reincarnation. On this rod was written the name of God, in order that Adam could remember from whence he came. Essentially, Adam could have gone forth carrying the Tree of Life within. But this rod was neglected, in other words, misunderstood in the physical world and thus it withered and broke into three parts. These parts represent the three that came from the one. The pieces are said to have budded once more, symbolising the unstoppable journey that always leads back to the Source. Even during the darkest of hours, this journey is kept very much alive by the power of resurrection. Without this connection, the rod of light, which is the spine, weakens through energy leakage, which in turn has a dissipative effect on all the endocrine glands and ganglia. The rod of Aaron may look incomplete but its top is as rooted in the sky as is its base in the earth.

The word manna means the food from heaven. This is the kind of food that is also gifted to line the stomach but here the emphasis is of Divine spirit, which provides the faith, vision and direction when one finds oneself lost in the wilderness. Therefore it is this that is 'our daily bread' from which Self should feed. The content of the Covenant is Divine Love, the making of mankind, designed for all and not just a few privileged persons in positions of authority. However, not all can look upon the contents of the Ark, for the soul has to be of equal measure and this practice is not for the uninitiated – the purpose of the forty-two names. One will only receive what is needed from the Ark depending on one's level. The qualification here is humility. This is provided by the Source, nourishment for the soul. This humility is a reflection of higher aspiration. Ask and you will gain. It is that which we digest, the quality of what is absorbed which we need as our daily input that sustains us. It is spiritual love.

In relation to the Ark, Blavatsky states 'the umbilicus is connected with the receptacle in which are fructified the germs of the race.' Just like the pyramids, the Ark is like a womb, the means by which humans reincarnate. With all the mystery and pageantry attached to the crown chakra, its simplicity comes down to that which is contained in the Ark, that which is venerated as the means to clear one's karma.

In relation to this reality, the Incarnating Ego does not actually move; only the surrounding existence or the experiences change. It is our imagination that maintains the illusion of movement, as in reality the Ego is expanding its influence whilst still fixed in what we call the higher planes. Imagination is the vehicle to explore, in the one and only true world. The Arc shows us how difficult it is to differentiate reality in what we think is the world by showing us this other world. Being here on Earth is not reality for the Ego, and thus it cannot surrender its movement to something that doesn't exist. This is similar to the Polestar, which represents one's position within the universe. Like Self, Polestars have to change with evolution through the Epochs. The Djed, which connects this star to the Earth and acts as the axis of the universe, is that of the human spine, along which the chakras are lined up. Along this axis, we can plot our station in the universe. This enables the Ego to construct its movement within imagination that navigates it through the obstacles of delusion within the Laws of Absolute.

In this notion of manifestation, the idea of matter and the existence within it has to be provided by the three Gunas. If the three principal Hindu deities are a representation of that which maintains existence, and which manifests in reality, they therefore cannot manifest

Chapter 7 ~ The Crown Chakra

an illusion. This is why they work collectively through the Gunas, the attributes that sustain the illusion necessary when spirit lies within matter. This is different when it comes to that which is at work within the highest triad, for it is not matter that spirit impregnates but form. Form is always present and is necessary in the construction of illusion. It is well written and generally agreed throughout the many spiritual philosophies that the three upper cosmic planes are formless, whereas the lower four are form producing. As one is born from the other there will be form, even within the three higher planes. However, it is so spiritualised that we can only associate it with the 'word', it being the formlessness, which is the radiation of cosmic will or the Logos. Hence it is the form of Self that is enabled when reaching the highest point of individualised self on Earth, to transcend and disregard its illusion, that of matter. Here the spirit of the individualised self is spiritualised wisdom.

It was between the twelfth and the fourteenth centuries that secrets held within the Church pertaining to such spiritualised wisdom started to become accessible to all humanity. Numerologically-speaking, this was inevitable. The release of information at this time was also the result of a backlash cleverly orchestrated against the cruel Theologian movement, which continued to use fear to instil its message. These centuries opened up the possibility to partake in the twelve virtues, the principles of harmony in the soul, which lead to a greater awareness of the significance of the resurrection – the amalgamation of the triad of fourteen. Of course the Vatican was strictly opposed to the masses gaining this choice or having any spiritual choice for that matter and attempted to stamp it out, a reflection of the mentality that had motivated the crusades. But the advent of the printing press enabled study and people were able to form their own interpretation of the scriptures. Information as to their meaning, other than that controlled by the Church, could also be published, but of course this was unsafe for a long time.

Desire for investigation and knowledge led to the expansion of more groups and more movements that dedicated themselves to the acquisition of wisdom that mysticism, rather than religion, had to offer. This culminated in the rise of the spiritualist movement in the seventeenth and eighteenth centuries. This movement developed originally from the need to deliver the first King – an opening to the accessibility of self-development. The crown chakra is all about revealing what is secret.

It was impossible for all of the spiritual teachings of the church to be swallowed up by the Theologians. Leaders were able, under the disguise of modest-looking practices, to retain a basic structure in which to pursue their spiritual beliefs. The Benedictine Rule was one such compromise; religion governed in a manner that could be considered monarchic, yet the Rule acted as a constitution under which all were protected as equal but separated by the level of mystical elevation. It was St. Benedict who developed such a system, but in secrecy, and using knowledge of teachings that had come before. This guide is part of a tradition that evolved in order to develop methods of being in the 'present' or at one with the Divine. Those early members of the Christian faith who were more spiritual than religious were so because they could encapsulate the connections between all faiths (such as St. Augustine of Hippo). This is the true role of sainthood, to be able to connect to universal love. Miracles are no more than the relinquishing of the hold of the physical plane over to the greater good of the higher planes.

To open up the crown chakra is to open up the Seventh Seal. This is not possible without first opening the previous six seals one at a time, and in their natural order. The Seventh Seal then allows Self to behold all the precious contents that can be found within. This is the state of Christhood, which is called the Lamb, which has two lots of seven – seven horns and seven eyes – a reference to that which is obtained at the end of the cycle, a truly awakened state. St. John used two letters from the Greek alphabet in order to illustrate this state, proclaiming to be Alpha and Omega. He stated 'I am the first and the last', which is to be complete – standing in the midst of the seven lights of the seven chakras. Of this light, the twelfth vibration is that of the soul. The fourteenth vibration is that of Self, hence without the completeness of the fourteen we may say that we are all in a sense lost souls, hence the difficulties in life that confront us. To be immortal in consciousness does not necessarily mean an end to physical life, but to have the ability to leave and re-enter the higher planes at will. Of prime importance in the description of the seventh seal is Fire. This is not the element of death but of enduring life, which is light, free of all worldly karma.

St. Augustus saw seven as the perfection of the Plentitude and whilst at his abbey he realised that at the crown chakra this number was doubled. In order to be at the level of the crown, one must realise, in light of the non-physicality, that here all is of the second vibration. This can only be witnessed and truly understood by not being attached to the

Chapter 7 ~ The Crown Chakra

physical world, for here nothing is material so is a reflection. By the very fact that all is a reflection, every vibration is doubled, i.e. through being a reflection it has doubled in its relevance. This reflection is a complete resonance of the original, whatever this may be, and so in the case of the seven chakras there is a full set of a reflected seven, making fourteen. To be in the crown chakra means the doubling of resonance has began which on Earth translates into consequence.

An object in the material world relies on its dense molecular structure to exist and function. At the crown there are no molecules, so all existence becomes a reflection, thus its vibration (its existence) is increased – or doubled to be precise. This is why construction in the physical world can only occur once outside the crown chakra. It also explains, when writing from the perspective of the crown chakra, why a sentence can make perfect sense to me, but when removed from this influence, I can see that in fact it makes no sense to anyone else and requires great expansion. The contradiction of reflection at the crown is that although all is energetically doubled, the vibration is refined, for in terms of light vibration this is a process of returning to the One in order to relinquish the physical. The Double vibration is more complete, and this is why the crown reveals everything, for here is the true reality. This is the same truth present within the structure of a homœopathic remedy.

Consequence that Self feels will be heightened, for Karma will also double here, it being a reflection. This means karma is a double double, as it's already a reflection of its original self; hence the crown is a very difficult place to deal with it. Here at the crown, karma manifests as already having happened twice – giving the candidate the experience of not knowing which reality they are in. Every action is an extension of several realities, or it is a response to one particular reality being played out in another. To balance this, one's perception is heightened in order to deal with being bombarded with significance equal to the rate at which one's karma is being investigated. To construct one's daily life and relationships amongst such a kaleidoscope of experiences gives one the feeling that one really does not know what will happen next. It feels like being detached from what is believed to be the real world, not being able to connect with events that one would normally be either able to control or have the time and space to gently adjust to. At the same time, as karma is so innately a part of each situation, here it is refined and because one is creating karma all the time, there is a sense that one already knows what is coming next but is helpless to avoid it. One can only hope it will turn out fine as the process is one of discovery! Such is the power of consequence and such is the nature of its clarity whilst on the crown chakra. The paradox remains, 'how does one work on the crown chakra whilst still having Earthly karma?' and the answer is 'very carefully'. This is to try and play out down here on Earth, a reflection of the two lots of seven or the Moon's reflection that when synthesised is immortality.

Blocks in this chakra are multidimensional. They are an amalgamation or the result of many different decisions from the past that have led to confusion, and present themselves in this life or the next like a fractured jewel, offering many sides of refraction on a single theme. This is because all human existence manifests by being drawn down from the crown chakra in order to be resolved by humanity in the physical realm or to be earthed. Clarity can only be achieved through choice, but may take time and a great deal of effort, as the associated negative karma is usually vast.

Blocks are presented at the crown chakra as big choices that need to be made in life. Each has many aspects, leading to more choices, having been created by many parts of negative and positive karma. Therefore these blocks form major crossroads and the differing directions come in the form of lifelong dilemmas. Here they cannot be ignored as they are presented with frightening persistence. The point is not to be alarmed but to acknowledge the mess in order that it can clear. To work on the crown is to accept that worldly karma will be resurrected in order to be changed. The short-term chaos is better for long-term growth, and knowledge of this will support the candidate, although those around will not necessarily see it in this way and judgement may be cast. This process is, however, more important than the constraints of trying to maintain your reputation. A negative reaction from others will usually only arise from those who are struggling with their own means to share in the transformation of karma. The reason for such work is the joy of becoming free of recurring consequence, perpetuated by the dilemma of trying to find a better day. The mess of these multidimensional blocks created by many layers over many lifetimes has to be undone before release can happen. We are, in a sense, laying down and then working through that which will build the reality from the illusion. This process will also contain the greatest dilemmas that Self has to face, so if accepted with trust then the crown chakra will provide safety. The secret to success in this work on the crown chakra is pace. This chakra is addictive: it holds one in a space that one does not readily release from, so the personality may become prepared to trade the experiences of this other world for the unpredictability of its consequence. What is required at the crown chakra is to apply the discipline learnt in the base chakra. One has to maintain a structure, in order that one can be reminded as to the limit that one can cope with. There is no rush, this will be profound so take your time - it requires a gentle pace.

HEALING THE SPIRIT WITHIN

Communication is of utmost priority at present as we go into the New Age and also the next epoch. There is a coming together and entwining of lives because people now need that connection and understanding. There is a global need to develop the crown chakra in each and every one of us. This is a process of breaking down and understanding Self's previous lives and thus changing past negative karma. We all are being asked to receive as a group now, for the priority at present is that the work has to be done down here on the Earth which is where the concentration lies at present. What is being received is for the good of the work we all have to do, but we cannot succeed in this without understanding and having a contact with above. This communication is acceptance for all that is presently at a state of change. There will be more and more information coming through which requires acceptance with open minds in order to do the work necessary down here where it is needed.

Individual development is so very important at present because this is the way in which we, as humans, heal. Change has always been imperative to this but now it is happening at such a vast and fast rate that we need to keep up with it. This is the freedom that humanity so desired and the weave, the network, that is also needed in order to structure the change in the physical world. Light will always be the answer and using it intelligently will solve preoblems and create many of the solutions. More people will ask for freedom, and much interpretation, before a selection can be agreed on which necessitates the solution of help – when true help can be provided. There will also be those who wish to hinder this progress but they will not succeed as this light is at a global level, far more powerful than before and the group is seeking it out. Just like grains of sand we all add up; so every positive action adds to the group energy. All that is on Earth has the solution, or contains it, and so all is provided for. It is perception that requires tuning into the signals that are provided on the higher realms. Trust.

Trust in the truth and maintain this trust in seeing it through, for this will surely be what your patients are attracted to.

Death and the fear of it, which is the fear of life, is so often the problem that lays behind pathology and this is more pronounced in the crown chakra than in any other centre. Connection with truth serves Self and the group as it expands outwards and touches the lives of each individual in the extended group. So that which is received should be spread. Reception is the elixir of life: it is each step on the staircase that takes Self up to a higher level when ready. It is for Self, and Self only, to be the centre from which, with the combination of Divine as well as personal will, we move forward from within: it cannot come from anywhere else.

The term 'spiritual healing' is simply healing, for it all filters through. What is important is not ignoring but recognising all the connections and especially the wisdom of knowing that a developed crown chakra is imperative. All of us use methods to enable this – as one changes, one treats more, one sees more, one develops more – it is the double connection, the Double Holy Seven. Only when one can give on all levels, then one will receive on all levels. For some strange reason, this is considered odd in homœopathy, even though the practitioner heals by healing, the spiritual significance of this is shied away from as it is in Western religion and perhaps there lies the link. To heal ourselves we need to look at our own spiritual content, so therefore, it makes sense that this is the same for healing our patients.

THE PINEAL GLAND

This gland is a source of much mystery and speculation. It is hidden deep in the brain and contains a paradox, as its expansion is much hindered by earthbound thinking and so its use is lost on those who ponder over its true significance. Those who are more open to loftier thought, are so because this gland is providing them with a helping hand, thus revealing its quality. This gland receives, reflects and distributes light and is comprised of cells that relate very much in form to those found in the two human eyes (which are also light receptors). But here light is

Chapter 7 ~ The Crown Chakra

of a higher octave, and is constant, hitting the receptors that reach from above the top of the head. The pineal may be compared to the thousand-petalled lotus flower in its capacity to absorb light.

The mystery of this gland is that here at the crown no form or organ has any means of existence. Like the Buddhi/Atman relationship, this gland in its physical form is very much of the head, and is able to relate, via its endocrine function, with the relevant sympathetic plexus of the physical body. In this sense it is associated with the brow chakra. But its mysterious function, that which has no form in the physical realm, pertains only to the crown chakra. Thus its elusive nature has in the past been described through the telling of stories, fables and metaphors and represented in religious works of art. Its unworldly significance has been, and still is, explored in rituals as well. This is because it is the link between objective and subjective states of consciousness. It is Divine beauty personified in function, and one can only gasp in wonder that its connection with the infinite is retained within the human aura.

The pineal does have its own auric field, for as well as receiving light it radiates light, in relation to the degree of luminosity being received. It is present strongly in those who have a deep spiritual connection, and can be detected by those who cannot see auras, evoking a response in anyone, regardless of their level.

In the physical realm the pineal gland holds back the pituitary gland until the time is right to undertake the transition into adulthood, the initiation known as puberty. Just how this happens is unknown to science, although it is known not to come from the secretion of melatonin (produced by the pineal and fed into the cerebrospinal fluid). It is though, via the directive of soul impulses – whatever the physical mechanism proves to be. It is therefore, a gland of childhood and after the seventh year, like the thymus gland, it atrophies. Being composed of phosphate and calcium, the gland slowly calcifies with age. This can also happen prematurely, when this gland is not used enough in the enhancement of intuitive reception.

In those who are mentally retarded, the gland remains underdeveloped. Damage to this gland, which usually comes in the form of a tumour, can bring on early puberty and the failure of it to atrophy delays the onset of puberty. Being light sensitive, it works with the hypothalamus in relation to the rhythms of the body that are governed by the cycles of the day and night, and also relates to the aging process, controlled by a greater cycle on the higher spheres. Thus it is associated with the quality of sleep patterns, and also seasonal disorders linked to a lack of light.

Reception of light is not simply via the retina or lungs, but also through the top of the crown. Because of its association with light, the pineal gland interacts with both nervous systems, and converts the signals of these systems to endocrine signals. Through the secretion of melatonin, the pituitary prepares us for times of reception or simply for being in a state of relaxation in order that calm and bliss can be enjoyed. This secretion is inhibited by daylight and increases considerably during the night hours, and levels are much higher in children under the age of seven years.

The level of intensity of daylight is 50,000 microwatt/cm^2, compared to that of moonlight which is only 0.3 microwatt/c^2. Hormonal output is influenced by seasonal changes; longer days increase fertility during the summer months. The administering of light in mid-cycle has been shown in experiments to have a regulating effect on the menstrual cycle. It is not the level of brightness (multiples of candle-light) that is important here but the frequency of radiation.

The Moon, by lowering the transmission of light, enables the soul to leave the body at night. Moonlight is still sunlight, but reflected. When it suits them, those scientists who doubt the relevance of cosmology are still prepared to pencil in factors that have been learnt through studying the influence of the Sun and the Moon. The pineal gland is very sensitive to highly-charged magnetic and radioactive fields. Ironically, the great increase in electro-magnetic fields used in modern mass communication is destroying the subtlety of the pineal gland function, for these methods are too earthbound.

Such electromagnetic fields also destroy the human aura, the protective layer which is imperative to life itself. Microwaves produced by mobile phone communication are tumour-forming. This interference with the human status quo begins at the crown chakra and in the function of the pineal gland.

The endocrine system demands more respect that the human race gives it at present. Health depends hugely on reception at the crown chakra, and many forms of illness can occur when this is disturbed, for it places chaos in the subtle bodies. For instance, lowered levels of melatonin in the blood have been found in breast cancer patients.

Chapter 7 ~ The Crown Chakra

(Incidentally, the cases of breast cancer are lower amongst blind women who as compensation produce more melatonin, possibly due to a more proactive third eye.)

It cannot be stressed enough that a well-developed and active crown chakra provides the utmost protection, enabling one to be guided in life. The lack of this protection allows disease easy access and external influences to breach the aura, creating such conditions like schizophrenia.

The reception of light should not only be reliant on the Sun, as it should also manifest from within. People who live in places that lack light are often introverted, and can appear quite bleak. Similar symptoms can arise in patients who struggle emotionally with the dark winter months, and require remedies like *Hornbeam*. This difficulty is of course due to karma, and the struggle between light and dark, as with the place where one chooses to be born. It is a state that necessitates the task of life in order for it to be resolved.

Remedies such as *Hornbeam* act by raising spiritual awareness in the crown by reaching out to the chakra above, and thus one can retain joy in the heart with only the smallest rays of elixir. This enables the soul to understand the purpose of the winter months, to embrace this celebration, enabling one to radiate light from within. This is why the production of melatonin coincides with the yearly seasonal cycle of growth and rest.

Energetically, the pituitary gland is male and the pineal gland is female. These two great forces combine in meditation so that their positive attributes amalgamate to enable reception at the third eye. When this happens, light connects through the crown, opening a channel, and this chakra acts as a bridge from the physical realm to the invisible one. This is only possible if this light is earthed by the light of the kundalini, and primarily by this gland being touched by the sushumna. This rainbow is said to extend over the Divine throne, so connecting it to the King on Earth. Behind this lies the reason why the pineal gland is associated with royalty.

Over the past few decades, a level of reception has been induced by the use of pleasure drugs. Originally, these drugs provided the means to astral travel by those consciously searching for a higher meaning. In recent times, however, they have been used by those who know no other way of leaving the constraints they feel in the physical world. The problem with these drugs – and this includes all hallucinogens – is that they damage the pineal gland, and interfere with the electro-connections that are so important in maintaining its communication with the chakras. Therefore using these drugs leads to consequences other than pure consciousness, and weakens the very apparatus of deep exploration. This is a damaging cycle, for these drugs end up limiting reception and the only means to maintain it is taking more drugs, leading to addiction. Meditation is the best way to develop receptivity but it does require discipline and patience.

As mankind continues to raise its level of consciousness out of matter and towards the Source, the relationship of the pineal gland and the third eye will become ever more apparent. We must be ready for this and pay attention to what is being asked, supporting those who are here to lead the way.

THE MOON AND PURPLE

There is a monthly phase to the Moon. Each day presents a different Moon, and its influence is also different in each month depending on the season of the yearly cycle. Hence the Moon influences us strongly, and the degree to which we are in harmony with our pursuits. The influence of the New and Full Moon cycles affects humanity on a daily basis and is reflected in the twenty-four elders (hours) who surround the throne. This influence is subtle, as the Moon evokes stillness, it not being of the physical realm. So to be at one with the Moon is to be free of emotional and mental constraints, as to be at peace renders the negative attributes of these functions inconsequential. Thus what is achieved through the Moon is the highest form of detachment. The significance of this detachment is conveyed on the image of the white flag with its gold edging, the white being the unification of all colours, of all chakras, that of truth and the gold representing the vision that gains wisdom through this unity. This flag represents the honour and peace received through an awakened crown chakra, and is a symbol of attainment. It is what all the secret societies worth any credit try to evoke.

The Moon's luminosity is that of a secret shadow; it is the afterthought of another world. Insight reveals this light to be more than simply a reflection of sunlight. On deeper contemplation, it reveals further secrets as to the nature of light in the higher realms. The luminosity here is said to be that of a hundred million Suns and having lost any form of crudeness, this light although intense is very refined. For we humans, this light represents the purest vibration, so subtle that it can

Chapter 7 ~ The Crown Chakra

only be absorbed by an equivalent reflective soul, light being the spirit's vehicle into matter. This refinement and receptivity is only possible in the stillest of stillness, provided only in the centre of the crown chakra, there being no limits here.

We have already addressed the various levels of light that act upon the human constitution, but here Self is in the presence of the light of the Logos, the amalgamation of the Holy Trinity, or the upper three spheroids of the tree of Kabbala. The key to the acceptance of this light into the human system is through the resonances that are the channels that the ray of purple creates. Being of the highest frequency of vibration and the shortest wavelength of all the visible light colours, it opens the gateway from Heaven to Earth and vice versa, and thus facilitates the transmission of light. When potentised, the colour *Purple* is the transitional remedy especially needed in assisting birth and death and has much in common with *Ayahuasca* in encouraging release through the crown chakra. *Purple* provides protection for this process and therefore its colour or vibration is the same as the soul of the crown chakra's aura.

Purple reveals the syphilitic miasm, for its vibration acts differently from all the other colours, and it can be used as a lamp in its pursuit (much in the same way ultraviolet is used to unearth hidden forensic evidence). This process has much to do with the circular motion of ascendance towards the Source around which life is structured, and which the syphilitic miasm has tried to copy in its pursuit of power. The syphilitic miasm acts as a vortex, pulling in and corrupting that which is around it (including the creation and evolution of the other miasms). This miasm is the centre of negative karma and in it rotates a swirling mass of negative energy that can be seen reflected in the biology of its physical disease state. The eye of this storm within the crown chakra facilitates all that comes in and goes out, so within it there is both the spiral of existence and that replicated by the syphilitic miasm but in reverse. They coexist, rotating in opposite directions, for they are the energetic motion of liberation and choice that Self has sought in being conscious and from which it enters and leaves physical existence. This aberrant rotation twists what would otherwise be the desire to aspire in the correct direction.

To use the colour purple in remedy form engenders much change and assists those who are overwhelmed by their vision and others who are trying to further theirs but are being held back by the past. Its relationship with the Moon is very simple; it converts the light of the logos into a frequency in tune with the brow chakra. *Purple* is therefore a converter, which explains why it raises hidden negative karma in order that it may be healed, enabling more light to come through. It also acts as a barrier between earthly karma and that of those souls working on cosmic karma on the higher levels. *Purple* thus strengthens the aura from the crown to the base and provides protection against those negative energies that are so keen to infiltrate Self. Without its resonance we would not be able to connect to spiritual power. It is very much a lifeline. It is the link to the authority of vision, which is truth. This colour requires true resonance within the being for purpose to mature and is useful in removing possessions and fixed negative states.

There is a point where the crown ends and the pineal gland begins, which is the Ayahuasca within. If seen, this appears as a great purple helix and makes up a part of the spiral of life. It is wound so tightly as it is under the constant forces of reception from which the three strands that are dissimilated from the one are channelled into Self as life force. Through this compression flows love from the heart and from above, and by this means the two can remain connected. This love is the route to all healing and its connection is imperative in changing debilitating negative karma.

The Moon has no means of radiating by itself. Its silvery luminosity is only a reflection of light on its cold, detached exterior. Hence its dead weight can obscure the open night sky, like the emotion that can block who we truly are. When the crown is used properly, the reflective properties of the Earth's mother and servant of the Sun take on a translucent quality, thus its presence truly becomes a portal to higher consciousness. Meditation makes invisible this mass that obscures our view so that light can be brought into the dark, the freeing of all obstacles in order to reach the unreachable. From this, the light of the Solar Logos is delivered enabling one to transcend karma. The Moon now acts as a filter, and by relinquishing its role as a reflector of light, it allows us to put into perspective that which we hold so dearly. The best time to do this is during a Moon Void-of-Course, as there will be no pressing tasks to clutter one's vision, created by major aspects to other planets in a particular sign, before the Moon moves on to the next sign.

To help to put these things into perspective, one's birth chart can indicate where the knots of the past (emotion and the female principle)

Chapter 7 ~ The Crown Chakra

have been governing our attachments (will and the male principle), and so reveals to us the means by which they may possibly be undone. These knots are the North and South Nodes, which in some systems are referred to mythically as the head and the tail of an immortal serpent or dragon. It cannot be emphasised enough that the Moon is the reflector of deep negative karma and this is revealed in order to provide the realisation of what can be accomplished. It acts as a filter only when this karma is ready to be discerned. A prominently placed South Node will indicate that the soul has much in the way of talented gifts to contribute in this life, which will often have a spiritual significance. The relationship between the Nodes is in fact the relationship between the Sun and the Moon. The Sun can never be taken out of the equation when it comes to the Moon, for it is the light of the Solar Logos that is being channelled at the crown.

It is because of this channel that the Moon has a dark side that never attracts the Sun. Esoterically, it can be said that this part of the Moon represents the negative part of oneself or at least this dark side that attracts no light – those secret desires that elude Self of any bliss. The Moon is the past, whereas the Sun represents the present. So working with these energies is the same as working up through the chakras to regain that which has been forgotten by making it conscious. Here karma is revealed in order to be healed or put another way the crown chakra is sunrise and the base chakra is sunset.

Where these Nodes sit in relation to the Sun and the Moon in the birth chart will reveal definable mental and emotional characteristics. This is because of the Moon's effect on the Earth's magnetic fields, as in its influence on the cycles of the oceans and on our own bodily flow, electrical or molecular. This is what connects a mother to her offspring.

The Moon maps out all of our cycles, which relate primarily to the Mother Goddess principle and which cannot exist without the Father and the Son. So within the scope of the Moon there is also contained this triad of Mother, Father and Son. The New Moon represents the Divine spark, the male, the monad, the idea. It is grown, nurtured and developed by the Full Moon, the creative female, that of the womb and the home, that of the soul, from which it is granted form. It is Earth or the son that is the destination and all that it brings to be played out, eventually finding its way into the personality. The agricultural cycle, the planting, picking and rest, refers to the same cycle and beginning something new will have most chance of success if timed to coincide with the New Moon.

The Moon is a filter from the past to the new, from what has been to that which is becoming. It is thus a gateway from negative into positive karma, and prescribing *Lunar, Purple* or *Moonstone* can assist in this process. The Moon is an evolutionary gatekeeper, but unlike Saturn it deals with the timeless. However, when it comes to karma, the Moon and Saturn always work very closely together as this combination is the means to Earthly existence. Their behaviour should be observed closely by the practitioner when it comes to trying to change the stuck cycles of the past.

The Saturn/Moon link is a very special one. Saturn orbits the Sun approximately every thirty years but remains in each sign of the zodiac approximately nineteen months. Whilst Saturn orbits the Sun, the Moon orbits the Earth. However, the Sun's gravitational pull influences the Moon's plane of orbit around the Earth, so the Earth and the Moon do in fact orbit each other as they dance around the Sun. The Moon's nodes are positions in which the Moon's orbit crosses the ecliptic (the plane of the Earth's orbit), either in a northerly position – the North Node, or dropping below as with the South Node. It takes about nineteen years for the Nodes to complete a cycle of 360 degrees backwards around the Earth. It is the mystical relationship that both Saturn and the Moon have with the number nineteen that links the two planets together. Nineteen or one plus nine that when reduced mark both the beginning and completion. This number is also achieved when the twelve astrological signs are added to the seven sacred planets.

The mathematical relationship between the Moon orbiting the Earth and them both orbiting the Sun is complex, the solution of which is highly sophisticated. Because of the Moon's relationship to Earth, its orbit is not fixed in Space. As it takes the Nodes nineteen years to complete a cycle, then roughly every nineteen years at the summer solstice the Moon rises and is placed at its most northerly direction, and at winter solstice, at its most southerly in the Northern Hemisphere. These two points of the nodes' lunar orbit are known as major and minor standstills, depending on whether they fall during an ascending or descending Equinox.

The Moon has around 27 standstills a year and the sun has two. In a major or minor standstill the Moon appears to hover for some time, creating the opportunity to see its universally still quality and feel its

Chapter 7 ~ The Crown Chakra

subsequent effect. The Moon's orbital axis around the Earth is practically the same as that of the Earth's around the Sun, there being only five degrees difference between each orbital plane. So at each major standstill, as seen from Stonehenge, the Sun and the Moon's orbits (but not celestial bodies) line up above one another. This is where the trajectory of the maximum Declination of the Moon is added to the maximum of the Sun. This is a powerful time, where all three globes stop in unison. A major standstill's influence on humanity can be compared to that of the task of the Lunar and Saturn returns but to a lesser degree; each being an opportunity to examine one's purpose after having undertaken much work. The unison of the three globes by enhancing positiveness helps to reaffirm that Self is on the right path.

At Stonehenge, there are thirty outer stones that represent Saturn's cycle around the Sun, and nineteen blue inner stones in the form of a horseshoe representing the Lunastice (standstills of the Moon) of the Moon's nodes. Between these two circles of inner and outer stones are five trilithons forming another horseshoe.

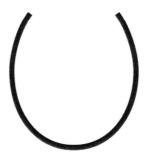

Figure 33. The Horseshoe.

These are the other five chakras that line up much in the same way their respective planets have influence on each orbit of all of the sacred planets. When in the upright position, the horseshoe is the vessel in which spiritual content can be captured and when in the downward position, the symbol of the womb – of giving birth to spiritual consequence in the material world. Together they are the regenerative powers of immortality, that of the Sun in the upward position to receive the seed and that of the Moon in its downward direction to provide the form. The two triangles that produce the Star of David have the same significance, as do the three pyramids in (see figure 31, page 327), for they all illustrate the birth of enlightenment. Therefore the deepest of karma can be summoned to be released when the Moon and Saturn are in the same conclusion. This is the winter fire that brings light into the darkness (Moon uplifting) or the summer sun providing the ultimate growth (Sun uplifting). It is the amalgamation of male and female that resonates as cosmic fire, constantly changing – the resonance of the Double Holy Seven.

Meditating on the Moon has always been approached with the respect and caution that such an activity requires. In the past, as it should be today, much preparation and cleansing was done before focusing on the crown chakra; particularly in regard to the previous six chakras. Also, profoundly spiritually aware people would have been called upon to assist in guidance and reassurance, for heightened receptivity can be a lot to bear depending on the levels of sensitivity. Receptivity also has much to do with the quality of the thymus gland and the heart chakra, both of which have to be of a certain resonance. This equation is equal to the required amount of sufficiently transcended earthly karma that enables Self to work through the instruction (unction) of the crown. To be brief, one has to be ready for the crown chakra. The brow also has to be prepared, for it will have the greatest of struggles if averse to such influence.

One's karma is paramount here, for the energy evoked at the crown works through all of Self. This isn't simply about speeding up karma, although it feels this way, but the making of decisions and subsequent actions that transcend rational thought. Further, karma arrives on one's doorstep at an alarming rate and the energy that it meets from above is also being received at an equally fast tempo. This can result in an enormous wake-up call, which can be felt to be too much; one might then prefer to hide or avoid this experience. In its extreme form, insanity can occur, as is often the case when the patient is heavily traumatised and is lacking any form of base which would allow such reception to work down through the other chakras, and be earthed and integrated. It is impossible to be directed solely by the crown chakra, as all the other centres have to be in order first.

On the positive side, the doors that have been closed for a lifetime or more and that lead off from the corridor in which Self has been patiently pacing, suddenly start to open up. Negative karma is often formed as a result of these closed doors, so it can be extremely uncomfortable when things start to open up. One has to confront the result of having had to

Chapter 7 ~ The Crown Chakra

compensate for such a long time, for all conscious knowledge as to the reason for this compensation has been lost through denial. It often feels like being under the supernatural control of another as one searches to think rationally what could happen next. One has to be extremely patient and extremely trusting. Trust is not only imperative here but is a lesson. The more one has lessened one's load of unfinished business, the easier it is to integrate what has been received.

One's truth is examined at the crown. Truths may be formed by many influences on the physical plane; this does not mean a jot at the crown chakra if they are not in concordance with Divine truth. Of course many aspects will concur, considerably so for some, but the Moon, being a reflector, will soon highlight that which is not the truth by delivering a bout of chaos. The truth will not let life off the hook.

The word 'lunacy' derives from the word lunar, being of the Moon, and is the result of leaving the body in an unsafe manner, the effect this night light has on enticing the soul. Caught unaware this feels as if going against one's truth. A much milder sensation can happen when the Full Moon pulls energy upwards from the body that is too much for the mind to handle. Truth relies heavily on the consciousness of Self, which falls upon the responsibility of the triadic relationship of the manas-buddhi-Atman. This includes the ability to cope with an influx of energy from the crown centre. Lunacy results from the inability to control the energy of this centre. There is no doubt that psychics have in the past been institutionalised because of this and probably will continue to be in the future. Truth is a very difficult concept to grapple with in life, and one has to have the complete confidence in Divine truth in order to work on the crown chakra and not become moonstruck.

Purple does much in nourishing the spleen, it being the organ that links Heaven and Earth, the dual relationship that constructs truth. In Traditional Chinese Medicine, all the other organs pertain to elements, but the spleen remains in the centre as a connection to them all. The spleen is etherically rooted in the soil of the Earth and is concerned with the conversion of nourishment in order to sustain the physical world. Both the spleen and the kidneys support the lungs that pertain to the process of reaching out to the heavens. So indirectly the absorption of light enables both ends of the human constitution to coexist. This is because the soul, being the spiritual bridge from Heaven to Earth, is that

Chakra Prescribing and Homœopathy

which holds the root information of the rainbow. The remedy *Rainbow*, if studied or taken, opens one up to the vast connection from the crown to the heart chakra and then to the base chakra.

Silver has long been associated with the reflectivity of the Moon and thus is the alchemical metal that symbolises it. It is one of the best conductors of heat and electricity and is used in the production of mirrors and photographic imagery, on account of its capacity to reveal. Silver was held in high esteem by the alchemists as one of the seven sacred metals. We have produced a homœopathic remedy, *Argentum*, from silver and its compound variants. Its power, when used by healers and magicians in its raw state, was varied, but great significance was placed on its ability to balance the body's electro-magnetic field, which is very susceptible to feelings of failure and lack of self-esteem.

Silver has long been a representation of second best, of being reminded that one is of the material world and even today winning is still rewarded with gold. In the making of jewellery, silver was considered to energetically address imbalance, rather than simply being used for its malleable qualities. It has of course been used extensively throughout history as an antibacterial agent, and its nitrates used to suppress syphilitic and gonorrhoeal suppuration. It has also been particularly useful in the draining of pus. As part of this history of having antibacterial properties, it has been used as a food preservative and purifier of liquids. Because of the fear of infections, royalty had eating utensils made from solid silver, including food containers. It is supposedly from this that they acquired the name 'Blue Blood', for their skin acquired a blue shimmer as a result of the accumulation of minute silver particles. Of course, through the homœopathic proving of this material we are privy to the damaging effect that its suppressive nature has on all the human bodies once it has entered the bloodstream. Being a heavy metal Silver plays havoc not only within Self's next life, but the future generations of its offspring. This is a reflection, literally, of poorly received instruction from the crown chakra. Even the Divine qualities of the Moon have a destructive nature if used inappropriately.

Silver, as an element of the Moon, also reflects its conductivity in relation to the temperature of the seasons. There is the Cold Moon in December and the Hunter's Moon, the solar silver of June. The Harvest Moon shines with a yellowy glow, helping to extend the daylight in order that the last of the crop can be reaped, which we know is also the

Chapter 7 ~ The Crown Chakra

harvest within Self.

It is by the silver cord that one remains attached to the physical world when the soul is exploring, anchored to the seed atom lodged deep in the left ventricle of the heart. The silver cord provides the strongest connection, fed by life energy during the reception of cosmic consciousness. The Moon is guide and failed mother of Earth, failed in its own evolutionary consciousness, and uses the element of silver for its alchemic connection to divert all efforts to her son. She is thus destined to follow in his path. Self relies on this connection, for it is very important to maintain some remnant of an Earth bond when travelling in the other world.

At Full Moon the Earth is situated in the centre of the Holy Triad and thus the son is under the most vibrant and positively radiant guidance of a harmonic pair.

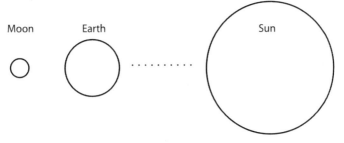

Figure 34. The Position of the Sun, Earth and Moon during a Full Moon.

The Full Moon is a time for great healing for planet Earth. The healing energy offered at this time has long been sought by white witches in their pursuit of group healing. A waxing Moon is the time in which these energies are gathered and stored before their release at Full Moon. This is intensified during a Blue Moon, on a cycle of about every two and a half years, in which there are two opportunities for this intensity to be expressed within one month. This is a time to be precise both with what one asks for and what one promises in return. It is at the crown chakra that the Moon holds one true to what is wished. It is always wise to be cautious when faced with the level of consequence that a Blue Moon evokes. The energy that the Moon gathers is received from the Sun, but each month these offerings are different according to the attributes of each sign of the zodiac.

The spiritualised intensity of the waxing Moon acts upon the consciousness of humanity, and from its release these fourteen days provide the radiance that has come to be known as the immolated Christ. Hence spiritualist groups and religions have devised their calendars around the significance of the Moon's cycles. For instance, Easter always falls on the first Sunday following the first Full Moon, and that occurs on or after the day of the Spring Equinox.

The New Moon that conjuncts the Sun is the most contemplative of New Moons and marks the time of Winter Solstice. This cycle is the same for the Sun, for as already mentioned the Sun and Moon cannot be seen separately. Therefore, the Autumn Equinox is under the influence of waning sunlight, and the Spring that of waxing sunlight. Along with the fullness of the Sun and the shortest day, both are related to the development of the soul, as are the four directions and the four elements. This is the principle behind the balance of spirit and matter. But it will be at the point of Winter Solstice that the soul will finally find itself free of this cycle and be at peace forever.

The 'Moon Period' of the Earth's planetary evolution was in effect the solidification of the universe from fluids and gases, and from which issued all the planets of the Solar System (including those yet to be discovered), the Earth and the Moon itself. This period in evolution, which also gave rise to the materialisation of humankind into its universe, naturally fell under the creative process of the Moon as representative of the Mother Goddess. She provides the means for that which is able to form matter by becoming conscious. Just as with the mother and child, the Earth and the Moon were at one stage a single unit – until the Moon expelled itself. The child, Earth, was ready to develop its own identity, its own ego, from its own Spirit.

As the Earth began to solidify, it was then possible for it to sustain humanity. The first integrated human forms were very fiery, as light attempted to gain physicality. Earth was primordially more light than solid, but the first Polar epoch, the first root-race of this present planetary cycle, began when the Moon relinquished the Earth's independence to the trust of humanity. This was subsequently followed by the Hyperboreic root-race and then the Lemurian, and so on. As things evolved, fire retreated inside and became stored in the blood. Becoming warm-blooded, human beings relied on Divine sustenance being provided by the Sun. This has always been a matter of degree, for human survival has always depended on the differing levels of light's radiation

Chapter 7 ~ The Crown Chakra

according to human evolution. This is because the various levels of light, as represented by the Arc, have a direct correlation to consciousness.

There is the central spiritual Sun, the heart of the Sun and the physical Sun that the human constitution mimics in its triad of monad, soul and personality. The spiritual Sun shines on the planets and then lastly reflects on the Moon. We are required to extend beyond the physical or solar Sun, to the spiritual light. This is why the influence of the heart chakra has its part in determining the function of the crown. Close down the heart and there will be very little in the way of contact for spiritual connection.

The light of the night can be so mysterious that a strong heart gives much in the way of support, for truth requires much faith. This is suggested by the glyph of this chakra, the half shaped crescent of the moon as if just caught in light, not crudely but gently caressed. With the aid of imagination its shape is just beginning to reveal the whole Moon and thus represents the subtlety of its wisdom. Make no mistake though, the strength of its pull is not subtle. This strength is the patience of its persistence and the repetition of its loyalty, the equilibrium of truth. It may be that we are no more than a receptacle for receiving and processing light, the luminosity of which is an important factor in the evolution of humanity. It is not a reflection of physical sunlight that creates this evolution but that which emanates light from within. This is the luminous arc of the lokas set against the shadowy arc of the talas, for they are both forces in the equilibrium of the truth of life and are contained within the heart of the Sun and so in the soul.

The frequencies and intensities of light emanation have evolved through the root-races, and carried forth the evolution of life. The more conscious we are, the greater our luminosity, which eventually takes root in the material world. The consciousness of the group can light up the planet through the vibration of all its living atoms. This vibration will increase the more Self's soul has been liberated, for it only pertains to the higher Self. The Spiritual Sun grants vision and is illuminated by Divine light by the means of the monad, as directed by the Solar Logos. This light is in the process of merging the Spiritual Sun with the Solar Logos but there is a long, long way to go. At least it has started in the pursuit for Absolute, or should I say Absolution. Absolution is to come from a place of unselfconsciousness in order to embrace cosmic consciousness, a state in which the candidate has no more to learn within this plane of existence, or the spiritual ego has no more to teach it. It is the amalgamation of the results of creativity or the three in one, The Father, Son and Holy Spirit (mother) that is the making of what is Divine in the Higher Self. At this point all is contained in the now, or the spiritual monad united with the Divine monad. However, together this pair encourage one to go beyond the notion of now, for everything that has manifested by creation is an extension of that which has come before, balanced by what will be or prophesy. Here the prophet is the Divine ego. All that Self has ever been can now be witnessed by it through cosmic consciousness, thus shedding the need for the astral plane. Therefore, it is to possess vision in order to state the future as seen through the Divine monad or the God within. Enlightenment is only the beginning, it will be this spiritual and Divine unity that inspires Self in its higher form to go on to greater things.

Heaven is a stop off point. It is a place from which one still reincarnates and a place where one still has to wrestle with the trauma of earthly karma. It is Self's task to relinquish the Atman from its buddhic ties and by using Christ (the Divine ego) as guide to cross this gorge, which is heaven. If one wishes to be free of reincarnation one requires the use of this prophet. Only here, or perhaps where the eighth chakra lies, can Self start its long journey in its true emancipation from the Divine ego. Nirvana is a state that differs from heaven, heaven being a locality and a place where the soul resides in a particular sphere that best suits it between reincarnations. This sphere will be appropriate to its position in its journey towards emancipation. There are very many spheres that make up the whole of heaven. The purpose of obtaining the triad (that is the three lots of fourteen stations or the forty-two points to transcendence) is to fully emancipate Atman in order that spirit can join the higher hierarchy of the cosmic planes: this is Brahman. Also contained within these planes will be the balance of the lokas and talas in order to manifest creativity but, just as in light and dark, they are so interconnected that, at these levels, they resonate as one. For the same reason that the soul is infused with spirit, Self has to sample all. Just as dictated by the chain of reincarnation (globe ego) and therefore that of the planetary chain of reincarnation (planetary cycle ego), all transcends to resonate with love, which Self knows in its awakened state is the true vibration of the Divine Soul. This is what 'to know', is truly about.

The first stage to the emancipation of the Atman is the attainment of

Chapter 7 ~ The Crown Chakra

the first set of fourteen stations of the Double Holy Seven, which also begins the process of gathering up all that is within the seven sacred planets. This is to relinquish the need for matter. Once this is achieved, the second set of fourteen stations is a process of becoming fully conscious of the consequence, in a Divine sense, as to the significance of holding this energy within. In effect, what it means for Self to be at this stage in relation to its own immortality. To understand this or to integrate with this inner power, one remains Earthbound and returns to complete a further set of fourteen stations. This is far quicker in Earthly work than the previous two. In doing so, Self is a representative of the higher planes and no longer a representative of his fellow human beings, for he has integrated sufficiently with his own divine monad in order to radiate it here on Earth during the incarnation. This manifests in the spreading of divine light. Therefore, this achievement replicates the pattern of creation: first the message is presented, then the boundary is laid in which it can manifest for humans to put into action.

It is the process of having made conscious the spreading of Divine light that instigates the final set of fourteen stations and completes the triad. This leads to the dematerialisation of all that is associated with heaven, and leaves the chosen spirit entwined with the process of beginning the next cycle of seven that joins the seventh cosmic plane to the sixth. This is no longer to find divinity within but to be universally Divine. The third set of fourteen stations and the final path to obtaining complete enlightenment is a path of the most wondrous compassion. It stems from the spiritual-intellectual body which is limited in its help for humanity, still consisting of what we have been taught and not what we 'know' to be so. Even though not completely disconnected from its ego, the spiritual-intellectual body is connected to the spiritualised body and therefore able to make this transition as they are both in direct cognition. The spiritualised body is not a state of nirvana but is the closest form to it without becoming it. So the work achieved on the crown in developing the spiritualised body is the making of compassion and the means to reach nirvana, that being a state in which all inferior aspects are completely reborn with positiveness on the spiritual monadic sphere. This readies the monad for its awaited release into the eternity of its hierarchy.

The last of these three sets of fourteen stations provides the opportunity for these spirits to help humanity during its various struggles in a particular root-race. We are never alone and though humanity is equipped with free will, even at times when it is at its most destructive, there are still representatives from the higher planes here to help oversee the construction of a greater solution. The work achieved during the last of the three stages of the fourteen stations is significant to that which has gone before and so is picked up and continued much in the same way that aspiration is passed on to the child through the parents. In fact, even on this higher level, something new can only be derived from that which has come before, as stated by the lokas and underlined by the father-mother-child principle. Here, though, during this last stage, the work determines that which will obtain nirvana and until this is completed, Self remains compromised or more specifically, Self has not fully manifested a divine state. This can be understood as not fully encapsulating the whole truth.

During the final stage of the Double Holy Seven, there is a choice to be made, which takes us back to the significance of the seven colours chosen to represent the seven chakras, the making of this book, which differentiate them from the rainbow system. The colours represent or signify the choice that is presented at this stage of Self's development, as do the sequence of the planets that run up the spine; for they empower Self with choice, the ultimate mastery over its separation from the Divine and creative partnership: this is to determine the fate of its own reincarnation.

Self now has the power to make the choice; to volunteer not to reach a state of nirvana but to choose to remain with planet Earth as the ultimate act of selflessness in order to serve in the support of humanity. This is to be a planetary spirit and, as signified by these chosen colours, is considered by many who are deep in such understanding to be a greater achievement than reaching a state of nirvana. The souls that use this system and some that have been attracted to this book will choose to work with these colours throughout their development of the forty-two names because of a selfless understanding as to their own fate and the respect given as to the integrity of their purpose. They are the ultimate healers destined to remain. Even though Self has chosen not to enter a state of nirvana, this too is a blissful state, one highly spiritualised and so attached to nirvana. It is also a state that can be touched upon by the most focused of initiates during meditation. The choice to remain as a planetary spirit is determined by Self refusing to discard its astral body, which is finally redeemed in obtaining a state of nirvana. Those who

Chapter 7 ~ The Crown Chakra

are destined to stay have already relinquished their dense and etheric bodies during the first two stages of the triad, for Self has no need for them when facilitating its new task. This task of healing is undertaken by accompanying and thus inducing direction within those souls that require spiritual guidance. It will be up to each soul on Earth whether they choose to receive it.